Reader's Digest **MEDICAL BREAKTHROUGHS 2005**

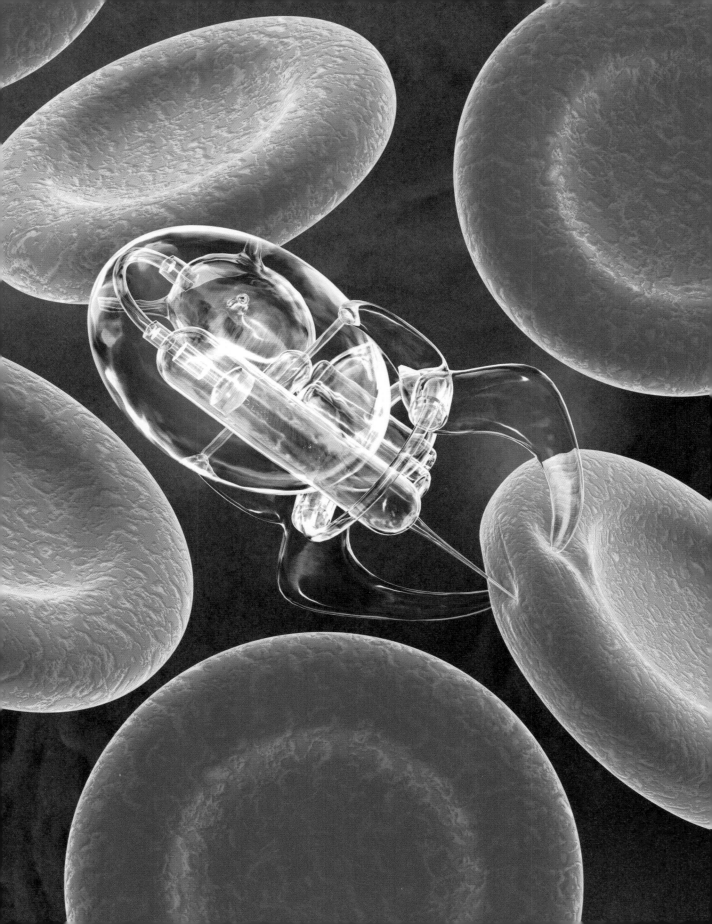

Reader's Digest MEDICAL BREAKTHROUGHS 2005

The latest advances and most important health developments

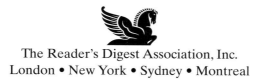

The Reader's Digest Association, Inc.
London • New York • Sydney • Montreal

MEDICAL BREAKTHROUGHS 2005

READER'S DIGEST PROJECT STAFF

Consultant
Sheena Meredith M.B., B.S.

Project editor
Rachel Warren Chadd

Art editor
Conorde Clarke

Assistant editors
Liz Clasen
Celia Coyne
Henrietta Heald

Proofreader
Ron Pankhurst

Indexer
Marie Lorimer

READER'S DIGEST GENERAL BOOKS

Editorial director
Cortina Butler

Art director
Nick Clark

Executive editor
Julian Browne

Picture resource manager
Martin Smith

Pre-press account manager
Penelope Grose

Origination
Colour Systems Limited, London

Printing and binding
Mateu Cromo, Spain

Medical Breakthroughs 2005 was originated by the editorial team of The Reader's Digest Association, Inc., USA

This edition was adapted and published by
The Reader's Digest Association Limited
11 Westferry Circus, Canary Wharf
London E14 4HE

We are committed to both the quality of our products and the service we provide to our customers. We value your comments, so please feel free to contact us on **08705 113366** or via our web site at: **www.readersdigest.co.uk**
If you have any comments or suggestions about the content of our books, email us at gbeditorial@readersdigest.co.uk

Concept code IE0088A/IC
Book code 440-203-01
ISBN 0 276 42960 5
Oracle code 250008623H.00.24

READER'S DIGEST USA PROJECT STAFF

Senior Editor
Marianne Wait

Senior Design Director
Elizabeth Tunnicliffe

Production Technology Manager
Douglas A. Croll

Manufacturing Manager
John L. Cassidy

CONTRIBUTORS

Editor
Jeff Bredenberg, Sheridan Warrick

Writers
Susan Arns, Kelly Garrett,
Debra Gordon, Joely Johnson, Eric
Metcalf, Ron Sauder, Marc Schogol,
Carol Svec, Rob Waters

Designer
Marian Purcell

Copy Editor
Jane Sherman

Indexer
Ann Cassar

Picture Research
Jeanne Leslie

MEDICAL ADVISORS

Charles Atkins M.D.
*Medical Director, Western
Connecticut Mental Health Network;
Assistant Professor, Yale University
School of Medicine, New Haven,
Connecticut*

Jacob Bitran M.D.
*Professor of Medicine, Finch
University of Health Sciences/The
Chicago Medical School; Section
Chief, Hematology/Oncology,
Lutheran General Hospital,
Park Ridge, Illinois*

Lawrence C. Brody Ph.D.
*Senior Investigator, Head, Molecular
Pathogenesis Section, National
Human Genome Research Institute,
National Institutes of Health,
Bethesda, Maryland (contributions
rendered as an individual, not in the
name of the U.S. government)*

Nicholas A. DiNubile M.D.
*Orthopaedic Consultant,
Philadelphia 76ers Basketball
and Pennsylvania Ballet; Clinical
Assistant Professor, Department
of Orthopaedic Surgery, Hospital of
the University of Pennsylvania,
Philadelphia*

Marygrace Elson M.D.
*Associate Clinical Professor of
Obstetrics and Gynecology,
University of Iowa Hospital and
Clinics, Iowa City*

Bradley W. Fenton M.D.
*General Internist, Clinical Associate
Professor, Thomas Jefferson
University Hospital, Philadelphia*

Joel A. Kahn M.D.
*President, WorldCare Global Health
Plan Ltd, Boston*

Barry Make M.D.
*Director, Emphysema Center,
National Jewish Medical and
Research Center, Denver; Professor
of Medicine, University of Colorado
School of Medicine, Denver*

Randolph P. Martin M.D.
*Director, Emory Non-Invasive Lab,
Emory University Hospital, Atlanta;
President of the American Society of
Echocardiography (for 2003)*

Vincent Yang M.D., Ph.D.
*Director, Division of Digestive
Diseases, Emory University Hospital,
Atlanta*

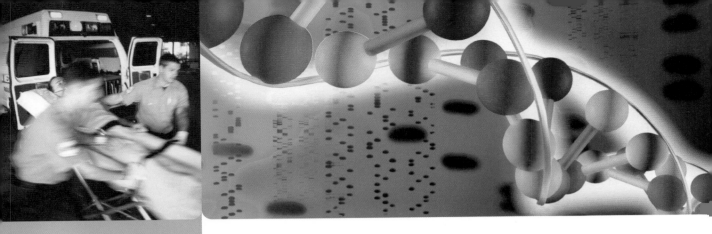

Contents

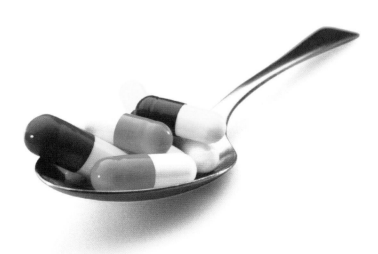

PART 3 : YOUR BODY HEAD TO TOE (continued)

Reproduction and sexuality 200-215

Respiratory system 216-227

Skin, hair and nails 228-233

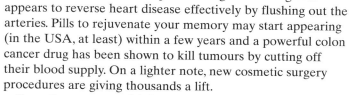

About **this book**

These days, your daily newspaper is likely to be filled with stories of war, heartache and woe. *Medical Breakthroughs 2005,* on the other hand, is packed from cover to cover with good news – hope in the form of new lifesaving drugs, faster cures and discoveries to help all of us stay healthy.

Among our top stories this year: scientists are experimenting with a drug that appears to reverse heart disease effectively by flushing out the arteries. Pills to rejuvenate your memory may start appearing (in the USA, at least) within a few years and a powerful colon cancer drug has been shown to kill tumours by cutting off their blood supply. On a lighter note, new cosmetic surgery procedures are giving thousands a lift.

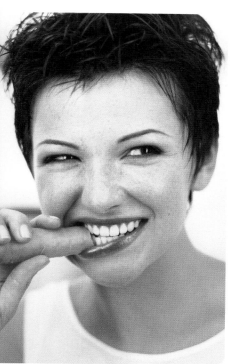

Even the most casual follower of medical news will find this book fun and inspiring to read. In these pages, you'll learn about bat saliva being used to dissolve blood clots that cause strokes, deep-sea sponges that yield cancer cures, and newly discovered healing powers of everyday substances such as coffee. You'll also read about an exciting future, a time when microscopic robots will be sent in to repair damage to cells and cure disease, when you'll get your medicine from needles that are too tiny to hurt, and when you'll use biological bandages that speed wound healing and pop a daily pill that could slash your risk of ever developing heart disease.

Medical Breakthroughs 2005 is organized to make the reading easy. Part 1, 'The year's top stories', is a series of in-depth articles on some of the biggest medical stories in the news. Part 2, 'General health', provides updates in chapters on Ageing, Children's health and Wellness. In Part 3, 'Your body head to toe', news about specific diseases is organized by body system – Brain and nervous system, Heart and circulatory system, Reproduction and sexuality, and so on.

As you read, you should bear in mind that many of the breakthroughs unveiled here are experimental and it could be years before some of these discoveries become available to the general public. In the UK, there is currently no easy way to find a clinical trial that might be suitable for you or someone close to you, although the Medical Research Council (MRC) is working with the NHS and others to develop registers of clinical trials with free access for everyone. The MRC's trials unit can be found at: www.ctu.mrc.ac.uk/ You should also remember that, in many cases, older, time-tested treatments may be the best approach for your particular condition. Talk it over with your doctor or health professional, who should be able to help. Meanwhile, we hope that this book will both encourage and inform.

As Sheena Meredith, our UK consultant, says: 'People today are encouraged to take more responsibility for their own health, and most of us are fascinated to hear of the latest wonder-drug or new medical procedure. Yet it can be difficult to be sure that we are getting accurate information. Reader's Digest's *Medical Breakthroughs* is full of easily understood, up-to-date information based on sound scientific studies, and offers an authoritative guide to the year's top medical stories.'

PART 1

THE YEAR'S
TOP
STORIES

SOME OF THE YEAR'S biggest health stories unfolded at
the microscopic level: viruses that pass from animals to
humans have scientists scrambling to prepare for the next
post-SARS killer outbreak – perhaps of a new strain of bird
flu. Researchers cloned the first human embryo and used it
to create a new line of stem cells, the controversial cells that
could one day be used to cure the major diseases of our time.
And scientists have developed unimaginably tiny particles
that bring the old sci-fi movie *Fantastic Voyage* a big step
closer to reality. In other major stories, researchers
accidentally discovered that a certain type of MRI may help
cure depression, and an experimental drug is unblocking
clogged arteries and saving lives.

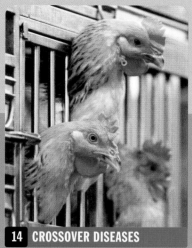

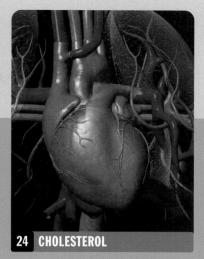

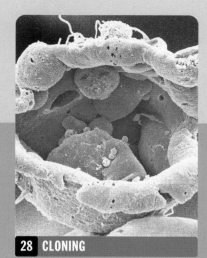

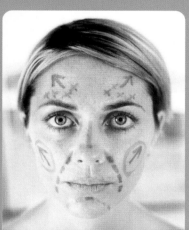

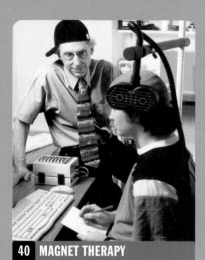

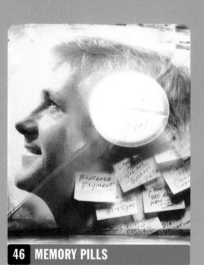

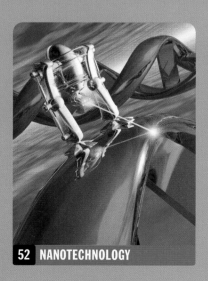

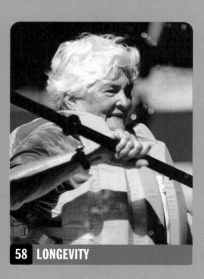

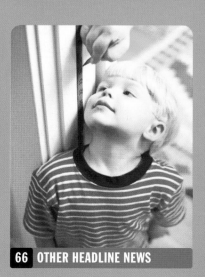

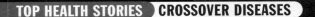

THE NEXT
KILLER VIRUS:
COMING YOUR WAY?

Thai soldiers carry off chickens that may be infected with a deadly strain of bird flu. Millions of chickens have been destroyed in Asian countries to protect the public.

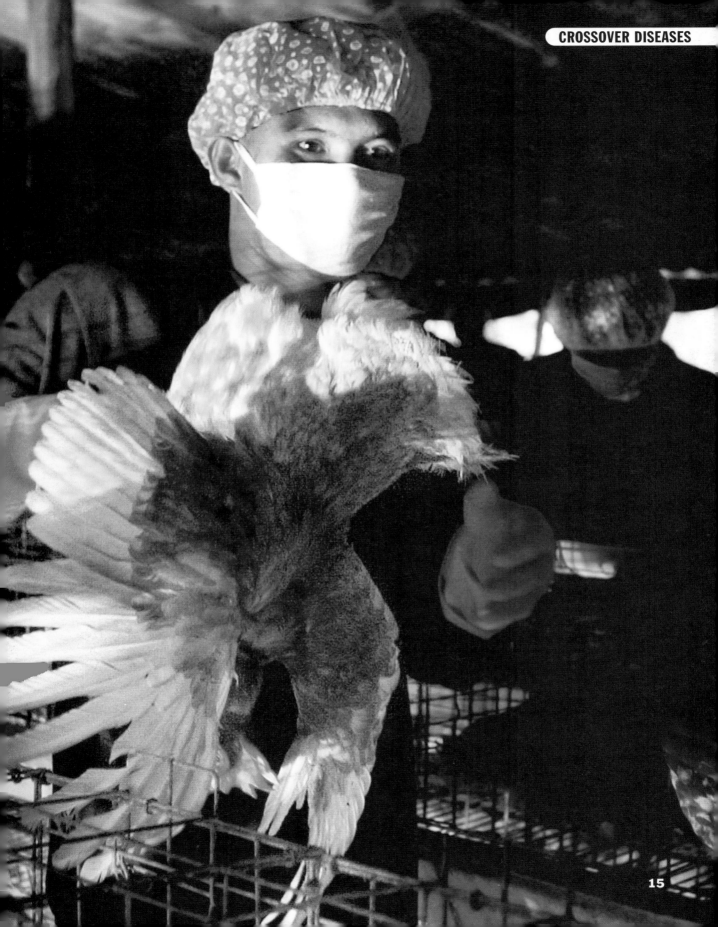

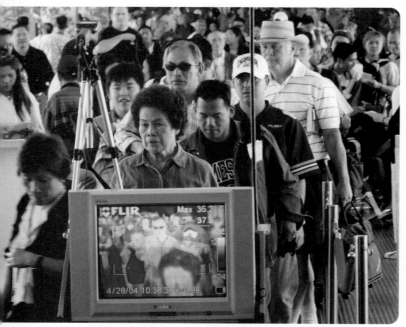

A fever-sensing scanner screens tourists arriving in the Philippines after suspected cases of SARS were reported in China in the spring of 2004.

acute respiratory syndrome (SARS), the virus that in 2003 spread through two dozen countries and infected more than 8,000 people? Or, worse still, could it be the start of the world's next pandemic?

From animals to humans

The question was not an unreasonable one. Experts on infectious disease are growing increasingly alarmed that a deadly new virus could leap national borders and, in a matter of months, reach every corner of the world. SARS is just one of a growing number of threatening diseases that have a particular trait in common: known as zoonoses, they begin among wild or domestic animals and spread to people. Animal-borne diseases that infect humans have existed for centuries. In fact, scientists believe that virtually all human viral diseases originated in animals, and that every species of bird, mammal or reptile is a possible source of new human illness.

'The universe of potential emerging diseases from animals is huge and is, to a great extent, unknown,' says Dr David Morens, a research scientist at the National Institute of Allergy and Infectious Diseases (NIAID) in the USA. 'Because we don't know how big it is, we don't know what's "behind the screen". It's difficult to get a handle on the exact scope of the problem.' Not every organism that infects animals is able to cross over to people, and an organism won't necessarily cause disease if it does. But the potential for a new bug to cause an epidemic is what keeps virus hunters on the alert.

One of the first recorded epidemics that may have originated in animals began about 430 BC during the Peloponnesian War, when an unknown illness killed about a third of the population of Athens.

Recent epidemics that are thought to have begun as animal diseases include Ebola haemorrhagic fever in Africa, which started in an unknown animal and transferred to humans in 1976 – since when it has killed 1,261 people. Another is acquired immune deficiency syndrome (AIDS), which is caused by the human immunodeficiency virus (HIV). Although HIV has been found retrospectively in samples from humans dating back to the 1950s, it was not until 1999 that scientists managed to trace its source to a particular species of chimpanzee in Africa. The disease had crossed over to people when hunters came in contact with infected blood. Even as

To mark his 79th birthday in the summer of 2003, Ed and his wife, Marie, a couple from San Diego, spent three weeks travelling in China. On the return flight to the USA, Marie felt iller than she had ever felt before. 'Some strange bug,' she said to her daughter on the telephone the day after they arrived home. The conversation was punctuated by Marie's deep, rasping coughs, and she complained of fever, chest pains and a runny nose. 'It feels like a cold and flu rolled into one,' Marie said. A couple of days later, Ed also fell ill.

Concerned about her parents' health, the couple's daughter Karen flew from North Carolina to look after them. Within a week, she was in her doctor's surgery. 'It feels like I'm going to cough up a lung,' she said when asked to explain her symptoms. The doctor noted a fever, then held a stethoscope to Karen's back. 'I don't think it's flu,' the doctor said. She picked up Karen's notes. 'Have you travelled outside the country recently?'

When Karen said that she had just returned from seeing her parents, who had become ill while visiting China, the doctor's eyes widened. She walked calmly to the sink and washed her hands, then reached into an overhead cupboard for a surgical mask. As she fastened the mask over her mouth and nose, the doctor asked, 'What part of China did they visit?' The unspoken question was, could this be severe scientists begin to gain an understanding of how to prevent or control these viruses, new diseases continue to appear – some of them deadly.

How viruses cross the species line

Most diseases infect only one species or a handful of species, which is why your dog or cat doesn't catch a cold each time you get one. Every now and then, though, through mutation or adaptation, an infectious agent gains the ability to cross the species boundary. The threat is bigger now than it has ever been before, for several reasons.

With more than six billion people on the planet, we have created a kind of global sprawl. All of us need somewhere to live. Moving onto previously uninhabited land brings us into closer and closer contact with the animal world, where viruses hide. We end up living side by side with exotic diseases that can strike swiftly and lethally.

All of those people also need to eat. Feeding billions means that, in general, domestic animals such as pigs, chickens and cows can no longer roam freely on farms. High production often entails packing in the animals so that they are side by side and nose to tail in high-density pens, where the viruses shed by a single sick pig, for instance, can potentially infect the entire stock – and the risk to human handlers rises with every infected animal.

In this way, animals that were previously regarded as 'safe' such as pigs or chickens, can end up causing diseases in humans. Depending on the strength and action of the virus, the individuals who become infected may experience no illness at all or only mild illness – or they may become very ill indeed and eventually die.

Scientists point to the rodent-borne disease called hantavirus pulmonary syndrome (HPS) as a prime example of what happens when people and wild animals compete for living space. Hantavirus is an old virus that was recognized only in 1993 when an outbreak of HPS occurred in the southwestern USA. In 1992, the rodent population in that area had grown so much that a large number of mice sought shelter in people's homes. Although mice are common in rural areas, the problem was worse than usual because it had been an exceptionally wet year – and some of the mice were carrying hantavirus.

Where there are mice, there are droppings – and infected mice leave infected droppings. After the rodents had left the houses, the droppings dried up and turned to dust. In 1993, as people cleaned out storage areas around their homes, they inhaled the virus-laden dust particles.

For 22 people that year, spring cleaning was fatal. The deaths were painful, marked by fever, aching muscles and so much fluid accumulation in the lungs that it must have seemed like drowning on dry land.

Scientists have since determined that about 430 species of mice can carry hantavirus, but only about 10 per cent of them are infected. It was the explosion in the mouse population that exposed people to this deadly disease.

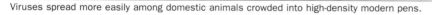

Viruses spread more easily among domestic animals crowded into high-density modern pens.

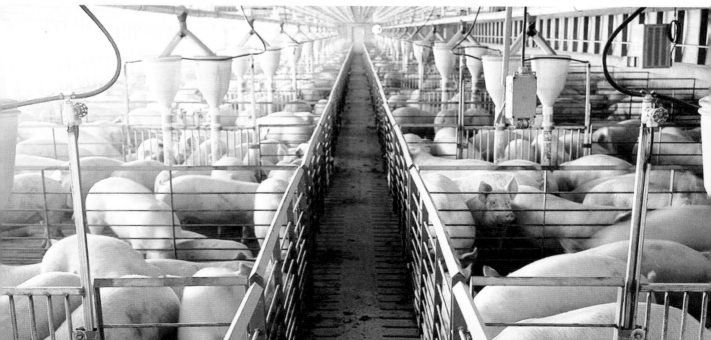

How epidemics evolve

Although diseases that jump from animals to humans are frightening, they are generally self-contained – that is, only the people who come into contact with infected animals become ill. For a virus to spread through the world, it must develop the ability to spread from person to person through mutation. Imagine, for example, a farmer who gets flu – nothing special, just the usual bug that goes around among humans every year. If he also contracts a virus from a sick mouse or chicken, he will have two different viruses in his cells at the same time. Viruses in such proximity may swap some genes, thereby creating a totally new virus that contains genetic material from both the original viruses.

How the new virus will behave depends on which genes have come together. It could end up being harmless – or, in a nightmare scenario, it could turn out to be both as deadly as Ebola and as contagious as the common cold. Meanwhile, just about anyone

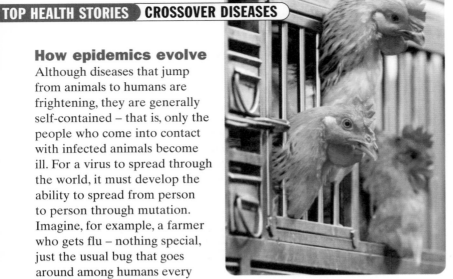

In Asia, a deadly strain of avian flu crossed from chickens to the humans who handled them.

can leave home and arrive in any city on the planet within 24 hours – even people who are extremely ill. 'All diseases are basically one plane flight away,' says Lyle Petersen, a director of the US disease control and prevention authority.

What that means in terms of illness and death depends on the type of bug being spread. If it is one of the quick-spreading varieties, scientists estimate that it could take only a few weeks before an outbreak becomes a worldwide threat – 25 to 40 per cent of the world's population could become infected.

The biggest threat: Asian flu

When the next worldwide outbreak occurs – and scientists agree that it will happen – the most likely source will be an influenza virus.

Dr Morens of NIAID admits that he is worried. 'Most people who have spent their careers working in infectious diseases, as I have, will put influenza at the very top of the list or very close to the top of the

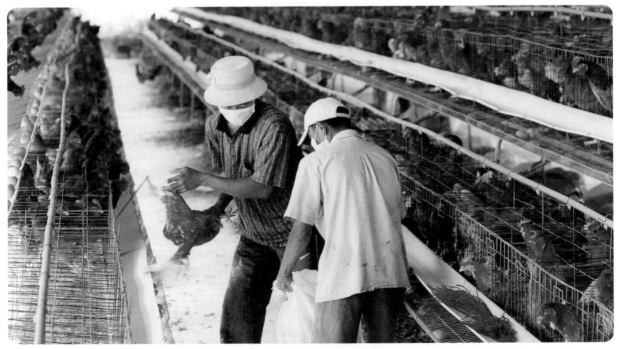

Workers place chickens into bags for burial in Ho Chi Minh City, Vietnam, to control an outbreak of bird flu.

list of Andromeda strains – really bad things that could, and probably eventually will, come out of the environment and cause a terrible epidemic. The 1918 influenza pandemic killed between 50 million and 100 million people. That's more than the Black Death of the 14th century. That's more, so far, than AIDS. There's nothing that we know to assure us that it cannot happen again.'

Although the exact cause of the 1918 pandemic is not known, genetic evidence found in tissue samples suggests that it started as a bird flu that spent time in another species – possibly pigs or horses – before becoming a threat to people.

The rise of a deadly strain of avian flu in Asia in 2003 was particularly worrying. The strain was 100 per cent lethal in chickens. When it began infecting humans, it became an imminent threat. By the spring of 2004, 34 people in Asia had contracted bird flu through touching, handling, butchering or being in proximity to infected birds. Of those who became infected, 23 died, reflecting a 68 per cent mortality rate.

Although the virus has not yet adapted to spread from person to person, the steep rise in the number of infections in chickens suggests that it may be only a matter of time until that lethal mutation occurs. In 1997 and 1998, about 1.4 million chickens died of the disease or were destroyed to prevent its spread. In 2001 and 2002, 2.5 million birds were killed. In 2003 and 2004, more than 100 million chickens in eight Asian countries had to be sacrificed to protect public health.

'It's clear that this virus poses a much larger risk than many other viruses,' says Klaus Stöhr, head of the World Health Organization (WHO) Global Influenza Programme. 'The virus is transmitted to humans. It replicates in humans. It causes disease in humans.'

If a human is infected with both this avian strain and a human strain, says Dr Stöhr, it is possible that the viruses could swap genetic material and create a more virulent strain.

The current concern is that even the most extreme precautions seem unable to contain the avian flu. Despite careful surveillance and immediate action when even a single affected chicken is identified, outbreaks of the disease have continued to occur, most notably in Thailand.

An epidemic arrested: SARS

Another new human disease that originated in Asia was SARS. It killed 774 people during its first major outbreak in 2003 and is also thought to have crossed over from animals.

In 2003 and 2004, SARS, which made its first appearance in the Guangdong province of southern China, had medical professionals around the world on red alert. Everything about it was a mystery.

'When SARS emerged, we didn't know what it was, we didn't know where it came from, and we

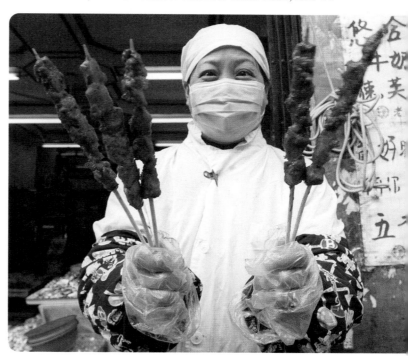

In China, a woman on a Shanghai street wears a surgical mask to protect herself from SARS in the spring of 2004.

didn't have any drugs or vaccines,' says Dr Morens. 'In the early stages, we didn't even have prevention measures that would allow us to stop it.' For a while, it looked as if SARS could be the virus to cause the next worldwide disease outbreak.

Although SARS is evidently a crossover disease, no one knows which animal was the original host. 'Traces of the virus were found in civet cats, which are a delicacy in the southeast part of China,' says Francois Meslin, a coordinator of zoonosis and food-borne diseases at the WHO. 'What we don't know is if SARS really originated from this animal species or if those civet cats were victims as much as humans.' What quickly became clear was that SARS was a coronavirus – one of the family of viruses that can cause the common cold – and that it could be spread from person to person. Once a disease no longer requires animal contact to be transmitted, it becomes a full-fledged human disease.

After much investigation, researchers learned that SARS can be spread in the same ways as flu – by breathing in virus-tainted droplets after an infected person sneezes or coughs, or by touching a person or a surface that the virus has contaminated.

That knowledge came too late for the nearly 800 people who died of SARS. Once the outbreak had been identified, health authorities in all 29 affected countries acted swiftly to isolate patients and anyone who had come into contact with them. Despite the highly contagious nature of the virus, medical staff managed to prevent it from spreading throughout the world. The toll could have been much higher.

Public health experts have become wiser since the SARS crisis. The WHO has issued regulations for preventing the spread of a virus within hospitals. These include guidelines on wearing surgical masks, gloves and eye protection, and instructions for the use of ventilation and air conditioning in rooms that house SARS patients.

'We now know what to do to prevent exposure to contacts of the patient and of the hospital staff who work with the patient,' says Dr Morens. 'It seems like simple knowledge, but it's a big step. I feel that if SARS breaks out again, we have the theoretical knowledge to contain any epidemics.'

Indeed, when a laboratory worker in China acquired SARS in early 2004, nine people – but no more – became infected before the outbreak was contained. No one knows whether SARS will return

soon but, just in case, a vaccine is being prepared. So far it has proved effective in protecting monkeys against the virus, and in May 2004 the first human tests began in China.

West Nile virus

The West Nile virus, discovered in northern Uganda in 1937, has probably been at large for thousands of years. It typically causes very mild, influenza-like symptoms with no long-term effects. But in the 1990s there were reports of outbreaks of West Nile in the Mediterranean region, Russia and Romania – but, this time, hundreds of people developed severe neurological disease in addition to the aches, pains and fatigue caused by the older strain.

According to one theory, a genetic mutation changed a relatively weak virus into one capable of causing meningitis (inflammation of the lining of the brain or spinal cord), encephalitis (inflammation of the brain), paralysis and death. That strain was the one that made its way to New York in 1999.

West Nile virus is capable of infecting numerous species, including birds, horses and dogs, but it is spread by mosquitoes, not by direct contact with the infected animal. When an infected animal is bitten, the mosquito sucks up the virus circulating in the animal's blood. The next time that mosquito bites, a small amount of the blood-borne virus is injected before fresh blood is removed. In this way, the tiny mosquito carries disease from animal to animal – or from animal to human.

Although not all mosquitoes carry West Nile virus, enough do to strike down even wary scientists. 'I got West Nile last summer,' says Dr Peterson. 'I just went out to my mailbox, thinking I would be out there for a minute. Then I ran into one of my neighbours, we started talking, and we both got bitten by a bunch of mosquitoes. Three days later, both of us got West Nile.'

No one knows how the virus reached the USA, says Dr Petersen. 'It probably arrived by an infected animal that was imported, or an infected person came, or possibly an infected mosquito hitchhiked on an airplane, which is actually fairly common.' Since it arrived in America, the virus has marched relentlessly across the country,

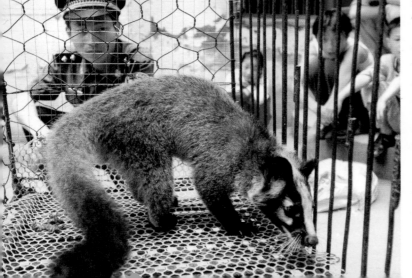

A policeman in central China guards a civet cat captured by a farmer. The cats are one possible source of the country's outbreak of SARS.

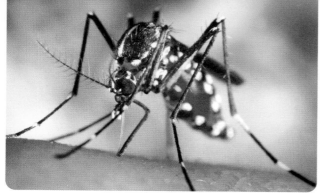

Call in the swat team: The *Aedes albopictus* mosquito can pass the West Nile virus from one animal to another – or to humans.

each year moving a little further west. In 2003, 9,858 cases of West Nile were reported in the USA. Of those, 2,863 people had severe forms of the disease that affected their brains and nerves, and 262 died. In 2004, the disease expanded its reach into Arizona, New Mexico and California. By 2005, West Nile virus will have reached all parts of the country. After that, no one can predict what will happen. 'Once the disease enters an area, it tends to stick around,' says Dr Petersen. 'West Nile virus will be a significant public health problem for the foreseeable future. Luckily, there's no indication that the virus is mutating to become even more severe than it already is.'

In July 2004 two cases of the virus were confirmed in Ireland; both of those infected had recently returned from the Algarve in Portugal. No case has yet been reported in the UK, but in May 2004 the Department of Health announced that, as a precaution, it had drawn up plans for dealing with an outbreak of the virus.

Preparing for the next global outbreak

Public health officials have to be vigilant. The first line of defence is surveillance and monitoring. Once a disease reaches a country with a sophisticated medical communication and reporting system, it cannot hide. In the UK, for instance, influenza outbreaks are tracked from various sources by the Communicable Disease Surveillance Centre while the Influenza Pandemic Plan would note potential cases of avian flu as well.

The best weapons against influenza are vaccines, which can prevent or at least lessen the effects of the virus, but vaccines take a minimum of six months to manufacture and distribute. Also, because the exact strain of virus causing a disease is not known until it establishes itself, a vaccine prepared in advance and stockpiled may not work against the strain that later appears. As Dr Stöhr says, it is like owning a gun for protection but having to wait until your enemy is shooting at you to make the ammunition. The virus will spread more quickly than we are able to make

FAST FACTS

ASIAN INFLUENZA

It started as a disease of wild waterbirds such as ducks but is now commonly found in domestic chickens in many parts of Asia.

Scientists believe that the virus is spread through the blood, faeces and mucus secretions of infected birds. This means that people who butcher live birds, or those who work without face masks in an area populated by infected birds, are most likely to catch the disease.

People do not become ill by eating infected chickens. Normal cooking temperatures kill the virus.

It is not yet transmissible from person to person.

SARS

No one knows which animal first spread the disease to humans.

No one knows exactly how the disease travels from person to person, although it appears to be spread in the same ways as the common cold.

Vaccine development began in 2004, but years of testing are required before vaccines can become available to the public.

It is not yet transmissible from person to person.

WEST NILE VIRUS

About 99 per cent of all cases are transmitted by mosquitoes, which pass the virus from birds, horses and other mammals to humans.

People in the western part of the USA may be at greater risk that people elsewhere in the country because the most efficient carrier – the culex species of mosquito – is prevalent there.

The disease can also be spread through blood transfusions. However, blood is now routinely screened for the virus, so the risk is minuscule.

The best preventive is to use an insect repellent containing DEET. When used as directed, this compound is considered safe for people of all ages. Insect repellents containing permethrin can be applied to clothing – but never to skin – for extra protection.

VARIANT CJD: **FEARS WON'T GO AWAY**

The world's most mysterious animal-borne disease reared its head again in 2004, when the agents that cause BSE, or mad cow disease, were found in sheep muscles – the parts commonly cut into portions such as chops or leg of lamb. Scientists used to think that these tiny infectious agents, bits of abnormal protein called prions, were found only in brain, nerve and lymph system tissues.

The discovery of prions in muscle means that the risk of mad cow disease may be greater than previously suspected. Scientists think that people acquire the human form of the illness, called variant Creutzfeldt-Jakob disease (vCJD), by eating meat from animals that had the disease. Until 2004, they believed that careful butchering could separate the tainted from the untainted meat, but the new study, published by researchers in France in June 2004, raised fresh worries.

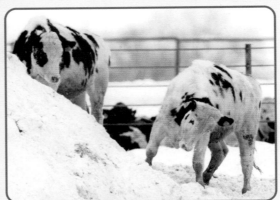

Cases of BSE continue to be found in Europe and the USA.

Although prions are fewer in muscle than in brain, no one knows how many are needed to cause disease. In fact, very little is known about prions. Unlike bacteria and viruses, they do not seem to contain DNA or RNA. They can survive heat, disinfectant chemicals, immune attack and ultraviolet radiation. In people and animals, prions act like toxic seeds that start a cascade of destruction.

Scientists believe that they proliferate by encouraging normal proteins in the body to mutate in imitation of the prions. When enough prions accumulate in the brain, cells die, leaving so many holes that the organ ends up looking like a sponge. People and animals lose their ability to think and control their bodies. Eventually, they become delirious, then fall into a coma before dying. In the UK, the country that has been worst affected by vCJD, there were 147 cases reported up to June 2004, of whom 142 had died. Some statistics suggest that the epidemic may already have peaked, but a study published in May 2004 raised the chilling possibility that there may be thousands of people in the UK who are carrying vCJD prions. The concern is that, even though these people may seem outwardly to be healthy, they may be able to transmit the disease to others through blood transfusions, organ donations or tainted surgical or dental instruments.

Many health experts believe that it is within our power to eradicate BSE from the countries where it persists, as long as we maintain vigilance in detecting sick animals and make sure we enforce strict regulations to protect herds and compliance by those who tend the cattle.

the vaccine. Antiviral medications are also effective for preventing influenza but extremely expensive, and the world's drug companies aren't currently set up to make the large amounts that could be needed in the event of a global outbreak. This means that, if a pandemic begins, antiviral drugs will become a hot commodity. 'They're completely out of reach for every developing country. They cannot afford it,' says Dr Stöhr. 'And developed countries may even start fighting for the very little which is available. There is no one who can produce enough.'

Once a pandemic is recognized, the goal will be to control it and minimize the number of infections and deaths. Success will depend partly on how fast we can produce vaccines and antiviral medications. 'Currently, we are not very well off in this part,' says

Dr Stöhr. 'The disease and the public will not forgive complacency.' He warns that the next pandemic will catch everyone by surprise unless governments, health agencies, and pharmaceutical companies devise innovative ways to make these therapies available. Some researchers are striving to shorten the vaccine production time by using genetically engineered viruses instead of growing actual viruses in eggs (the current procedure). Because these techniques are new, though, extensive testing will be needed before they are finally approved for use.

Ideally, we would prevent emerging diseases instead of merely reacting to them once they strike. To do so, however, would require international cooperation on an unprecedented scale – as well as some economic sacrifices. The virus hunters'

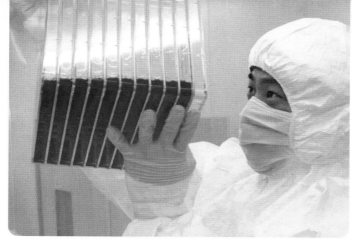

A Chinese scientist examines a SARS vaccine being developed for human use.

'wish list' includes keeping rain forests, wetlands and other undeveloped environments safe from human intrusion; developing rules for importing and exporting wildlife; and changing farm practices so that animals have more space. 'We need to consider the continuum from animals to humans with respect to the infectious diseases,' says Dr Meslin, 'not divide this [issue] into small sectors, saying wildlife diseases are not our problem because our problem is domestic animals, or our problem is public health. We have to look at all beings as one – including the infectious diseases – and realize that whatever is done in one sector affects all the other sectors.' Agriculture, industry, housing, countryside and pollution policies are all part of the same tangled public health issue.

Crisis averted for now

Such matters were far from the thoughts of Marie and Ed from San Diego and their daughter Karen as they endured the flu-like symptoms of the 'strange bug' picked up in China. It turned out that they did not have SARS; they had an unidentified infection that never spread beyond the family.

Had it been SARS, everyone on Marie and Ed's plane from China would have been exposed, as well as everyone they met or talked to in the airport or in the week after they arrived home. Similarly, everyone on Karen's plane back to North Carolina would have been at risk, plus everyone in the doctor's surgery and in the supermarket she visited on the way. And all the people those people came into contact with might also have had the potential to catch the disease. A once-in-a-lifetime holiday could have turned into a regional or national disaster. When the laboratory worker in China was exposed to SARS in 2004, about 1,000 people were quarantined to keep the disease from spreading. No one is sure what will happen next time. Maybe a more virulent strain of virus will sweep the globe faster than doctors can react – or maybe the experience of dealing with SARS taught us enough.

'We have learned a lot,' says Dr Stöhr. 'However creative nature is in producing new pathogens, I believe we will be even more creative to stem those outbreaks, to control them.'

How bird flu vaccine is made

A technique called reverse genetics allows scientists to mix and match genes from different viruses. This should allow them to create a harmless flu virus that triggers immunity to a pandemic strain.

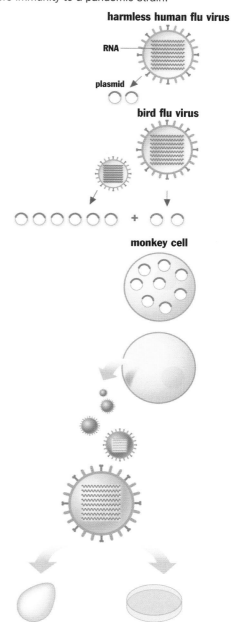

The traditional way to make a vaccine is to inject the virus into eggs. After a few weeks, large quantities of virus can be harvested for vaccines.

NEW DRUG FLUSHES OUT ARTERIES

A scientific mystery that dates back a quarter of a century to a small group of people in an Italian lake resort may have produced a powerful and unexpected new weapon that could revolutionize the fight against heart disease, Britain's single biggest killer.

Infusions of a special, bio-engineered version of 'good' cholesterol can shrink plaque in the arteries in a matter of weeks, putting heart disease in reverse.

Back in the 1970s, doctors began scratching their heads when they came across a curious family in Limone sul Garda, a picturesque Italian village. Blood tests showed that three people, a father and two of his children, had very low levels of HDL (high-density lipoprotein, or 'good' cholesterol, the kind that protects against heart disease) and very high levels of dangerous blood fats called triglycerides. The combination was a recipe for heart attacks, yet their arteries appeared to be perfectly healthy, and they all lived long lives remarkably free of heart disease. What could account for the paradox?

Research revealed that they had a 'mutant' form of HDL that made it extremely effective at cleaning up LDL (low-density lipoprotein), the 'bad' cholesterol that clogs up arteries. About 40 people in the town were eventually

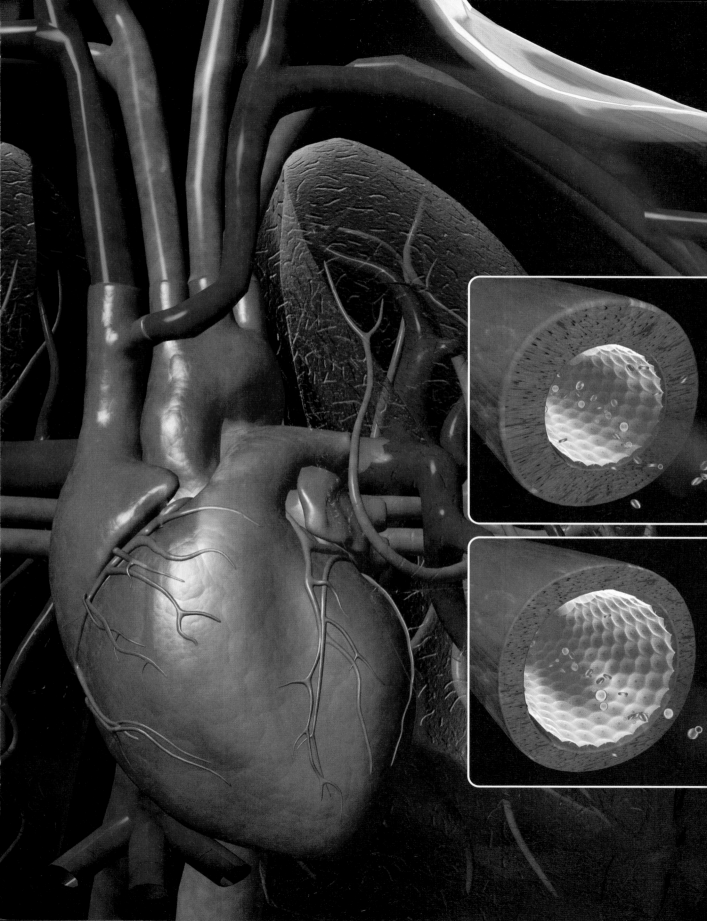

found to have this unique type of HDL and all had lower-than-expected rates of heart disease. The altered HDL responsible for their heart health was eventually named ApoA-I Milano, after the region where it was found.

Eventually, a bioengineered version of ApoA-I Milano was created, and when scientists fed it to rabbits and other laboratory animals over a period of 10 years, the results were remarkable: The plaque build-up inside the animals' arteries stopped and the existing plaque shrank.

Scientists know that what works in animals does not always work in humans, so when doctors at the Cleveland Clinic in Ohio and nine other sites gave ApoA-I Milano intravenously to 36 patients with coronary artery disease, they were astounded at the outcome. Both the speed and the scale of improvement were impressive. After five weekly infusions, intravascular ultrasound scans showed that the plaque in the patients' arteries had shrunk by an average of about 4 per cent. By comparison, in patients treated with an LDL-lowering statin drug and niacin over a three-year period, the reduction in plaque was less than 0.5 per cent.

A SUPER HDL SUCCESS STORY

Since taking part in an ApoA-I Milano study two years ago, Bob Garrison, a retired postal services manager in his seventies from Oklahoma City, has been largely free of heart disease symptoms, including chest pain. Garrison, who currently takes atorvastatin (Lipitor), one of the cholesterol-lowering statin drugs, was 59 and about to embark on a fishing trip when he had his first heart attack. Over the next decade, he had a second heart attack and multiple angioplasties. But now his story has changed. 'I haven't had any problems. I haven't had to have any more angioplasties. I used to have pain in my chest every once in a while, but I've had hardly any pain. I haven't had anything go wrong with me since I took that.'

Garrison is very aware, however, that the super HDL needs to be tested for several years before it can be approved for use by the general public. 'The only thing I dislike about it,' he says, 'is that at my age, it may take so long to get out on the market that I may never get to use it."

'Good' cholesterol can clear plaque

Infusions of a synthetic component of 'good' cholesterol, or HDL, reduced artery disease in just five weeks in a small study that could have bigger implications for treating the nation's leading killer.

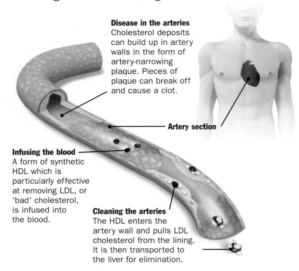

Disease in the arteries Cholesterol deposits can build up in artery walls in the form of artery-narrowing plaque. Pieces of plaque can break off and cause a clot.

Artery section

Infusing the blood A form of synthetic HDL which is particularly effective at removing LDL, or 'bad' cholesterol, is infused into the blood.

Cleaning the arteries The HDL enters the artery wall and pulls LDL cholesterol from the lining. It is then transported to the liver for elimination.

The implication is huge. Some day in the foreseeable future, heart disease could be treated not with invasive bypass surgery or angioplasty (an artery-opening procedure) but with a drug that would actually reverse the disease.

Professor Sir Charles George, medical director of the British Heart Foundation, welcomed the findings. 'ApoA-I Milano variant is of considerable interest since some people with it seem to be protected from coronary heart disease,' he told BBC News Online. 'The small study shows that this modification could have positive effects on treating patients.' But he also made it clear that 'more research is needed to prove the effectiveness of this treatment'.

The role of 'good' cholesterol

The normal HDL in most people's blood helps to protect them against heart disease by removing the build-up of LDL ('bad' cholesterol) from arteries. That is why high levels – more than 40mg/dL – of HDL cholesterol are good. (Losing weight and taking more exercise are two ways to boost your HDL levels.) Other benefits of HDL include possible roles in fighting inflammation (now considered a major contributor to heart disease) and offsetting the tendency of blood to clot.

The Italians in the Milano region had HDL that was only slightly different from what most of us have. In one of the main proteins making up their HDL, apolipoprotein A-I, the amino acid cysteine was substituted for the amino acid arginine. The chemical switch seems to make the protein unusually good at its job of latching on to LDL molecules, lifting them out of artery walls and carrying them to the liver for disposal.

Scientists also discovered that the 'super' HDL appears to have especially strong antioxidant properties, meaning that it helps to prevent damaging molecules called free radicals from oxidizing LDL particles and making them more likely to stick to artery walls. (Similar to the process of rusting, oxidation occurs when cells are attacked by free radicals, which are by-products of body processes that involve oxygen.)

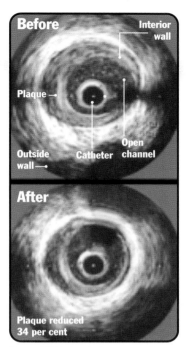

'Super HDL' shrank dangerous plaque, visible in this cross-section of an artery before and after treatment.

Liquid drain cleaner for the arteries

The biggest potential benefit of ApoA-I Milano may be its ability to act on the whole circulatory system at once, flushing out the arteries like a liquid drain cleaner. In heart disease, the arteries are narrowed due to the accumulation of plaque. If a plaque is unstable, it can burst, spewing its contents into the artery. The body sends chemicals that trigger a clotting response, and if the resulting clot blocks the artery, it can cause a heart attack.

Most people with heart disease have plaque in more than one place, says researcher Dr Muhammad Yasin of Integris Southwest Medical Center in Oklahoma City, who was involved in the study. 'You look at the arteries with ultrasound – they are studded with plaques,' he says.

Angioplasty, the catheter-based surgical procedure that is commonly used, opens only one area of an artery at a time. ApoA-I Milano, on the other hand, unclogs the whole plumbing system.

In the future, when someone is diagnosed with unstable angina (chest pain caused by narrowed arteries) and is clearly at risk of having a heart attack, a drug such as ApoA-I Milano might be used to stabilize the patient long enough to allow other treatments, such as an LDL-lowering statin drug, to get him or her out of danger.

Esperion Therapeutics, the small company that made ApoA-I Milano, was bought for £700m ($1.3 billion) by the giant drug company Pfizer in December 2003. Pfizer will need to invest in several more years of drug trials to prove the effectiveness and safety of ApoA-I Milano before it can be approved for use. And as an editorial in the *Journal of the American Medical Association* noted, ApoA-I Milano has yet to be tested head to head against regular HDL to prove that it is better at fighting heart disease.

Yet the study results are 'very promising', says lead researcher Dr Steven E. Nissen of the Cleveland Clinic. 'It produced a lot of excitement. How far can we go with this? What happens if we give it for 12 weeks? There are many things we don't know. All we know is that it was a big surprise – a large effect, occurring rapidly – and we hope that it will be proven to be very beneficial in larger studies.'

What does it mean to you?

ApoA-I Milano must undergo several years of further testing before it can earn approval by for use in combating heart disease in the USA or the UK. Nonetheless, if the results of future studies support the earlier findings, the 'super HDL' may be part of a trend in new drugs and therapies aimed at controlling coronary artery disease chemically rather than surgically. The potential advantages are:

■ Super HDL may buy time for patients clearly at risk of having heart attacks, giving them the chance to let treatments, such as LDL-lowering statin drugs, get them out of the woods.

■ Unlike angioplasty and stents, which open just one or two blocked arteries at a time, super HDL acts on all plaques simultaneously, providing a much more efficient, clean-sweep approach to reducing artery-clogging plaque.

HUMAN EMBRYO CLONED:
DEBATE IGNITED

'Cloned human'. The two words that appeared side by side in a research paper published in the journal *Science* in February 2004 captured world attention. Indeed, the report generated a flurry of ethical, legal and religious debates that almost eclipsed the scientific achievement.

South Korean scientists, using human eggs and human DNA, had created human embryos through cloning. But they had no plans to make babies who would grow up into genetic replicas of the women who had produced the eggs. Instead, the scientists extracted stem cells from the microscopic balls of dividing cells.

Embryonic stem cells have the potential to develop into any type of human tissue. The hope is that healthy cells derived from stem cells could one day offer treatments or cures for damaged or diseased organs, spinal injuries, diabetes, Parkinson's disease, multiple sclerosis and other conditions.

By successfully extracting stem cells from a cloned human embryo, the South Korean scientists made a breakthrough in therapeutic cloning – that is, cloning to yield stem cells for research or treatment of disease.

Their announcement, though, renewed calls for a worldwide ban on all forms of human cloning – both therapeutic and reproductive. One reason for such a reaction is that the two strands of stem cell research, therapeutic and reproductive, are very similar in the early stages because both involve

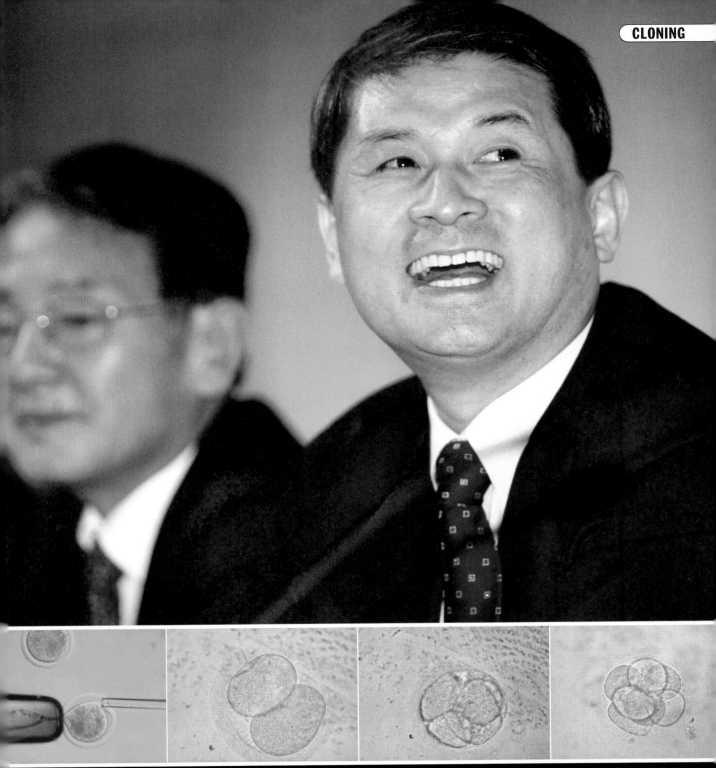

Dr Woo Suk Hwang *(top right)* and Dr Shin-Yong Moon *(top left)* of Seoul National University in Korea were the first in the world to clone a human embryo. Above, the cloning process.

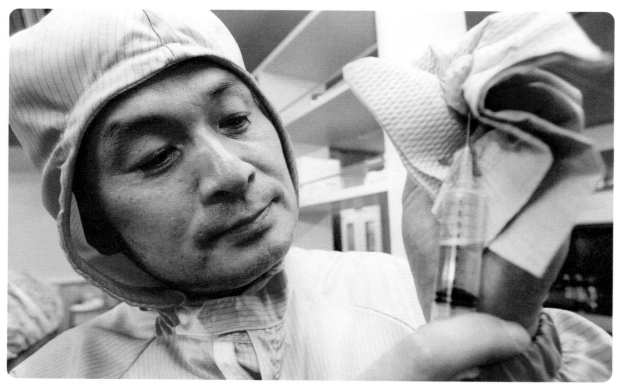

Pioneer Dr Woo Suk Hwang, shown in his Seoul laboratory, is working to make therapeutic cloning a reality. A veterinary medical researcher, he has also cloned cows and pigs.

the artificial creation of embryos. But there the similarity ends. In therapeutic cloning, the embryo is destroyed after a few days, as soon as the stem cells have been extracted. In reproductive cloning the embryo is implanted into a female and then allowed to develop into a baby. The fear is that the perfection of the science involved in the early stages of cloning could be exploited by those involved in reproductive cloning.

The egg cell division problem

Of course, someone, somewhere was bound to attempt human cloning, an event the world has been simultaneously anticipating and dreading. So why from the birth in 1996 of Dolly the sheep, the first cloned mammal, created by scientists from the Roslin Institute in Scotland, did it take eight years to clone human cells?

Blame the egg. That's the view of Gerald Schatten Ph.D., professor and vice chair of the department of obstetrics, gynaecology and reproductive sciences at the University of Pittsburgh School of Medicine and a leader in the world of cloning and stem cell research. In fact, in a paper published in *Science* in

April 2003 – only 10 months before the South Korean scientists' achievement – he predicted that human cloning might never be possible.

Dr Schatten and his team adopted the same process, known as nuclear transfer technology, that was used to create Dolly and other mammals in their own efforts to clone rhesus macaque monkeys. But after 700 attempts, they failed. The problem, he says, has to do with the way that monkey and human eggs divide. Removing the DNA from one of these eggs, which is a critical first step in cloning, effectively 'paralyses' the egg, rendering it unable to divide into the multiple cells that form an embryo.

The South Korean researchers eventually solved the cell division problem. They first 'harvested' eggs from 16 volunteers, using classic in vitro fertilization (IVF) techniques (the women were given drugs to stimulate their ovaries to produce multiple eggs, which were then harvested through an outpatient surgical procedure). Then they replaced the nuclei in the eggs from each woman with nuclei from cells in the woman's body (nuclear transfer technology), thereby exchanging the eggs' incomplete DNA for the woman's complete DNA. Ordinarily, an embryo has two DNA sources, a woman's egg and a man's sperm, and it is the fusion of the two that triggers cell division, notes lead researcher Woo Suk Hwang D.V.M., Ph.D., of Seoul National University in South Korea. In this instance, the eggs were given a chemical bath to kick-start their division.

A key reason why this cloning attempt succeeded where others had failed was that the South Koreans used eggs at an earlier stage of development. Researchers have long known that egg cells possess special 'motor' proteins, which, as the cells divide, pull apart tight packets of DNA, or chromosomes. Removing the DNA at the start of the cloning process also removes the motor proteins, preventing further cell division and bringing the cloning process to a halt. The South Korean researchers, however, used very fresh eggs in which motor proteins were still positioned at the edges of the cell and had not yet gathered around the DNA, so they remained in the egg after the DNA was removed.

The South Korean scientists had another advantage. They had collected 242 eggs from the 16 volunteers, so they could experiment with

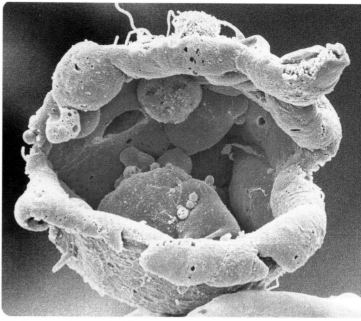

This human embryo, at the blastocyst stage, has been opened to reveal the inner cell mass, where stem cells can be harvested. Stem cells can be coaxed into becoming virtually any kind of tissue, making powerful new therapeutic treatments possible.

A new path to stem cells

South Korean researchers have created cloned embryos and grown them for about six days, until they formed blastocysts – balls of about 100 cells. At that stage, stem cells, perhaps useful for treating disease, can be extracted.

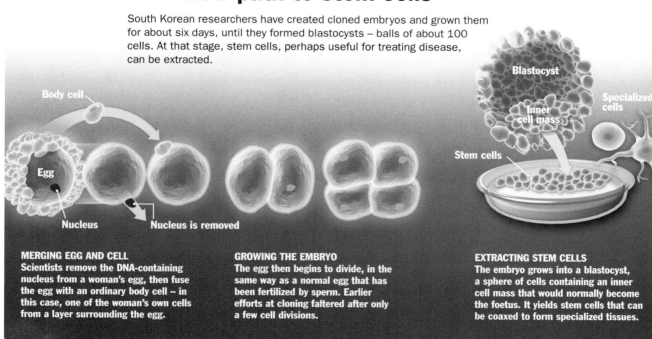

Blastocyst

Specialized cells

Inner cell mass

Stem cells

Body cell

Egg

Nucleus

Nucleus is removed

MERGING EGG AND CELL
Scientists remove the DNA-containing nucleus from a woman's egg, then fuse the egg with an ordinary body cell – in this case, one of the woman's own cells from a layer surrounding the egg.

GROWING THE EMBRYO
The egg then begins to divide, in the same way as a normal egg that has been fertilized by sperm. Earlier efforts at cloning faltered after only a few cell divisions.

EXTRACTING STEM CELLS
The embryo grows into a blastocyst, a sphere of cells containing an inner cell mass that would normally become the foetus. It yields stem cells that can be coaxed to form specialized tissues.

different techniques until they found one that worked. They succeeded in cloning 30 blastocysts – early-stage embryos each composed of only 100 cells, with an inner cell mass containing the all important stem cells – from which they harvested a single colony, or line, of stem cells. The rest were destroyed, as were the embryos.

Using this procedure, the scientists managed to dodge one major ethical issue in embryonic stem cell research: they did not have to use embryos left over from attempts at IVF. The eggs they harvested were identical to ones that the women would normally have lost during their menstrual cycles. Also, since the eggs were never fertilized, biologically speaking, there was no conception. The cells the scientists made were identical to those of each egg donor.

That is important when it comes to creating stem cells for therapeutic use, says Dr Hwang. A doctor attempting to treat a spinal injury can transplant cloned stem cells into the egg donor, and her body will welcome them as its own. Cells derived from another person could be rejected.

A workaholic at the cloning academy

Dr Hwang is exceptionally focused. He and his team have already cloned cattle resistant to mad cow disease and pigs that could be used for human organ transplants. He is at his laboratory – dubbed the cloning academy – by 6.30am seven days a week, 365 days a year. It took him just a couple of years to succeed in his therapeutic cloning efforts.

Dr Hwang's drive is fuelled by his own vision of what successful stem cell research would mean. In fact, he and his partners have structured the patents for their work so the doctors receive no financial rewards. 'I'd like to find the way to treat patients with degenerative disease,' he says. 'I'd like to bring therapeutic cloning into real life.' When his research flagged at one point, and he became frustrated, he met a couple just back from their honeymoon, during which the man had fallen

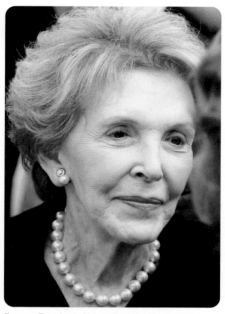

Former First Lady Nancy Reagan has become an outspoken advocate of stem cell research.

and been paralysed. Dr Hwang realized his work in the lab had the potential to enable the young man to walk again.

Although South Korea bans reproductive cloning, it allows therapeutic cloning in certain circumstances. At the same time, in common with most Asian countries, it does not allow organ transplants. Cloning to create stem cells that can develop into hearts, lungs and other organs is the only hope for people in these nations who need transplants. Additionally, Dr Hwang's religious beliefs – he is a Buddhist – support his actions. 'Buddhist faith is that all living things are given new life after they die,' he says. 'Cloning also means new life.'

Protest, politics and progress

Despite his successful results, Dr Hwang's work set off a storm of protest in the USA and elsewhere, including the UK, largely because even this means of therapeutic cloning involves the destruction of

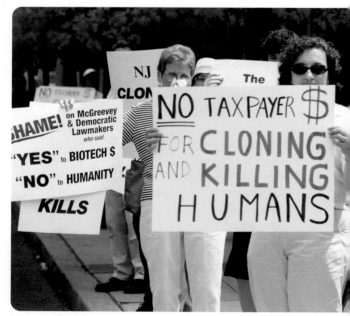

In New Brunswick, New Jersey, protesters gather outside a forum on the state's stem cell research initiative.

embryos created, which some view as human life. The US government now restricts federal funding for stem cell research to batches of embryonic stem cells that already existed in 2001, when the policy was announced. Those stem cell lines, of which about 18 remain, were created when the techniques were not well established, and they offer limited potential for furthering this field. In addition, human cloning of any kind is banned in many US states, including Pennsylvania, where Dr Schatten has his lab. The US stalemate leaves many scientists frustrated.

By contrast, Britain, where reproductive cloning is banned but therapeutic cloning is legal under strict conditions, is becoming a front-runner in this area of research. In August 2004 scientists at Newcastle University became the UK's first to be licensed by the Human Fertilization and Embryology Authority (HFEA) to clone human embryos for medical research. Professor Alison Murdoch, the team's co-leader, said the research should give valuable insight into the development of many diseases, although 'realistically, we have at least five years more of laboratory-based work before we move to clinical trials'.

The world's first stem cell bank opened in May 2004 inHertfordshire, with government funding of £2.6 million. Based at the National Institute for Biological Standards and Control (NIBSC), it will accept embryonic cells as well as those from adults and foetuses, and will store, characterize and clone cells and distribute them as required to researchers around the world. 'It's a very exciting development,' said Colin Blakemore, chief executive of the Medical Research Council (MRC). By making stem cells widely available, the cell bank will help to over-come the problem of extracting stem cells from early-stage embryos .

Ironically, the scientists who are using cloning to obtain embryonic stem cells are the ones calling most loudly for a worldwide ban on cloning for the purpose of creating babies. They are urging world governments to officially support therapeutic cloning, the kind of work done in South Korea. While that debate is aired, the next crucial step is to discover if newly created stem cells will actually be

> Scientists who are using cloning to obtain embryonic stem cells are the ones calling most loudly for a worldwide ban on cloning for the purpose of creating babies.

useful in medicine. Research from Sheffield University reported in 2004 found that human embryonic stem cell lines grown in the laboratory over months may have genetic abnormalities. Also, no one yet knows whether embryonic stem cells can generate the many types of cells the scientists want.

In South Korea, Dr Hwang's team are exploring whether the stem cells they retrieved will in fact produce specific cell types, such as nerve cells and pancreatic cells. They are also working to develop artificial eggs that could be used for cloning in nations where politics slams the door on embryo research. They have voluntarily halted new cloning of human eggs while the world debates the issues.

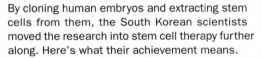

What does it mean to you?

By cloning human embryos and extracting stem cells from them, the South Korean scientists moved the research into stem cell therapy further along. Here's what their achievement means.

■ Scientists can now create their own batches, or lines, of stem cells. They no longer have to use human embryos left over from in vitro fertilization (IVF) attempts in order to get embryonic stem cells.

■ Cloning allows scientists to create embryos that genetically match the person who needs the therapy. Most likely, this will improve the chances of successful treatment.

■ Researchers hope one day to use stem cell therapy to treat conditions such as Alzheimer's, Parkinson's disease, diabetes, multiple sclerosis, heart disease, and spinal injuries, among others.

■ The technique remains controversial. In Britain, human cloning for medical research was made legal under strict guidelines in 2002, and in August 2004 scientists at Newcastle University became the first in the UK to be licensed by the Human Fertilization and Embryology Authority (HFEA) to clone human embryos for medical research. May 2004 saw the world's first stem cell bank opened in Hertfordshire, funded by a government grant of £2.6 million. But it is likely to be several years before medical treatments are developed for use.

THE NEW FACE OF
PLASTIC SURGERY

While watching television one evening, Doris Newton decided she was fed up with disliking her appearance. 'It always looked like I had a wrinkled polo-necked sweater on,' she says – and it was time to do something about it.

Doris Newton was not watching a romantic film starring gorgeous women and hunky men who make the rest of us feel plain and ordinary. The show was one of the new wave of 'reality' makeover programmes, which follow people as they receive everything from plastic and reconstructive surgery to injections of the latest 'line fillers' that plump out wrinkles.

Although Doris Newton is no spring chicken (she would not divulge her age but admitted to having three grandchildren), she decided there was no reason to look any older than necessary. So, brushing aside the old moral judgment – that plastic surgery strictly for the sake of appearance is foolishly vain – Doris had a facelift and a few other cosmetic procedures. It was not quite an extreme makeover, but it was definitely a change. Looking in the mirror afterwards, she says, 'I feel better about myself. I do look younger, but I don't look artificial. My face doesn't look tight. I look just

Doris is among millions of Americans who have been queuing up for treatment since television shows such as *Extreme Makeover* erased the stigma of cosmetic surgery.

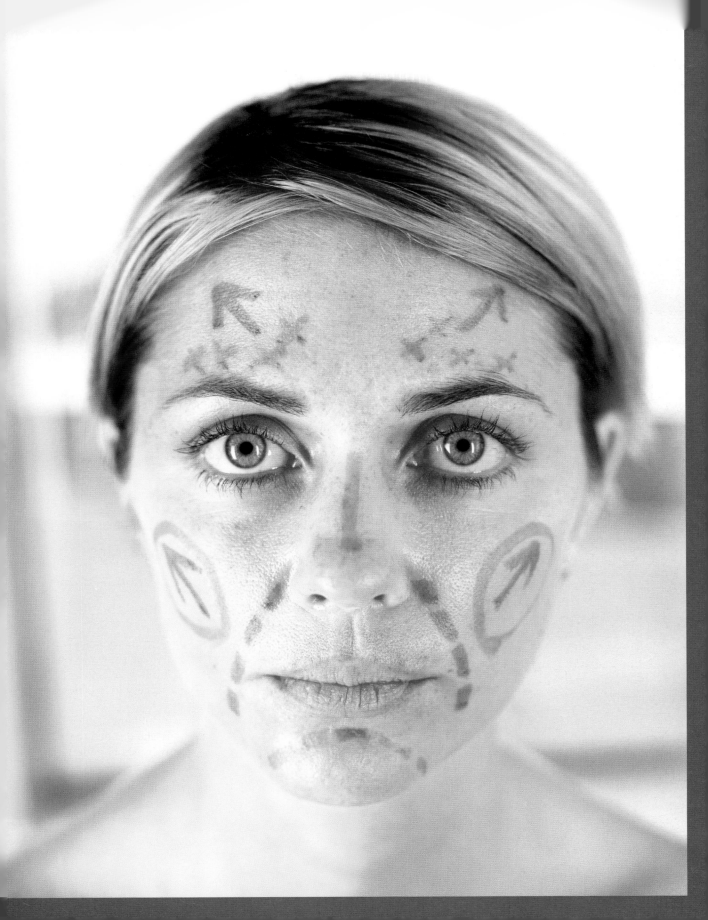

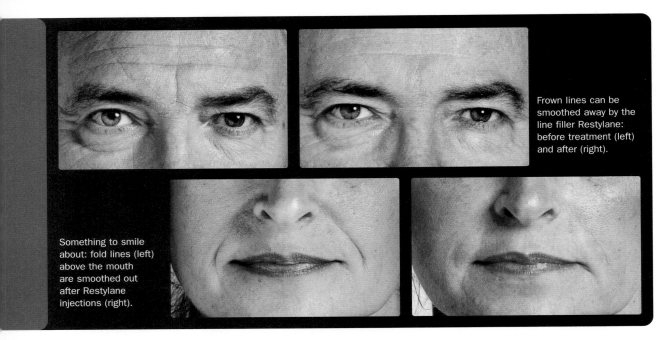

Frown lines can be smoothed away by the line filler Restylane: before treatment (left) and after (right).

Something to smile about: fold lines (left) above the mouth are smoothed out after Restylane injections (right).

like an ordinary woman.' Doris Newton is only one among millions of Americans in the past couple of years who have watched Cinderella-like, top-to-bottom transformations on programmes such as *I Want a Famous Face* and *Extreme Makeover* and then rushed out to have makeovers of their own.

The British Association of Aesthetic Plastic Surgeons (BAAPS) has expressed concern that programmes such as *I Want a Famous Face* and the drama series *Nip/Tuck* prey on the vulnerabilities of a society that is increasingly obsessed with physical perfection. They have warned people not to have cosmetic surgery to try to gain celebrity looks. 'Wanting to look exactly like a celebrity is a classic example of unrealistic attitudes,' says Norman Waterhouse, president of BAAPS. While he and other doctors fear that such programmes create an unrealistic picture of plastic surgery, people are voting with their feet – and their faces, breasts and stomachs. 'I have a waiting list as long as your arm,' says Dr Lori Saltz, a plastic surgeon in La Jolla, California. By the middle of 2004, she says, her business was up by 60 per cent compared with 2003.

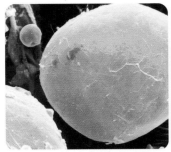

Microscopic view of collagen, part of the connective tissue in skin.

This is despite the high cost of the procedure: a top-to-toe revamp costs more than £100,000. In all, more than 8.7 million cosmetic surgery and related procedures were performed in the USA in 2003 – a 32 per cent increase from about 6.6 million the year before, according to the American Society of Plastic Surgeons. The patients are still mostly women, but a growing number of men are also going under the knife or needle. Following the arrival of *Extreme Makeover* in the UK this year, a similar trend may take hold in Britain.

The new wrinkle erasers

Television programmes are not the only thing that is driving the trend. Cosmetic surgery is in fact getting easier. The new era began with Botox, a toxin that is injected to paralyse the tiny muscles that give us crow's feet and laughter lines. Botox has become a household word in the past few years because of all the celebrities who have reportedly used it.

But, as Dr Brent Moelleken, a plastic surgeon who has been featured on *Extreme Makeover*, explains, 'We are now realizing that a tremendous

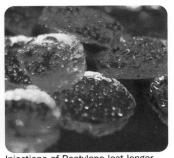

Injections of Restylane last longer than collagen injections.

component of ageing is loss of volume – the face is actually shrinking and facial fat is atrophying.' This can be counteracted by injectable line fillers such as Restylane and Hylaform. The basic component of these fillers is hyaluronic acid, a substance occurring naturally in the body (Restylane has no animal derivatives, but Hylaform is derived from cockerel combs). Hyaluronic acid pads tissue by attracting and binding water molecules to the skin. When natural levels of the acid fall as the years pass, skin becomes less resilient and looks older.

Three types of Restylane are currently available in the UK: the original Restylane, used to treat nose-to-mouth lines, lips and lines between the eyes just above the nose; Restylane Touch, which is used to smooth out fine lines around the mouth, brow lines and crow's feet; and Restylane Perlane, used to treat deeper lines and folds, creating full lips and cheek enhancement. In early 2005 a new type of

Restylane, called SubQ, came onto the market. It is based on a gel with a much larger particle size than its predecessors, making it suitable for facial sculpting and contouring to restore facial volume (rather than filling in wrinkles) – for example, injections to enhance high cheekbones or plump out cheeks after weight loss.

Other fillers that have proved popular include an individual's own fat cells plus collagen, a fibrous protein that is a constituent of the connective tissue in skin and tendons, but the life span of fat injections is unpredictable. Classic collagen – derived from cows – may cause allergic reactions, requiring time-consuming pre-injection testing, says Dr David Bank of the department of dermatology at Columbia Presbyterian Medical Center in New York City. New laboratory-grown strains of human collagen give better results, says Dr Bank, but he is an advocate of the hyaluronic acid fillers, which have only recently

A GROWING DEMAND FOR **SURGERY TO CORRECT OBESITY**

Severely obese people who are desperate to lose weight have been queuing up for stomach-shrinking surgery to curb their appetites. Demand has grown to such an extent that it led in 2004 to the opening of the first hospital in the UK dedicated to the treatment of the clinically obese. The private Dolan Park Hospital, at Bromsgrove in Worcestershire, hopes to perform more than 2,000 operations in its first year. 'We need to take a radical approach to obesity,' says Phil Thomas, the gastric surgeon who conceived the idea for a specialist obesity unit. 'Otherwise we will have millions of our citizens dying prematurely, having lived a life of chronic debilitation.' The procedures offered by the clinic range from gastric bypass surgery to implanting a pacemaker that tricks the brain into thinking that it has eaten enough.

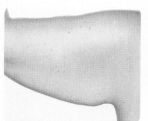

Losing large amounts of weight can leave sagging skin under the arms and elsewhere.

In the USA, such operations have proved so popular and successful that they are resulting in a boom in another kind of surgery – procedures that reshape the folds of skin left behind after massive weight loss.

Plastic surgeons are performing more and more 'body-contouring' procedures after stomach-shrinking surgery to

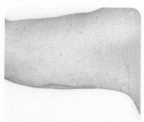

Having your 'wings' clipped: arm-lift surgery removes excess skin.

give a lift to the figure front and behind and to trim sail-like expanses of skin. They report a surge in the number of bottom lifts, upper-arm lifts, thigh and lower-body lifts, tummy tucks and face jobs. And they expect to do even more in the future. Skin-tightening surgical procedures are getting better as well as more frequent. For example, one procedure often done after gastric bypass surgery corrects an excess of skin that looks like a bat's wing between the elbow and the chest wall.

Previous techniques to restore a normal shape to this area often left unsightly scars that did not heal well because those methods failed to take into account how skin is pulled when an arm is flexed and extended.

Dr Berish Strauch, a plastic surgeon who is the author of a study on new arm-contouring techniques, says that such scars can be made less visible by making incisions on the underside of the arm. Using an S-shaped incision allows the scar to expand and contract with the arm's natural movements and heal better as a result. New, improved procedures also allow the skin to settle back into the armpit as naturally as it did before.

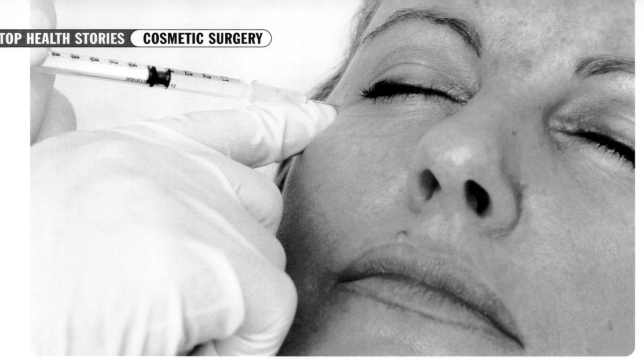

Better than Botox? While Botox injections (above) paralyse facial muscles that cause wrinkles, line fillers actually plump out the skin, padding tissue by attracting and binding water molecules to the skin.

become available in the USA. 'People can walk in and say, "I'm going to a special party this weekend, and I really want this corrected," and we can do it on the spot,' he says.

Although they are quick and relatively cheap, the treatments are not permanent. The body eventually absorbs the added material, and then new injections are required. Collagen injections generally last for about four to six months, Hylaform for six to nine months and Restylane for up to a year.

In 2003, medical trend watchers in the USA saw a 41 per cent increase in these so-called minimally invasive procedures over the previous year. Collagen treatments rose by 30 per cent and Botox injections shot up by 157 per cent. The Botox injection, which involves getting rid of wrinkles and lines by injecting a form of the botulinum toxin just under the skin, is the most popular cosmetic surgery procedure in the UK. The second most popular operation is the injection to plump up wrinkles and lips. Third on the list is laser skin resurfacing, in which dead skin is blasted away to reveal a clearer complexion. Some 50,000 Botox injections were given in Britain in 2003 and another 30,000 Restylane injections were performed to fill out lips and lines.

The 'minimalist' approach to surgery

There are still many people, however, who want the kinds of makeovers they have seen on television such as facelifts, nose reshaping, liposuction, eyelid

surgery, breast augmentation, breast and bottom lifts, tummy tucks and lip augmentation. According to the health insurance organization BUPA, up to 75,000 cosmetic surgery operations are performed in Britain each year. The most popular cosmetic procedures for women are breast enlargement or reduction, liposuction and rhinoplasty (nose surgery), while men mostly opt for liposuction and penis extensions. But virtually every part of the body can now be 'improved'.

To keep up with demand, plastic surgeons are 'minimalizing' many of those procedures. They are using smaller incisions and stitches for facelifts (which people increasingly want done on only certain parts of the face). For a traditional facelift, surgeons make a big cut, lift the skin and tissue beneath it, and use multiple stitches like bridge cables to pull it all up. Recovery takes weeks. With a new method, sometimes called a feather lift, a surgeon can thread barbed stitches through a small incision to lift and anchor underlying slack tissue. Recovery takes days instead of weeks, which means it is a procedure people can practically have done in time to get ready for an important occasion.

Also revolutionizing facelifts is endoscopic surgery, in which tiny instruments and cameras are inserted through small incisions. 'Instead of doing long incisions ear-to-ear, we make three small incisions at the hairline,' says Dr Rod Rohrich, president of the American Society of Plastic

Surgeons. Small incisions heal faster and allow patients to resume normal life sooner, he says. For breast augmentation, Dr Rohrich says, incisions below the breast are being replaced by small endoscopic incisions under the armpit, through which the implants are inserted and then filled.

The endoscopic facelift, which is also available in the UK, is most suitable for patients who are relatively young and whose facial ageing problems do not involve much excess skin.

Like fillers, surgery does not necessarily last for ever, but the less invasive procedures last as long as the original treatments. The life span of a facelift is still seven to ten years.

Is cosmetic surgery really needed?

Cosmetic surgery remains a controversial issue. Everyone agrees that plastic surgery is justifiable in the case of those who have suffered body damage – accident victims, for instance, or cancer patients. Proponents of cosmetic surgery also argue that extremely unsightly features, such as a large or misshapen nose, can seriously damage a person's professional and personal life and cause such intense self-loathing that life does not seem worth living. Anecdotal evidence suggests that cosmetic surgery can transform many such lives. The controversy arises when surgical procedures are performed on people who do not suffer from these disadvantages.

Critics say that the preoccupation with cosmetic surgery diverts attention and resources away from plastic surgeons' primary concern, which is function rather than appearance – in the UK, only 15 per cent of plastic surgery involves cosmetic procedures. Great advances in the field of tissue engineering, coupled with the prospect of scar-free healing, means that in future there will be more and more complaints that can be treated by plastic surgery.

Fuelled by exciting scientific advances, cosmetic surgery will doubtless continue its inexorable rise, but experts warn that it should not be seen as the solution to all ills. 'Many people want to change their appearance in some way, such as altering a feature they've always disliked,' says Dr Annabel Bentley, BUPA's assistant medical director. 'The way someone feels about their appearance affects self-esteem and confidence. But they should consider their reasoning carefully and surgery should not be seen as a quick-fix. Cosmetic surgery alone will not solve any personal problems or land you a dream job'. Furthermore, like any surgery, plastic surgery

carries risks. There are complications and, in rare cases, fatalities. For instance, on 16 January 2004, the American novelist Olivia Goldsmith, author of *The First Wives Club*, died of complications from surgery to remove loose skin from her chin.

Urging people who want cosmetic surgery to make every effort to find properly qualified plastic surgeons for advice and treatment, Dr Rohrich says, 'I have witnessed plastic surgery disasters where someone tried to look like someone else. '

British experts also counsel caution, pointing out that in the past 13 years more than £7 million in compensation has been paid out in the UK for cosmetic surgery mistakes.

What does it mean to you?

A wide range of procedures are now available in the UK but, if considering cosmetic surgery, make sure you are fully informed and aware of any risks and complications. To find out if a surgeon is on the General Medical Council specialist register of plastic surgeons, enquire at www.gmc-uk.org (020 7915 3638). To find a qualifed cosmetic surgeon, check with BAAPS at www.baaps.org.uk. BUPA says that, before making a decision, you should ask the following questions about the surgery, the specialist who will perform it, and the medical establishment where it will take place.

■ What qualifications does the specialist have? What experience does the specialist have in performing your procedure?

■ To what organizations does the specialist belong?

■ How much cosmetic surgery does this hospital or clinic perform each year?

■ What quality standards does the hospital or clinic have?

■ How can you best prepare for the procedure?

■ What results can usually be expected?

■ What are the side effects and potential complications of the procedure?

■ How long will it take to recover and what will this involve? How much scarring is there after the procedure? Will it change over time?

■ How long will the improvement last?

■ Is there a cooling off period between consultation and surgery?

■ What if anything goes wrong?

MAGNETS CAN RELIEVE DEPRESSION

A young woman at McLean Hospital, near Boston, USA, had bipolar disorder and was so depressed she could barely speak. She responded to questions with one-word answers. She made no eye contact. Then she lay on a platform and disappeared into the tunnel of a magnetic resonance imager, or MRI. Forty-five minutes later, she emerged, seemingly a new person.

'Something had changed,' says Aimee Parow, who was then a research assistant for a study of bipolar patients and is now a medical student. 'She was talking, she was sociable.' After the scan, Parow and the patient walked together to another part of the hospital, with the patient chattering away.

Parow thought the woman's mood shift must have been a fluke and dismissed it. Then she scanned another patient, a middle-aged woman whose depression took a different form. 'She was cranky, irritable and

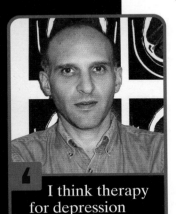

" I think therapy for depression is really going to be effective when behavioural treatments are combined with electrical ones.'

Dr Eric Wassermann

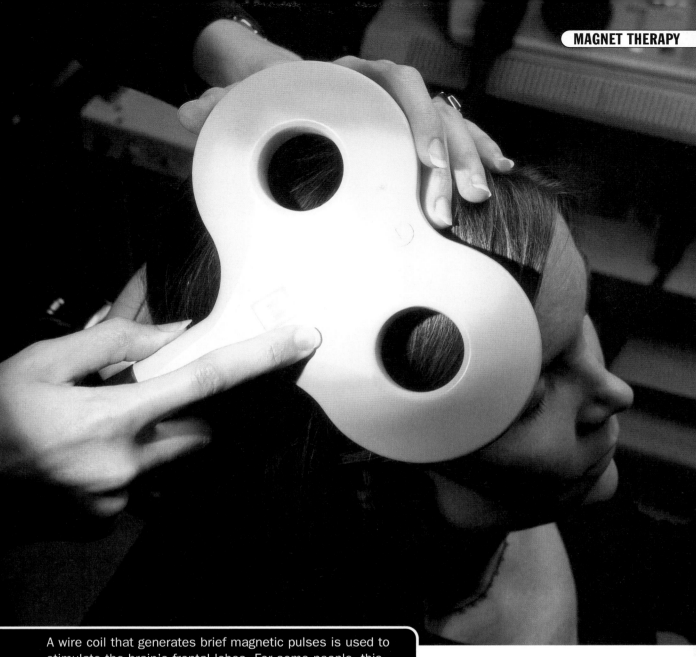

A wire coil that generates brief magnetic pulses is used to stimulate the brain's frontal lobes. For some people, this transcranial magnetic stimulation (TMS) relieves depression.

really didn't want to talk to me,' Parow says – but she came out of the machine smiling and cracking jokes.

Parow was baffled and excited. The MRI scans, using a special imaging method known as spectroscopy, were designed to measure patients' responses to antidepressant medications but it seemed that the scans themselves might be having an effect. Next morning, she told her boss what had happened and the study was quickly redesigned to measure patients' moods before and after their scans.

Over the following year, 30 patients with bipolar depression were given the same type of scan, a series of magnetic pulses delivered much more rapidly than in standard imaging MRIs. Afterwards, 23 of the patients said their moods had brightened. Meanwhile, among 10 patients who received sham scans, only three felt relief.

The study, published in the *American Journal of Psychiatry* in 2004, provided tantalizing support for an idea that could have come from an old sci-fi film:

that an electric coil poised over the skull could zap a person's brain with magnetic energy and improve the way it functioned. In fact, scientists have been exploring magnetism's power over the brain for many years. While an MRI had never been known to have this effect before the McLean Hospital study, a therapy called transcranial magnetic stimulation (TMS) has been tested widely on people with depression – and with some success – on both sides of the Atalantic. In recent US studies TMS was used on patients with Parkinson's disease, obsessive-compulsive disorder and even chronic pain; while recent UK studies have used TMS to treat spinal chord injury, epilepsy, stroke and neuropsychiatric disorders. Momentum is building, and these treatments may well make the transition from science fiction to everyday therapy for people with psychiatric and neurological disorders.

A magnetic idea takes off

The first uses of magnetic energy to trigger activity in the brain date from the 19th century but the early devices produced magnetic fields just strong enough to make volunteers see flashes of light. It was not until 1985 that Anthony Barker Ph.D., a medical physicist at the University of Sheffield, built the first effective TMS device, a single, doughnut-shaped coil

Brain mapping

Scientists were able to map out functions of the brain by aiming magnetic pulses at different sections.

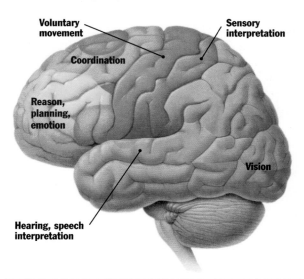

Voluntary movement

Sensory interpretation

Coordination

Reason, planning, emotion

Vision

Hearing, speech interpretation

> After the treatment, two of the patients showed what the reseachers called 'robust' improvement, and another had complete freedom from symptoms for the first time in three years.

of wire. When powered with electricity, it created a short-lived magnetic field. Dr Barker's device delivered a single pulse of magnetic energy and the magnetic field it created was weak and diffuse.

Within a few years, however, designs of the devices improved. Figure-of-eight-shaped coils created a more targeted magnetic field, and scientists were able to deliver a flurry of very brief pulses – up to 50 a second. At that stage, TMS was being used as a diagnostic tool. Much as a doctor might tap a knee with a mallet to test a person's reflexes, researchers used magnetic pulses to stimulate areas of the brain's motor cortex, causing patients' legs to kick and their arms to jerk.

As the technology improved and researchers began to aim magnetic pulses at brain structures beyond the motor cortex, they found that they could briefly block or inhibit certain brain functions. For example, by stimulating areas of the cortex known to control speech or vision, they could prevent people from speaking or perceiving some images.

From research tool to treatment

Before long, some researchers began to envisage TMS as a tool not only for mapping the brain but also for healing it.

In 1994, Dr Eric Wassermann, a neurologist and neurophysicist at the US National Institute of Neurological Diseases and Stroke, was using TMS for brain mapping. He was approached by Dr Mark George, a psychiatrist and neurologist at the National Institute of Mental Health, who had noticed that the PET scans (diagnostic scans using a short-lived radioactive 'tracer') of some depressed patients showed that their frontal lobes were inactive, and he wondered if this might be a cause of their depression. Dr Wassermann agreed to a trial TMS treatment on the frontal lobes to see if it relieved their depression.

'The prefrontal cortex is the part of the brain that is uniquely human,' says Dr George, who now directs the Brain Stimulation Laboratory at the

SWITCH ON YOUR **CREATIVITY**

Imagine sitting under a machine that resembles a hair dryer, flicking a switch, and suddenly possessing the extraordinary abilities of an autistic savant – hearing a piano sonata just once then being able to play it perfectly, for instance, or recalling a page of phone numbers.

That possibility is not so far-fetched. Allan Snyder, Ph.D., a physicist turned neurobiologist who directs the Centre for the Mind in Sydney, Australia, believes that a device sending magnetic pulses to the brain can greatly enhance powers of perception.

He has persuaded dozens of people to undergo transcranial magnetic stimulation, or TMS, aimed at the left-front temporal lobe, the grey matter just under the left temple. The aim is to temporarily shut off higher brain functions and give free rein to the detail-obsessed 'perceptual' brain, mimicking the brain damage in autistic savants and people with left-brain injuries, who sometimes develop

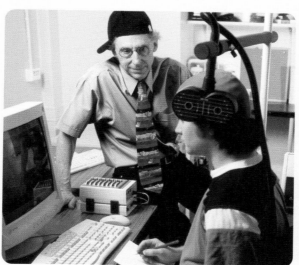

Allan Snyder Ph.D. uses magnetic pulses to simulate brain damage in a volunteer to see if savant-like skills emerge.

savant-like skills. The perceptual brain takes in a wealth of accurate raw information but in most of us the conceptual mind processes and simplifies all the details.

While TMS had no effect in seven volunteers in his most recent study, it created a change in four others. They drew more realistic pictures of animals after glancing at photographs or were more likely to notice a subtle mistake when asked to proofread a sentence. According to Dr Snyder, these seemingly small differences amount to a sharper, more perceptive view of the world. And one day, he says, we may be able to focus such heightened powers of observation and recall on challenging creative tasks, such as writing memoirs or painting landscapes.

A recent study at Flinders University, Adelaide, in which TMS was used to switch off the frontal lobe, found that 'savant skills' – memory, maths and art – improved in 5 of the 17 volunteers, supporting Dr Snyder's theory.

Medical University of South Carolina in Charleston. 'It does nothing in particular but a lot of things in general – it helps us to plan and hope and dream. And we also think that it helps regulate some of the deeper emotional parts of the brain.' His idea was that magnetic pulses aimed at the lobes of the prefrontal cortex (the area just above the eyes) could create changes in the cortex or in its relationship with deeper brain structures. The goal, he explains, was 'to reset mood regulation and treat depression'.

The two scientists used TMS on six depressed patients who had not improved with numerous trials of antidepressants. After the treatment, two of the patients showed what the researchers called 'robust' improvement and another had complete freedom from symptoms for the first time in three years. These results generated a lot of excitement among

neurologists and psychiatrists and led to dozens more studies, although most have been quite small. With no drug company paying the bills, most of the studies have been government funded and the largest one to date included only 70 people.

The results have been encouraging but not stellar. Overall, a minority of patients found their moods greatly improved, but most experienced relatively little change. Still, taken together, Dr Wassermann says, the studies suggest that TMS does help many people with depression.

Altering brain chemistry without drugs

The big question, of course, is why would TMS improve mood? Studies with other high-tech machines show that magnetic stimulation affects blood flow and sugar use in parts of the brain. But most researchers think that TMS may work for some of the same reasons as another poorly understood treatment: electroconvulsive therapy (ECT), better known as shock therapy. With ECT, doctors jolt the brains of anaesthetized patients with electricity, inducing seizures. Many ECT patients show significant improvement, although these gains often come at a price: cognitive problems, including a sometimes profound loss of memory, that scientists believe are caused by zapping the hippocampus, a key centre of memory formation. In the early days of TMS research, the powerful magnetic fields also induced seizures in some patients. That has not happened for many years, Dr Wassermann says, because researchers follow protocols governing the place, length, strength and timing of treatments.

According to Dr George, TMS amounts to electrical stimulation without the electrodes. 'We're electrically stimulating the cortex but we're using the magnetic field as the trick to get past the skull,' he says. As the magnetic pulses penetrate past hair, skin and bone and reach brain cells in the cortex, on the surface of the brain, they cause the nerve cells to electrically discharge and send a signal in the form of electrons flowing from cell to cell. As this signal spreads through the brain, it triggers changes in neurotransmitters – brain chemicals that are the target of antidepressant medications.

Dr George believes that depressed people have problems in the mood-regulating circuitry of their brains, centred in the prefrontal cortex. He thinks that ECT, perhaps by inducing a seizure, interrupts the normal flow of electrons and 'resets' the regulatory circuit. 'My idea with TMS is that instead of inducing a generalized seizure, we could reset that circuit with daily, gentle nudges,' he says.

But Dr George's theory does not explain the improvements that Aimee Parow saw in the MRI patients at McLean Hospital. That is because the low-frequency magnetic fields emitted during the MRI scans were too weak to make neurons fire and send a signal, says Michael Rohan, the physicist who led the study.

He speculates that the unique sequence of magnetic pulses in his spectroscopic MRIs somehow altered the chemistry of the brain cells without causing them to fire. 'We think we've hit some kind of a magic spot in the timing', so the pulses are synchronizing with processes taking place in the cells and correcting some kind of chemical imbalance. 'It's a mystery to us, but the effect was rather profound,' Rohan says.

Pulse of the future

Rohan and his colleagues have designed a tabletop device that emits the same kind of pulses as their specialized MRI. They hope to replicate the results of their first study.

Meanwhile, other medical scientists are exploring the effects of TMS on a range of psychiatric and neurological disorders. Working with schizophrenic patients who hear voices, Dr Ralph Hoffman, a Yale researcher, has applied low-frequency TMS to the auditory cortex (the part of the brain that processes and interprets sound) and discovered that the patients' auditory hallucinations declined markedly.

Moreover, French researchers have reported that stimulating the motor cortex seems to give relief to people with chronic pain. However, results have been mixed in studies using TMS to

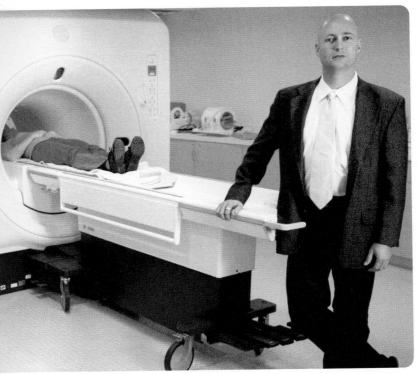

Physicist Michael Rohan explored the antidepressant effects of a special MRI in a study conducted at McLean Hospital near Boston, USA.

Transcranial magnetic stimulation

When a transcranial magnetic stimulation (TMS) coil is turned on close to a patient's scalp, a powerful and rapidly changing magnetic field passes safely and painlessly through skin and bone. The shallow, precisely focused magnetic pulses stimulate brain cells to start signalling.

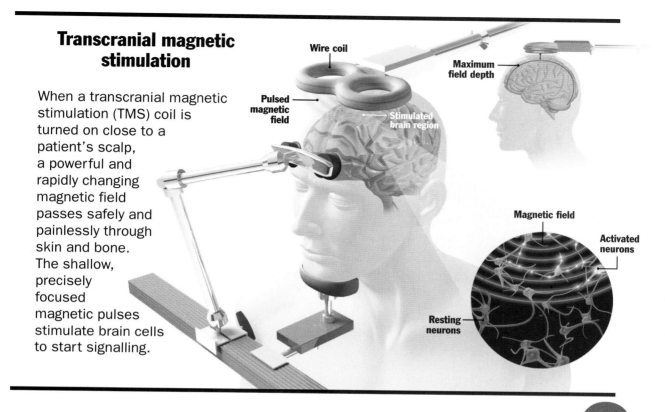

relieve the palsied movements of Parkinson's disease and seizures caused by epilepsy.

'Most pathological and neurological disorders are related to deeper structures in the brain,' says Abraham Zangen Ph.D. While at the USA's National Institutes of Health (NIH), he developed a coil that may be able to penetrate farther into the brain than standard TMS devices. Dr Zangen, now a consultant for an Israeli-American company that bought the coil's patent from the NIH, hopes that it may be used to treat autism, Parkinson's disease, addiction, obesity and depression. He is organizing a study of several dozen depressed patients.

In the UK, TMS is being used experimentally to treat depression, with recent trials in hospitals in London, Newcastle and Edinburgh. 'It's still early days,' says Declan McLoughlin, senior lecturer at the Maudsley Hospital, London. 'More research is needed into the extent and duration of the effect and how best to administer the treatment.'

What does it mean to you?

Using magnetic energy to treat brain disorders is not as far fetched as it may seem. The technique called transcranial magnetic stimulation (TMS) has the full attention of brain researchers and psychiatrists, who see it as a noninvasive way to treat a number of different problems.

■ Treatment of depression holds the greatest promise. Overall, numerous studies suggest that TMS can help relieve the symptoms of many depressed patients.

■ Experts believe that TMS may act in ways quite similar to electroconvulsive therapy (ECT), but without causing seizures or impairing patients' memories.

■ Scientists also believe that TMS may help relieve the shaking experienced by people with Parkinson's disease, reduce the scary voices sometimes caused by schizophrenia, and bring some relief to people with chronic pain.

■ In both the UK and the USA the technique is still being tested. More research is needed before TMS will be routinely available in the UK.

SHARPER MEMORY FROM A PILL?

Can a pill sharpen memory dulled by age or even disease? Several promising drugs are currently being tested in humans.

Most people accept reading glasses as a bothersome but bearable accompaniment to maturity. When they keep forgetting where they left the blasted things, though – well, that's when they start to worry. Three-quarters of people over 50 complain of memory lapses – the name that won't come to you, the bafflement as to why you're in a room you just entered, and, of course, the 15-minute search for those specs that were perched on top of your head the whole time. While a degree of memory loss is a natural consequence of ageing, don't tell that to these middle-aged and older people; they are not amused by what some like to call 'senior moments'. A big part of what it means to be alive and to be yourself is being taken away, and there really ought to be a pill to stop it.

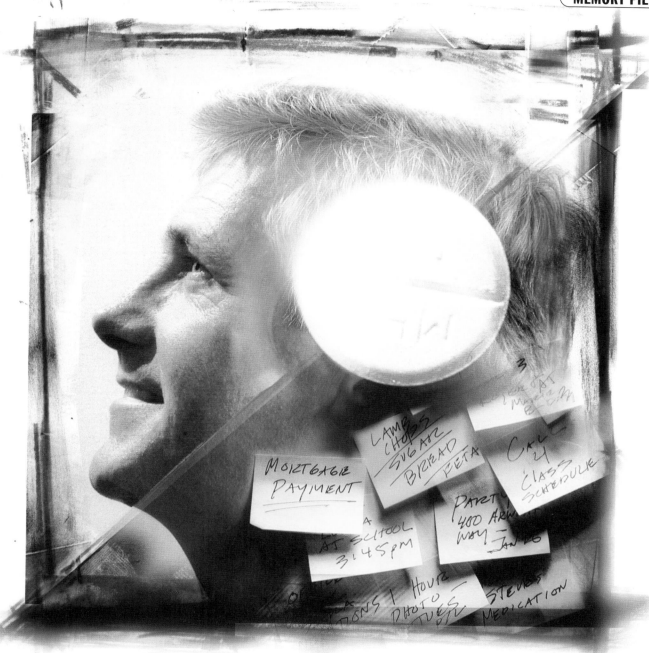

In fact, dozens of memory-enhancement drugs are now being tested, and in 2004 many showed enough promise to advance into new phases of human trials. The first memory pills may be available in just a few years. Even better ones will follow.

The drugs are arriving just in time as the world's population is ageing rapidly. In the UK, 23 million will be 50 or older by 2014 – which means some 18 million potential memory problems. One in 10 aged 65-plus have a persistent memory problem severe enough to interfere with daily routines and 15 per cent of these develop dementia each year.

'Hanging on to memory is important for quality of life,' says Axel Unterbeck Ph.D., chief scientific officer of Memory Pharmaceuticals in Montvale, New Jersey, which is developing several drugs.

Memory impairment makes daily tasks harder. It impedes communication, which can contribute to depression. And as you lose the ability to form memories, you lose part of what makes you, you.

The promised pills are not mere refinements of the modestly effective medications prescribed since the early 1990s to slow the memory decline of Alzheimer's disease. They spring from far-reaching studies of exactly how the brain takes in sights, sounds and scents and stores them as memories.

'These new drugs work on different mechanisms in the brain from anything previously,' says Tim Tully Ph.D., a pioneer in the memory-enhancement field who oversees development of some of the drugs at the Helicon Therapeutics biotech lab in Farmingdale, New York. 'They directly upgrade the biochemical process of memory storage.'

Gary Lynch Ph.D., a pioneer of memory-enhancing drugs called ampakines and scientific adviser for Cortex Pharmaceuticals in Irvine, California, notes that the act of storing a new memory causes chemical and physical changes among the brain's billions of nerve cells – changes that scientists are now learning to manipulate. Memory-enhancing experiments in animals have been very successful. Dr Tully, for example, created memory-enhanced fruit flies that performed 10 times better than normal fruit flies in tests such as learning to remember – and avoid – sources of electric shocks.

How memories are made

To understand what the new drugs can eventually do for you, it helps to understand how memory works.

'Memory is a process, not a thing,' says Dr Tully, 'and it's not one process but many.' First comes alertness. If you're not paying attention to what's coming in through your eyes or ears or other senses, the memory-forming interplay of chemical reactions in the brain never gets started. Can't remember the name of a person you just met? Perhaps you never actually listened in the first place.

Forming a memory and calling it up (retrieval) are also distinct processes. Improving retrieval is a low priority in memory research for the simple reason that calling up existing memories is much less of a problem for older people than forming new ones. An 80-year-old, for example, can probably tell you what she was doing on VE Day, some 60 years ago.

Likewise, separate processes control the two main types of memories. Short-term memories are the many temporary, everyday impressions – such as the location of your reading glasses – that help you to get things done but are soon discarded. Long-term

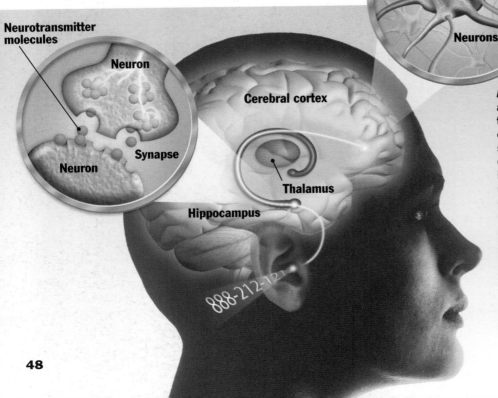

Neurotransmitter molecules

Neuron

Neuron

Synapse

Neurons

Cerebral cortex

Thalamus

Hippocampus

A human brain is more efficient at storing memories than the fastest super-computer , constantly reconfiguring cells to store new memories and purge old ones. There is no one place in the brain where memories are stored. As new information comes in, nerve cells (neurons) capture it as a pattern of electrical signals and transmit it to the hippocampus to be processed. Messenger chemicals called neurotransmitters carry the information across gaps (synapses) between neurons. A group of neurons band together to store a long-term memory.

memories consist of information that you are able to recall days, months or decades later.

Sensations entering the brain create short-term memory by triggering a multi-chemical cascade that causes changes in the junctions (synapses) between brain cells (neurons). New or altered connections give memory a physical structure. Since any two of your billions of neurons may have thousands of synapses, there is no shortage of storage space.

These changes are temporary unless another chemical sequence is initiated. To convert an experience from a passing event into a long-term memory, the identical cascade must run many times, forming a permanent point of contact between neurons where nerve impulses can pass. That's why you know what 9 times 5 equals – because you repeated your times tables over and over again.

The new drugs don't promise you more memory per se but instead help new memories to lock themselves in. When you take one of these pills, memorizing poetry is no longer a lost ability from your youth but an achievable objective.

So is remembering that new acquaintance's name. While sharpening long-term memory is the primary effect of most memory pills being developed, short-term memory is also improved. That's because the processes, although distinct, 'speak to each other', as Dr Tully puts it. 'Conversion to long-term memory depends on short-term memory, or otherwise there would be nothing to convert,' he says. 'Anybody with short-term memory deficits will benefit from the drug as a secondary effect.'

Help for those with Alzheimer's

Creating smarter humans has a certain futuristic appeal, but it is not what is driving the new research into memory drugs. The goal is to make sick people better – to help those whose memory has been impaired by clinical conditions. The most serious of those conditions, of course, is Alzheimer's disease, which is where Helicon, Memory, Cortex and other memory drug developers are focusing their efforts.

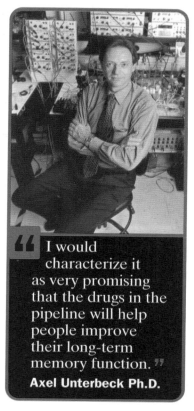

" I would characterize it as very promising that the drugs in the pipeline will help people improve their long-term memory function. "
Axel Unterbeck Ph.D.

Among those taking part in final Phase III trials for an Alzheimer's drug called Alzhemed, which helps to prevent the formation of the amyloid plaques believed to contribute to memory loss, is the Kingshill Research Centre, at Victoria Hospital, Swindon, a leading UK establishment in the field of memory and dementia.

But, even if a drug to halt the disease is found, says Dr Tully, you'll still have to give patients back some of the memory they have lost. 'That's where our drugs will be effective.'

And Alzheimer's accounts for only a small percentage of people with failing memories. About 50 per cent of people over 65 clearly suffer from some degree of impairment, but the figure may be significantly higher (evidence is not conclusive). Most have either mild cognitive impairment (MCI) or age-associated memory impairment (AAMI).

The symptoms of both conditions run the gamut from episodes of forgetfulness to a noticeably reduced capacity to form short and long-term memories. However, MCI is a far more serious diagnosis than the more common AAMI because about 80 per cent of those who have it develop Alzheimer's within seven years.

That makes MCI a prime target for the memory drug developers. 'If we can help MCI sufferers to postpone their progression to Alzheimer's disease by even a year, it would have a hugely beneficial impact on their health and the economy,' Dr Unterbeck says.

Meanwhile, there's also good news for the memory-challenged masses with AAMI. 'These drugs are potentially extremely effective in restoring memory with age-related impairment,' says Dr Unterbeck.

The new drugs take the test

Drug developers are focusing on three main types of memory pills, all of which are being tested now.

Ampakines These manmade molecules boost the electrical signals that trigger the memory-forming chemical exchanges that occur between neurons.

Since those signals weaken with age, memory impairment is in part a problem of power supply. An ampakine turns up the power by attaching itself to a protein on the brain cell surface, called an AMPA receptor, and helping it to respond to the hormone glutamate – a response that generates most of the electrical signals running through brain cells. 'It's surprisingly simple,' says Dr Lynch. 'All ampakines do is help the AMPA receptor's function to increase the current. It's like turning up the dimmer on a light switch.'

Ampakines were the first memory drugs to undergo trials in the 1990s and were predicted to be the first to be approved for use. But after cross-national trials in the USA and Europe conducted by Cortex Pharmaceuticals and the French company Les Laboratoires Servier, the drug developers were forced to abandon testing of an ampakine that was chosen for its safety but proved too weak to consistently deliver the desired effects in humans (although some study subjects still showed marked improvement). 'The concern with any of these drugs is to make sure they don't cause brain damage,' Dr Lynch says, 'so we were very cautious.'

In January 2004, Servier, France's largest privately owned pharmaceutical company, renewed its research collaboration with Cortex for a further two years, and both are conducting trials on more powerful ampakine drugs, with the working names CX717 (Cortex) and S-18986 (Servier). CX717 has proved safe in humans. In 2004, it entered Phase II studies, in which its efficacy is tested on 100 or more memory-impaired volunteers with some taking the drug daily and others taking a placebo. The next step, Phase III, repeats the testing but in a much larger pool of memory-impaired volunteers. Success in that phase could lead to approval of the drug. Servier's S-18986 has completed Phase I and was expected to enter Phase II trials by the end of 2004. The Kingshill Research Centre is also involved in these new Phase III trials.

CREB enhancers These drugs are perhaps the most eagerly awaited because they deliver to humans essentially the same benefits that gave Dr Tully's fruit flies their super-powered memory. The drugs boost the amount of a brain protein called CREB (cyclic AMP response element binding protein), which plays a major role in memory formation.

Like a shop foreman, CREB organizes the other chemical workers involved in memory formation. When its levels are raised, the process moves into high gear. CREB enhancers achieve that effect by blocking the action of another protein that normally keeps CREB levels in check.

Higher CREB levels make the brain much more efficient at creating permanent connections between synapses – and the faster those connections form, the fewer times you have to repeat the words of a

New help for fading memory

Dozen of drug developers are testing different approaches to memory enhancement. Here are three of the most promising types of memory drugs and when they might come to market.

DRUG	EXAMPLE	ACTION	OPTIMISTIC ARRIVAL DATE
Ampakines	CX717 (Cortex Pharmaceuticals)	Speed and strengthen the formation of new memories by boosting the electrical signals between brain cells.	2007
CREB enhancers	HT712 (Helicon Therapeutics), MEM 1414 (Memory Pharmaceuticals)	Bolster cell-to-cell connections in the brain by raising levels of the protein CREB, a key organizer in memory formation.	2009
Calcium channel modulators	MEM 1003 (Memory Pharmaceuticals)	Optimize levels of calcium inside and outside of each brain cell, which counteracts memory decline by making cells more responsive to incoming signals.	2008

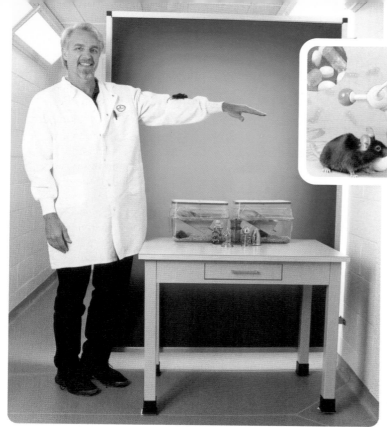

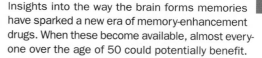

Say 'cheese': Dr Tim Tully's memory-impaired laboratory mice benefited from new drugs under development.

At his Helicon Therapeutics lab, Tim Tully Ph.D. oversees development of drugs that will improve memory storage.

The race to market

It is possible that memory drugs will be generally available in five to ten years, although ampakines may well arrive sooner. 'There's no way to predict exactly how long it will take,' Dr Tully says, 'but it's a question of when, not if.'

Meanwhile, a new study at Edinburgh University shows that a liquorice-based-compound which reduces levels of the stress hormone cortisol in the brain improves memory in older men. Study leader Jonathan Seckl says it could be available for the elderly in five years.

song or poem to store them for good. Take a daily CREB enhancer, and you may find that you can talk about the details of that novel you read last month instead of struggling even to recall the title.

Both Dr Tully's Helicon Therapeutics and Dr Unterbeck's Memory Pharmaceuticals are working on CREB enhancers. Helicon's main drug, HT712, was due to begin Phase I testing (mainly to establish human safety) by the end of 2004. Phase II, to test effectiveness, could begin in 2005. 'So maybe by the summer of 2006, we'll know if HT712 does what we think it will do for memory,' Dr Tully says. Phase III trials would follow, 'so we're talking at least five years from 2004 if all goes well.'

Memory Pharmaceuticals' version, called MEM 1414, is slightly further along in testing, with Phase I trials nearly complete. Memory has an alliance with the Swiss company Roche in developing these drugs.

Calcium channel modulators At Memory, another drug, dubbed MEM 1003, is entering Phase II of testing. It's a calcium channel modulator that improves memory in patients with Alzheimer's and MCI (but not those with AAMI) by restoring the balance of calcium inside and outside the neurons.

What does it mean to you?

Insights into the way the brain forms memories have sparked a new era of memory-enhancement drugs. When these become available, almost everyone over the age of 50 could potentially benefit.

■ Alzheimer's patients will be able to slow or even reverse memory decline with drugs that are much more effective than those currently available.

■ Although memory drugs themselves will never cure Alzheimer's (which involves much more than memory loss), they will play a major role once a drug that stops the disease is found. Recovering Alzheimer's patients will take the pills during 'brain rehabilitation' to restore memory capacity that the disease took away.

■ People with mild cognitive impairment (MCI) – a memory disorder that often leads to Alzheimer's – will be able to repair memory loss and slow or perhaps prevent the progression to Alzheimer's.

■ By taking once-a-day memory pills, people over 50 who are bothered by increasing memory lapses and declining ability to form new long-term memories – a condition known as age-associated memory impairment (AAMI) – will restore their recall to near-peak levels.

NANOTECHNOLOGY
HUGE HOPES
FOR TINY MEDICINE

A mere flaw in your DNA is no match for an astoundingly tiny, laser-armed repair robot, as depicted in this artist's impression of the future.

Last year, while a dogged little spacecraft dodging the rings of Saturn sent back photographs to awestruck outer-space scientists on Earth, inner-space scientists received astounding images as well. They used manmade particles a million times smaller than a pencil dot to do what most people never dreamed was possible: take live-action movies of genes at work inside living cells.

The researchers were actually able to watch the same cellular events that are targeted by some anti-cancer drugs. Being able to observe these processes may one day allow experts to create new and more finely tuned cancer treatments. Meanwhile, scientists working with similarly minuscule particles devised new ways to track – and curtail – the spread of breast cancer and even to kill tumours.

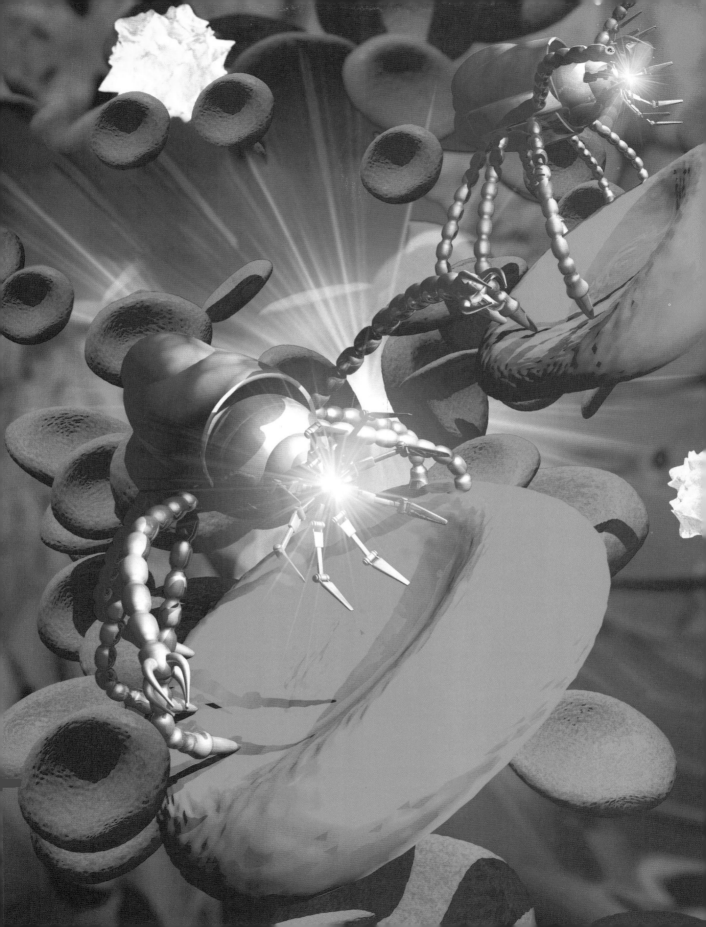

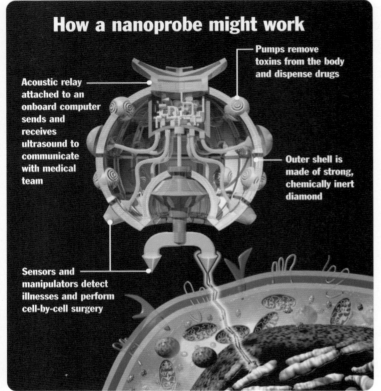

How a nanoprobe might work

Pumps remove toxins from the body and dispense drugs

Acoustic relay attached to an onboard computer sends and receives ultrasound to communicate with medical team

Outer shell is made of strong, chemically inert diamond

Sensors and manipulators detect illnesses and perform cell-by-cell surgery

Welcome to the new world of nanotechnology, a science that puts the arcane and bizarre discoveries of particle physics to work on real-life problems. Nanotech researchers are especially excited by the many opportunities in the world of medicine. These include tumour detection and eradication; crystal-clear imagery of blood vessels and tissues hidden deep within the body; medical tests that provide instant results; and revolutionary methods for defeating cancer, Aids and other major diseases.

Professor John Ryan of the Bionanotechnology Centre at Oxford University, looks forward to precisely targeted drug delivery, individualized therapy and nano-engineered cochlear implants. Hip joints made of biocompatible materials, intelligent clothing that measures pulse and respiration, and even medical sensors to monitor our physical state 24 hours a day, are all real possibilities.

What makes such progress possible is the outlandishly small size of the tools employed in nanotechnology (*nano-* is from

the Greek word for dwarf). Nanoscientists work at a scale a million times smaller than a pinhead, using materials and devices that are engineered at the scale of atoms and molecules. A nanometre, one billionth of a metre, is the width of 10 hydrogen atoms lined up in a row. In comparison, a red blood cell is a veritable giant, measuring 8,000 nanometres.

That is the scope of nanotechnology. Using a variety of techniques – such as vaporizing carbon and letting it condense in an inert gas to produce crystals – scientists are able to produce unimaginably tiny tubes, spheres, shells, snowflakes and other complex 'nanoparticles'. Several much-heralded nanotech advances in 2004 may help drug companies to develop new cancer drugs and therapies more quickly.

Tiny weapons against cancer

In one study, according to a report in *Nature Biotechnology,* researchers at Germany's Max Planck Institute used fluorescent nanoparticles called quantum dots to make the first movies of the signalling mechanisms and chemical processes that control genes.

Quantum dots, known as Qdots, glow in various colours when 'excited' by a light source, such as a laser. They can be customized to link up with, or tag, specific proteins that perform key tasks inside cells. Unlike existing imaging tools – such as fluorescent dyes, which fade away in seconds – Qdots can provide extended, real-time images of healthy and diseased cells at work.

According to the Quantum Dot Corporation in California, which created and manufactures Qdots, such live images will provide better understanding of how cell processes work and may allow researchers to observe closely as cells react to medications and treatments, including some used against cancer.

In a related experiment, scientists at Carnegie Mellon University in Pittsburgh gave quantum dots a special coating that enabled them to enter lab animals' tissues and send back trackable signals for many months. Without the new coating, the Qdots are too fragile to function in the body for more

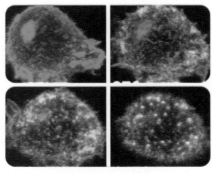

Scientists used minuscule 'quantum dots' to make the first movies of signalling within cells.

than hours or days. Eventually, these particles could be treated with substances that seek out specific tumours and then be injected into the body, tracked by laser technology and tiny microscopes called nanoscopes, and used to pinpoint and illuminate tumours so doctors can remove them with greater accuracy and with greater likelihood of getting all of the cancer. They could even be used to deliver antibodies or drugs.

Such possibilities no longer seem fanciful. In 2004, researchers at Rice University in Houston reported that in preliminary tests, 'nanoshells' had proved effective at eradicating tumours in laboratory animals. Twenty times smaller than a red blood cell, a nanoshell consists of a silica core covered by a thin layer of pure gold. Because of their small size, nanoshells are able to pass through the poorly formed blood vessels of a tumour and collect inside it. When near-infrared light is aimed at the tumour, it passes harmlessly through soft tissue and strikes the nanoshells' gold coating, raising its temperature just as sunlight heats a car's roof. The concentrated heat destroys the tumour.

'The results of these first animal studies are very promising,' says Naomi Halas Ph.D., professor of electrical engineering and chemistry at Rice. 'While we don't yet have a target date for our first human trial, our team is working hard to make this treatment available to cancer patients as soon as possible.'

Women may be among such technologies' earliest beneficiaries. At Carnegie Mellon, Byron Ballou Ph.D., a research scientist at the Molecular Biosensor

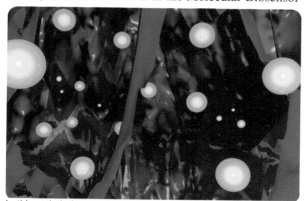

In this artist's impression, gold-covered microscopic particles called nanoshells cluster inside a tumour. When near-infrared light strikes the shells they heat up, destroying the cancer.

and Imaging Center at the Mellon College of Science, believes that the first medical use of nanotech tools will be against breast cancer. That disease spreads

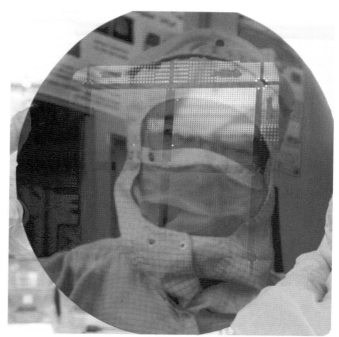

A technician at the New Jersey Nanotechnology Laboratory holds a disc printed with an etched pattern used to make nanotechnology devices.

through the lymph nodes, which must be removed along with the tumour if they have been affected by the cancer. When surgeons perform breast cancer surgery, Dr Ballou says, the vital question is, 'When should you stop taking nodes? The trick is to find out which nodes you should be taking.'

Currently, he says, surgeons inject radioactive dyes to try to locate 'sentinel nodes' – those closest to the tumour that show signs of the cancer's spread. Such detection methods can be slow and inexact, but injecting Qdots instead of radioactive dyes would give surgeons a quicker, more precise picture of where the diseased nodes begin and end. Armed with that knowledge, Dr Ballou says, they could operate with greater success.

New arsenal of disease fighters

Cancer is just one of many medical conditions that nanotechnologists are targeting. In 2004, researchers at Philadelphia's Drexel University reported progress in developing a device the size of a cell phone that would permit people on blood-thinning (anticoagulant) medication to take their own blood-clotting readings at home. The researchers say that the device, which is able to analyse submicroscopic particles, would take readings by targeting proteins involved in the clotting process. Determining the right anticoagulant dose has always been a process of trial and error, but the new method would more exactly calculate the required dose.

Nanotechnology is also improving genetic testing and gene therapy. For instance, researchers are exploring ways to test embryos for inherited cystic fibrosis (CF) prior to in vitro fertilization, using nanoparticles that glow when they encounter compounds produced by the CF gene. Other scientists are testing the feasibility of compressing healthy DNA strands from about 200 nanometres to less than 25 nanometres in order to slip healthy genes through the cell membranes of people who have CF and other genetic disorders. The healthy genes would force the cells to perform normally.

Meanwhile, researchers who are hoping to build better artificial joints and implants are trying their luck with rolled-up sheets of carbon atoms called nanotubes. Studies have found that, among other things, bone cells called osteoblasts bond to titanium coated with nanotubes better than to uncoated titanium. Among the potential benefits is a reduced chance that the ball and socket of a surgically implanted artificial hip joint will work loose.

Even the war on Aids may receive a boost from nanotechnology. In late 2003, the US Food and Drug Administration (FDA) approved early, small-scale human trials to determine the safety of an anti-HIV vaginal gel developed by the Australian nanotechnology firm Starpharma. The gel, which is inserted prior to sex, contains a protein that prevents the virus from infecting healthy cells. The nanotech components of the gel are dendrimers – minute snowflake-like molecules to which medical substances can be attached for special delivery. Dendrimers, too, are being tested as cancer fighters.

Nanotechnology has even reached the shelves where everyday health and beauty aids are sold. The

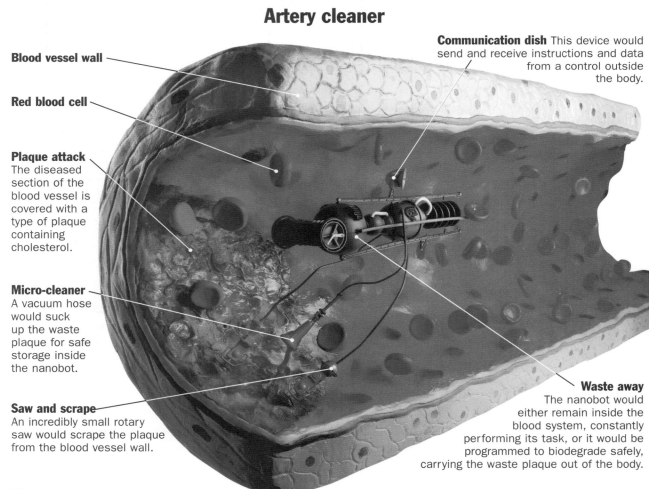

Artery cleaner

Blood vessel wall

Red blood cell

Plaque attack
The diseased section of the blood vessel is covered with a type of plaque containing cholesterol.

Micro-cleaner
A vacuum hose would suck up the waste plaque for safe storage inside the nanobot.

Saw and scrape
An incredibly small rotary saw would scrape the plaque from the blood vessel wall.

Communication dish This device would send and receive instructions and data from a control outside the body.

Waste away
The nanobot would either remain inside the blood system, constantly performing its task, or it would be programmed to biodegrade safely, carrying the waste plaque out of the body.

new products include high-protection sunscreens made with zinc oxide particles so tiny that they go on clear instead of chalky white, as traditional zinc oxide creams do. According to experts, zinc oxide offers superior protection from the sun because unlike other commonly used sunscreens, it provides protection from both ultraviolet A and ultraviolet B rays.

A micro-syringe could deliver drugs to precise targets – blood cells, for instance.

The truly fantastic voyage

What's the ultimate potential of nanotech therapies? Limitless, say some scientists, who foresee nanobots – nano-size molecular 'machines' – with propellers, gears and built-in power tools. Others caution that only time will tell if these dreams will come true.

'Gaining molecular-scale control is extremely relevant to medicine,' says Christine Peterson, a director of the Foresight Institute in Palo Alto, California, which promotes nanotechnology. Disease begins with molecular-level damage. If we can send in nano repair kits for such breakdowns, including cancer, 'the medical benefits are immense,' she says.

The focus is not only on disease but also on the ordinary ravages of time. 'We don't know a lot about ageing,' says James R. Von Ehr II, head of a Texas nanotechnology company called Zyvex, 'but it seems that the process is caused by cellular degradation – the little nanomachines inside our cells start to break down. If we had other nanoscale machines that could go in and repair some of those breakdowns, in principle, we could repair them. And if we can repair the cell to the state it was in when it was young and healthy, we might be able to repair the organism.'

Dr Ballou agrees – up to a point. 'The future hope is to be able to go in and replace or fix biochemical machinery,' he says.

There are also questions about possible harmful effects of nanotech particles and matter. Qdots, for example, are made from the heavy metal cadmium, and researchers from the University of California, San Diego, reported in early 2004 that under certain conditions, the Qdots proved to be acutely toxic. Other researchers say this danger can be countered by coating the dots with protective substances.

In the UK, an independent report released in July 2004 stressed that the emerging science could bring huge benefits. It proposed tighter UK and European regulation over some aspects of nanotechnology, and more research into nanoparticles and nanotubes, which should be treated as 'new chemicals' to allow for appropriate safety tests and labelling. It added that £6 million a year should be dedicated in the UK to researching potential health risks. Welcoming the report, the science minister, Lord Sainsbury, said that the government response would come by the end of the year.

The US government allotted $847 million (£470 million) in 2004 for the National Nanotechnology Initiative. The government of Japan, which for decades has been at the forefront of the miniaturization movement, is also heavily funding nanotechnology research. When such investment will pay off, no one can say.

In 1965, the movie *Fantastic Voyage* told of a microscopic submarine full of medical experts shrunk to cellular size. Their mission: to navigate the body of a dying scientist and save his life. It was science fiction then, but no longer. That fantastic voyage is actually happening.

What does it mean to you?

Most research in the UK is currently focused on commercial applications of nanotechnology and the biological research is very much at the stage of basic science. But if nanotechnology lives up to its promise, in the foreseeable future doctors will be able to:

■ Detect diseases, such as cancer, in their earliest stages and devise treatments to stop them in their tracks. Nanoparticles such as Qdots and dendrimers would reveal tumours that could be either destroyed by the nanoparticles or removed by precise surgery.

■ Locate signs of genetic susceptibility to health problems and fight bad genes with good. Researchers are exploring ways in which to detect a predisposition to cystic fibrosis – or the disease itself – in embryos and eliminate the problem with genetic treatments.

■ Make giant strides towards understanding and countering the ageing process where it begins – inside the body's cells.

COMING SOON: ANTI-AGEING DRUGS

Inside a San Francisco laboratory, some very special worms recently celebrated their 120th day of life. It was no ordinary birthday. For one thing, 120 days is about six times longer than any of these millimetre-long creatures would normally live. Even so, they looked and acted like budding youths.

There's more. The researchers who genetically altered the worms, making their astonishingly long lives possible, had an extra reason to celebrate. They had just unlocked the secret of the worms' ultralongevity, revealing the details of the life-expanding process that the gene manipulation had triggered – and they think they can duplicate that process in humans. In fact, they're working right now on an anti-ageing drug to do just that.

This isn't wishful thinking. Many people reading this article have a much better chance of happily reaching a healthy 100th birthday than they did just two years ago. The 'Methuselah worms' are part of the reason, but so is another breakthrough that occurred in 2003 and 2004, when researchers identified two human gene variations that are partially responsible for the

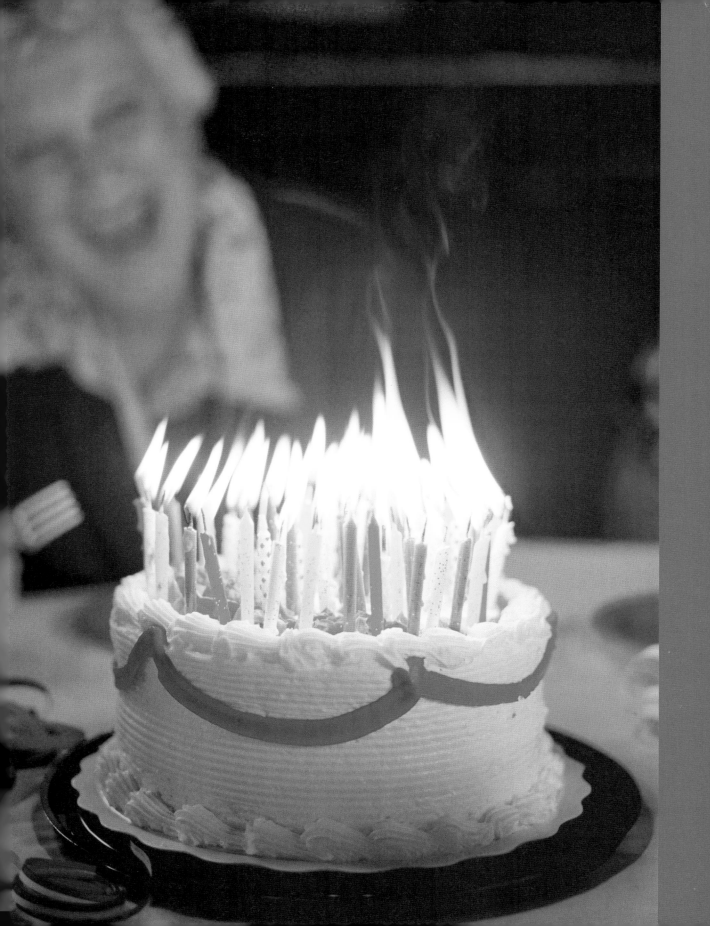

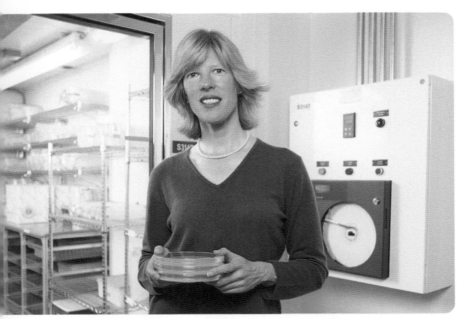

Worm experiments by Cynthia Kenyon Ph.D. turned scientific thinking on its head. No longer considered inevitable, ageing may be more like a disease that can be cured.

Dr Kenyon's work in 1993, when she coaxed some of the current worms' ancestors into living twice as long as normal. That alone was head-turning, but how she did it was revolutionary.

'Basically, we got worms to live much longer and stay very healthy by changing just one gene,' says Dr Kenyon.

This was so remarkable that it raised doubts about a concept of ageing that has held sway for thousands of years. 'People always thought that we just wore out like an old car, and there was nothing to be done about it,' Dr Kenyon says. 'But now we think ageing may be more like a disease with a cure.'

That cure, many researchers are convinced, is hidden in our genes. Some, like Dr Kenyon, believe that a single gene may hold the key. By 2004, manipulating that one gene had extended not only worm life but also the lives of fruit flies and mice.

The gene is called DAF-2. Its usual role is to give instructions for producing a hormone receptor – in this case a protein that sits on cells and grabs insulin, the sugar-delivery hormone, as it passes by. Under certain conditions, DAF-2 initiates a series of chemical events that allow the organism to live longer. It does this by causing another gene, called DAF-16, to order up a special protein that activates scores of other genes with widely varying roles. Alone, no single one of these secondary, or 'downstream', genes is life extending, but together they can potentially keep an organism up and running for as long as the genes are switched on.

Some of those genes make antioxidant proteins that protect cells from destructive oxygen molecules known as free radicals and from the age-

long lives of centenarians. The discovery of these 'longevity genes' could lead to a drug that duplicates the genes' life-extending effects.

The science of longevity has moved ahead so rapidly in recent years that many experts now consider it a matter of decades before sprightly, mentally sharp 100-year-olds will be too common to cause a raised eyebrow. The really interesting folks won't be mere centenarians but rather people who are pushing 150 without a health problem worth complaining about.

Ageing: now just another disease

Intrigued? So is Cynthia Kenyon Ph.D., a biologist at the University of California, San Francisco, who was one of the first to liberate anti-ageing medicine from the ranks of questionable 'miracle' products and bring it into the sober world of science. Much of today's optimism about the potential for longer, healthier human lives can be traced back to

Earlier worm research showed the roles of the DAF-2 and DAF-16 genes in the suppression of fat storage. (Fat storage is suppressed in worms B and C.) It may be possible to make drugs that have a similar effect in humans.

related diseases those free radicals hasten, such as heart disease. Other genes hold blueprints for antimicrobial proteins that guard against infection. Still others control fat storage, cholesterol transport, insulin output and other metabolic tasks.

Using a favourite metaphor of gene researchers, Dr Kenyon describes the group of genes as an orchestra. 'The hormone-receptor gene DAF-2 is the master regulator – the conductor,' she says, while the longevity gene DAF-16 is the first violin.

'The antioxidant genes would be the violins, the metabolic genes would be the cellos, the antibacterial genes the French horns, and so on. Each one contributes in its own way, and together, [they] produce a very big effect on life span.'

Harnessing the body's own powers

Dr Kenyon and others have shown they can toy with genes and proteins to force the conductor to play the 'Longevity Symphony' on demand. Of course, their success so far has been limited to rather humble members of the animal kingdom. Is there a DAF-2 equivalent in humans? Dr Kenyon thinks so. Before you believe her, though, you may want the answer to an obvious question: if animals really do have a gene that can help them to stay younger longer, why isn't it active all the time?

The explanation begins with evolution's preferred strategy for keeping species from becoming extinct. Our biological imperative is reproduction, not longevity. Once we've had time to procreate, our genes don't bother much with keeping us alive.

Put another way, death is the price we pay for sex. A cruel trade-off? Perhaps. If you're a parent, though, ask yourself if you'd have given up having children if that meant you could live for ever. In that light, evolution's choice seems more acceptable, doesn't it? But it turns out that we may be able to have it both ways – children and longer lives. How? By exploiting an exception clause in the death-for-sex contract.

Gerontologists have long known that when animals eat just enough to survive, they extend their life spans. As a longevity strategy, such calorie deprivation isn't likely to be a big hit, because who

wants to buy extra years by leading a life of near starvation? Even so, the longevity effect of calorie deprivation confirms that deep in our genes, there is an emergency back-up mechanism geared toward keeping us alive rather than producing more mouths to feed. It may be, the theory goes, that the DAF-2 chain of events is one such mechanism that's just sitting there, waiting for us to trick it into action.

'It makes perfect sense from an evolutionary point of view for organisms to retain a system for slower ageing at the expense of fertility during times of famine, when fertility's not such a good idea anyway,' says Aubrey de Grey Ph.D., a British longevity researcher. 'And, of course, anything that's evolved has some genetic structure to it that can be manipulated.' Dr de Grey is keen that the scientific community should adopt a more proactive approach to extending the healthy human life span 'sooner rather than later'. To this end he has set up a Strategies for Engineered Negligible Senescence (SENS) website, inviting comment (www.gen.cam.ac.uk/sens).

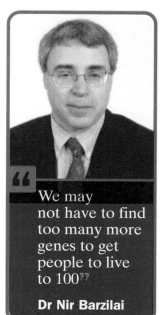

" We may not have to find too many more genes to get people to live to 100"

Dr Nir Barzilai

A real longevity pill?

Still, Dr de Grey doubts that DAF-2 or any similar genetic master conductor exists at the human level, at least not in any way that can extend life. Many agree with him, including Dr Nir Barzilai, a researcher at Albert Einstein College of Medicine in New York City and discoverer of one of the two recently announced human longevity genes. 'The idea that a single gene mutation can increase life span is an important research model,' Dr Barzilai says, 'but to get results in worms and apply them to humans takes a big leap of faith.'

However, Dr Kenyon and others have enough faith to see a chance that with the help of drugs, humans are genetically capable of unleashing a DAF-2–style response that will keep us alive and healthy into our hundreds.

'We think the human equivalents of the DAF-2 and DAF-16 genes are the genes that encode the insulin receptor and another protein called insulin-like growth factor, or IGF-1,' Dr Kenyon says. 'So maybe we can tweak the insulin/IGF-1 systems in humans like we did with the worms.'

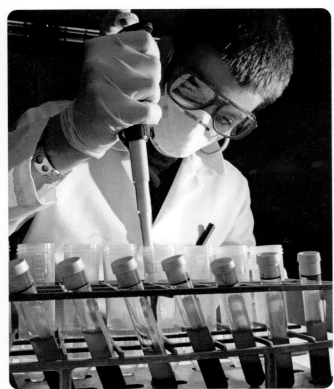

A researcher extracts DNA from the blood of centenarians at Elixir Pharmaceuticals, which is working to develop an anti-ageing drug.

She and like-minded colleagues recently set up a laboratory called Elixir Pharmaceuticals in Cambridge, Massachusetts, to develop a human anti-ageing drug. In 2004, testing was well under way in mice, a necessary step before trying out the drug on humans. The researchers won't reveal much until the study is done, perhaps in 2005, but Dr Kenyon does say, 'The early results are very promising.'

How would this longevity drug work? Rest assured that the researchers at Elixir are not trying to mutate a human gene to induce the DAF-2 longevity effect, as in worms and flies. Instead, their target is the proteins for which the genes carry instructions. 'What we're doing is creating a molecule that will bind to a protein and change it so it acts as if we had changed the gene's instructions,' Dr Kenyon says. 'That will lead to turning down-stream genes on and off the way DAF-16 does.'

If all goes well and the drug works safely in humans, pills that work on this principle and add 20 healthy years to the typical life span could be available within a decade. 'Whether it's in the next 10 years or 100 years, we really are going to be able to live longer, healthier lives,' Dr Kenyon says.

Why centenarians thrive

Even researchers who are sceptical of Dr Kenyon's single-gene approach agree that drugs to produce longer, healthier lives are on the way. For those scientists, the recent identification of two human longevity genes validates the intensive genetic studies of centenarians that began in earnest at the turn of the new century. Simply put, we can now be sure that people who live to be 100 are more likely to have certain variations of particular genes that predispose them to long life.

While we've long known that having the right parents improves your odds of making it into your eighties, a healthy lifestyle and a generous dose of good luck are equally important factors. But for ultra-longevity – that is, living to 100 or more – nothing matters except the right gene profile.

'I'm telling you, I studied 300 centenarians, and I didn't have a single yoghurt eater, not a single vegetarian, not even anybody who exercises,' Dr Barzilai says. 'On the other hand, 30 per cent of them were overweight or obese and one 104-year-old woman was celebrating her 95th year of cigarette smoking. These people have a unique genetic component that makes lifestyle insignificant for longevity.'

The two longevity genes are mutations of normal genes. Neither gene variation on its own accounts for more than perhaps 18 per cent of centenarians' longevity potential, but Dr Barzilai thinks it's just a matter of time before the rest of the genetic puzzle is filled in. 'And we may not have to find too many more genes to get people to live to 100,' he says. 'Just a few more might do it.'

The next step would be for researchers to create drugs that duplicate the biological processes unleashed by each of these genes. Interestingly, one of the genes turns out to be the exact equivalent of one of Dr Kenyon's worms' 'downstream' genes. It has the same name (metasomal transfer protein, or MTP) and the same function of regulating lipids, or blood fats.

The other gene, discovered by Dr Barzilai and called CTP, also controls lipids. Specifically, the version of the gene found in centenarians creates higher levels of the beneficial cholesterol known as

> **We can now be sure that people who live to be 100 are more likely to have certain variations of particular genes that predispose them to a long life.**

HDL. More importantly, it ensures that the molecules that carry cholesterol through the bloodstream, called lipoproteins, are larger than usual. Small lipoprotein particles are more susceptible to damage from free radicals and are more likely to embed themselves in artery walls.

'Everyone who has diabetes, heart disease, or hypertension has the smaller lipoprotein particle size,' Dr Barzilai says. 'I've also found evidence that I haven't published yet that the large lipoprotein particle size is associated with much better cognitive function, so CTP may also be protecting the brains of centenarians, which is extremely important for longevity.'

When will scientists develop drugs to mimic these genetic benefits? The process requires identifying molecules that will get the job done, testing them in animals for toxicity and effectiveness, and seeing how they work in humans via a series of rigidly controlled studies. Assuming that pharmaceutical companies immediately jump on the opportunities offered by the recent discoveries, we're again looking at a five to ten-year process before the first longevity drugs of this type are available.

Nevertheless, thanks to some medical serendipity, we may have a drug that will provide at least some of CTP's benefits much sooner. For reasons unrelated to Dr Barzilai's research, a pharmaceutical company is developing a drug that will simultaneously raise HDL levels and increase lipoprotein particle size. 'It does just what the CTP gene mutation in centenarians does,' Dr Barzilai says.

The drug is already in the advanced stages of human testing, so it could be available in 2005 or 2006. It's not meant as a longevity drug per se but rather as a way to reduce the risk of age-related diseases that are in part a consequence of cholesterol imbalance, such as heart disease. The question is: what's the difference?

From one perspective, not much. Except for possible master genes such as DAF-2, DAF-16 and a few others being explored, all of the human and animal longevity-associated genes discovered so far have to do with protecting against disease – through larger lipoprotein particles, special antioxidant proteins, infection-

fighting agents and so on. The logic is obvious: if you delay the age-related diseases that can kill you, you'll probably live longer.

'There's a really powerful medical potential in that,' Dr Kenyon says. 'We may be learning how to combat a lot of different diseases at once.'

The next milestone: 150

The anti-ageing drugs of the future should be able to do more than promise better ways to treat age-related diseases such as diabetes, cancer, heart disease and Alzheimer's. Longevity researchers hope they will alter the behaviour of certain genes so such diseases are out of the question for people 100 and older, just as they are for most 25-year-olds.

'We're approaching things from a whole different direction,' Dr Barzilai says. 'Many scientists have been studying people with specific age-related diseases and looking for the genes that cause them, but we're studying people who don't get these diseases and finding the genes that cause such long, healthy lives.'

Can there also be hidden in our genes a mechanism that doesn't just keep us disease-free but is also able to retard the ageing process? Many longevity researchers think so. Dr Kenyon sees such a possibility in the DAF-2 effect, or something like it. Others point out that women who give birth in their forties are four times likelier to live to 100,

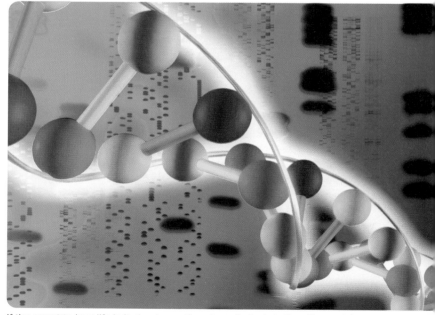

If the secret to long life is in the genes, then drugs that mimic the effects of those genes – such as creating more beneficial HDL cholesterol – could extend our life spans.

CAN A THOUSAND CANDLES FIT ON **A BIRTHDAY CAKE?**

Live to 120? Child's play, says Aubrey de Grey Ph.D. The British gerontologist from Cambridge University is convinced that medical know-how will soon keep human beings alive for hundreds, if not thousands, of years. 'Our ultimate goal,' he says, 'is the availability to the entire human race of technology that will restore them to whatever degree of youth they desire and keep them there for as long as they want.'

The way to do that, Dr de Grey says, is not by duplicating the action of selected longevity genes, as many leading anti-ageing researchers advocate. 'Tricking the body into doing what it already knows how to do will get you maybe 20 more years,' he says. 'My approach is to do much better than what evolution has given us.'

How? Basically, by getting under the hood and fixing whatever can possibly go wrong. Dr de Grey, who's also an engineer, has narrowed down the 'components of ageing' to just seven. He's also identified the 'fixes' for all of them, many of which are already found in laboratories. Here are Dr de Grey's keys to ultralongevity. Whether all seven will be available in 20 years (possibly) or 100 (quite probably), he can't say.

1 Restock the cell supply

The killer: Ageing brings an ultimately fatal net loss of cells in heart, brain and muscle tissue because more cells die than are replaced by new ones.

The solution: Coax all-purpose stem cells to convert in the laboratory to the cell type you want, then deliver them to multiply wherever they're needed in the body for a never-ending supply of new tissue. Such 'stem cell therapy' has already worked experimentally.

2 Really cure cancer

The killer: Malignant cells break free from the usual limits on their proliferation, so there's nothing to stop the tissue damage they cause.

The solution: Use periodic gene therapy to reprogram all of the body's cells so that the natural cell death mechanism can't be overridden. It's an ambitious (some would say audacious) but feasible plan to control cancer that has already been partially successful in mice.

3 Move mutating genes to a safer home

The killer: Mitochondria are power-producing units in a cell that induce ageing because the 13 genes they contain – the only genes found outside the nucleus – are not well protected from the consequences of mutation. Their unchecked mutations create damaging toxicity.

The solution: Use existing gene therapy techniques to duplicate the codes of the mitochondria's genes and relocate them permanently to the nucleus, where safeguards against runaway mutations are already found.

4 Clear out junk inside the cells

The killer: White blood cells that don't divide regularly accumulate a variety of unwanted molecules that can't be broken down and eliminated. Over time the piled up waste prevents the cells from working properly.

The solution: Genetically reprogram adult stem cells in the blood to include instructions for making a special enzyme that will break down material, then deliver these housekeeping cells via a bone marrow transplant.

5 Clear out junk outside the cells

The killer: With age, protein deposits called amyloids accumulate between brain cells, destroying brain function – not just in Alzheimer's patients, but eventually in everybody.

The solution: A vaccine to stimulate the body's immune system to get rid of these deposits has already been tested. Dangerous side effects halted progress, but safer versions are being explored.

6 Get rid of unwanted cells

The killer: Too many fat cells in the abdominal cavity create life-shortening metabolic problems, including diabetes. Also, ageing and useless (senescent) cells accumulate in the joints' cartilage tissue, where they become toxic.

The solution: Inject drugs that will either seek out and kill only the unwanted cells or induce the immune system to do the selective killing.

7 Loosen up the arteries

The killer: Arteries become stiff with age because of a process where unneeded proteins and sugars that surround the cells of the vessel walls eventually bond to each other. The process is called crosslinking and the result is high blood pressure, heart disease, or stroke.

The solution: The first drug to break down such crosslinks is currently in the advanced stages of testing in humans. More drugs need to be found, though, because there are many different types of crosslinks, which will require different drugs.

which may be an indication that some people have genetic structures that allow life events, including getting old, to unfold more slowly.

Dr Barzilai found more hope for such an age-slowing mechanism as he looked at the characteristics of the centenarians in his study. While tumours were rare in the group, people with the CTP variation were just as likely to have them as those who didn't have the variation – but they developed their tumours an average of ten years later. 'That implies that CTP may combine with other genes to actually slow ageing,' he says.

Is super-longevity worth it?

What can we really expect from these latest strides? Nobody knows for sure, of course, but the consensus among those doing longevity research is that within a decade there will be drugs that middle-aged people can take to boost their chances of staying healthy to the age of 100. Improved versions will soon follow that could make centenarians common. We may also see a gradual increase in the maximum life span, from about 12 decades to 13 or 14.

Some people have misgivings about these developments, the most common being that delaying death cheapens life. Dr de Grey, who envisions life spans measured in centuries, is convinced that people will drop their concerns once longer lives become a reality. 'They just don't want to be disappointed,' he says.

Dr Kenyon sees life extension as advancing well-established medical goals. 'We've always put a lot of effort and money into treating diseases to keep people alive,' she says.

'That's wonderful, but all that's been offered them is not being dead. What we're talking about now is prolonged health, the opportunity to enjoy the benefits of youth longer.'

If it all comes true, society will have to adjust to the skewed demographics brought on by so many centenarians. Population control will be even more urgent than it is now, and having full retirement and health benefits kick in at 65 may no longer be economically feasible.

For longevity researchers, these and other challenges pale in comparison to the priceless gift of life. As Dr Barzilai points out, the lucky few who have passed their 100th birthdays have lived some two and half times longer than their life expectancy at birth, which was about 40 at the time. Maybe it's time for the rest of us to share their good fortune.

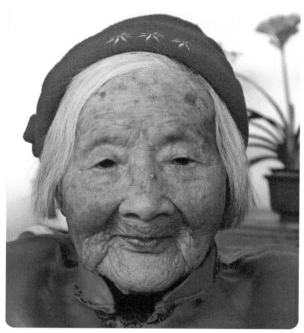

Ding Yushen of Rugao, China, made it past 100. You may, too – the first longevity drugs should arrive within the next decade.

What does it mean to you?

Advances in genetic research on animals, along with the discovery of human gene variations responsible for centenarians' long lives, have prompted researchers to test anti-ageing pills. These drugs could one day give everyone a shot at the extra years that centenarians now enjoy.

■ Drugs that mimic the results of a certain gene that increases worms' life spans by sixfold are currently being tested in mice. Such drugs could lengthen human lives by 20 years, and the first of them could be available within 10 years.

■ Pharmaceutical companies are expected to start work soon on drugs to mimic the disease-delaying benefits of two gene variations recently found in centenarians. The genes give special cholesterol-managing instructions that protect against heart disease, diabetes and brain deterioration.

■ If enough new longevity genes are discovered in centenarians in the next few years, those who develop drugs could have the insights they need to protect humans from all the major diseases of ageing, including cancer.

The new low-carbohydrate foods: welcome or worrying?

Food options for Britain's estimated 3 million low-carbohydrate dieters soared in 2004 as products designed especially for them gobbled up more and more shelf space in supermarkets.

Shoppers can now fill their trolleys with a growing range of low-carb goods from beer to bread. Even items that are difficult to regard as diet foods have been added to the mix. In late 2004 Nestlé Rowntree developed low-carbohydrate alternatives to two of its bestselling chocolate confectionery products – Kit Kat and Rolo. Weight Watchers from Heinz have added low-carb frozen ready meals to their range, and Nimble bread now has a low-carbohydrate version called Carb So Low.

Even so, the British market is less than a third of the size of that in the USA, where an estimated 10 million people follow a low-carb diet and sales of low-carb foods were set to reach $30 billion (£16.6 billion) in 2004 – double the sales of 2003.

A hunger for new options

'Consumers are looking at ways to control their carb intake,' says Stephanie Childs, a spokeswoman for the Grocery Manufacturers of America, 'and it's the consumer demand that has sparked the introduction of the low-carb products.'

Food companies have reduced the carbohydrates in these new foods mainly by replacing wheat flour with soya flour and sugar with sugar alcohols. Measure for measure, soya flour contains half the carbohydrates of wheat flour and several times as much protein. Sugar alcohols, including erythritol, maltitol, mannitol, sorbitol and xylitol, are lower in calories and can be used to replace sugar in baked goods, ice cream and other foods. The advantage of these sweeteners is that – unlike ordinary sugar, white bread, white flour and other foods such as potatoes – they do not cause a sharp rise in blood sugar. Such a rise causes a rush of the sugar-handling hormone insulin, which in turn can send blood sugar levels plummeting and make you hungry again.

People on the Atkins Diet and other low-carb diets are encouraged to avoid those carbohydrates known to boost blood sugar quickly. At the same time, they are told not to worry about carbohydrates from sugar alcohols and fibre, the indigestible roughage in whole grains, fruit and vegetables. But some of the supposedly 'Atkins-friendly' sugar alcohols do contain calories and may cause wind, diarrhoea or other digestive problems. And when you put one of those foods in your supermarket trolley, be aware that it may not be much lower in carbohydrates than its everyday counterpart – and yet it may be as high or even higher in calories.

Consider, for example, Kit Kat. An ordinary two-finger Kit Kat has 109 calories, 5.7g fat and 13g carbohydrate. The new low-carb Kit Kat has only marginally fewer calories and more fat – 92 calories, 6.6g fat and 5.9g carbohydrate (net carbs 4g). While an ordinary 57g tube of Nestlé Rolos contains 258 calories, 11.8g fat and 34.3g carbohydrate, the low-carb version contains 200 calories, 15.2g fat and 5.9g carbohydrate (net carbs 3.5g).

Under European labelling laws, manufacturers are required to list the total number of carbohydrates on the label, but manufacturers of low-carbohydrate foods often also list 'net carbs'; this figure is reached by subtracting so-called 'healthier' sugar alcohols from the total carbohydrate. For example, an Atkins Advantage chocolate hazelnut crunch bar contains 17.4g carbohydrate, but has a net carb value of 2g.

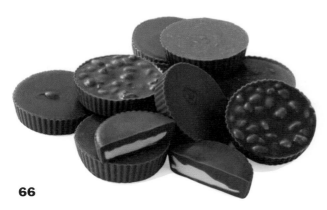

Low-carbohydrate biscuits such as these may not be the answer for people who want to lose weight.

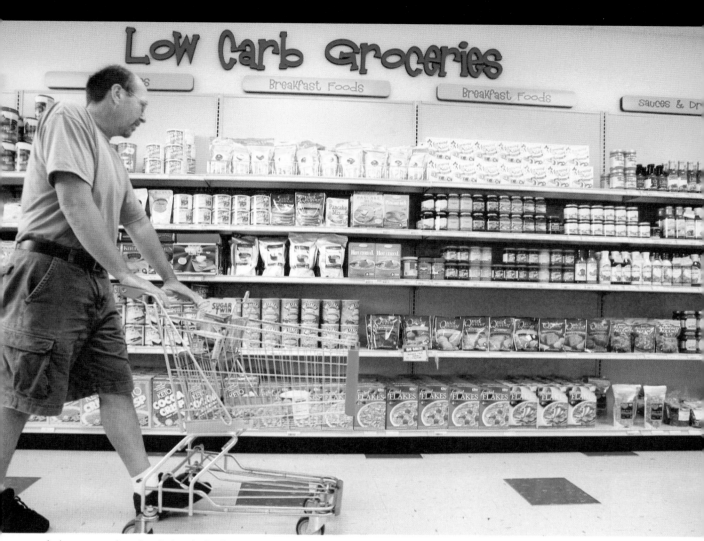

A shopper examines the shelves in the Castus Low Carb Superstore in Fremont, California. Owner Rick Schott started the small chain in 1999 after losing 45kg (7st 2lb) on a low-carbohydrate diet.

What really counts

The confusing information available to consumers has raised concern among some nutritional experts about low-carb products. 'Low-carbohydrate doesn't necessarily mean good nutrition or low-calorie,' says Amanda Johnson of the British Dietetic Association. In other words, shoppers who become too focused on carbohydrates may in fact be sabotaging their efforts to lose weight.

On the positive side, despite many warnings about the shortcomings of the low-carb approach – the weight loss is due to your body shedding water, and the diet is typically high in animal fats, which are known to heighten the risk of heart disease –

low-carbohydrate diets have recently earned some respect from the medical establishment. Studies published in top medical journals in 2003 showed that people could lose at least as much weight on low-carbohydrate diets as on other types of diet and at the same time improve their levels of 'good' HDL cholesterol. A 2004 study found similar results – and noted that the drop-out rate among study volunteers after six months was lower on the low-carbohydrate diet than on the low-fat diet.

Low-carbohydrate diets may be winning hearts and stomachs in the Western world for now but, for your health's sake, most medical experts would still advise cutting calories and avoiding saturated fats.

Antidepressants prompt warnings on aggression

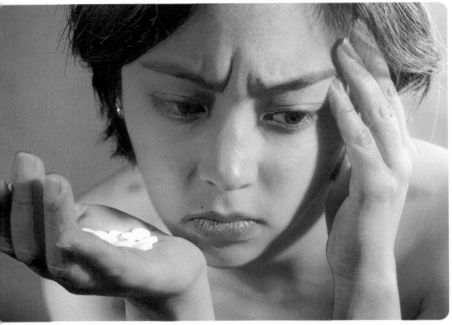

Teenagers taking antidepressants have something new to worry about. If the drugs don't make them feel suicidal, they may encourage feelings of hostility and aggression.

'hostile'. 'There is clear evidence for all the SSRI group of drugs that, in addition to making people suicidal, they can make people homicidal or seriously aggressive,' says Dr Healy. Separate trials in children with depression, social phobia or obsessive compulsive disorder showed that those taking Seroxat were 17 times more likely to become aggressive than those on a placebo. Dr Healy says that the MHRA has failed to act on the evidence.

This news came hot on the heels of a ruling by a committee of the US Food and Drug Administration (FDA) that all antidepressant drugs must carry the strongest possible public warning that they could cause children to harm themselves or commit suicide.

The ruling has more far-reaching implications than the action taken in December 2003 by the MHRA in Britain, when they warned that Prozac was the only SSRI that should be prescribed to children. For people under 18, other drugs in the same class – including Seroxat, escitalopram (Lexapro), fluvoxamine (Luvox), citalopram (Celexa) and sertraline (Zoloft) – carried risks that outweighed their benefits, the regulators said. Prozac was excluded because it appeared more effective than the rest of the class, which showed little improvement in the condition of depressed children when compared with a placebo.

However, Prozac was not exempted from the ruling by the FDA in September 2004 that all SSRIs should display health warnings – a decision that took account of recent research showing that Prozac was just as likely as the other drugs in its class to trigger suicidal behaviour.

Adults also warned

The concerns regarding a possible link between antidepressants and suicide did not stop with children. After holding committee hearings on the matter in February 2004, the FDA warned

In the latest of a series of shocks for individuals who depend on antidepressants such as paroxetine (Seroxat) and fluoxetine (Prozac), there are warnings that the drugs may make people aggressive and even homicidal. The alarm was sounded in September 2004 by David Healy, an expert on psychiatric drugs from north Wales, whose warnings that the drugs could cause suicide had prompted a major inquiry by the Medicines and Healthcare Products Regulatory Agency (MHRA). This led in 2003 to the entire class of drugs known as selective serotonin reuptake inhibitors (SSRIs) except Prozac being banned from use by children.

Dr Healy says that even some perfectly healthy people who volunteered to take part in early safety trials of the drugs became unaccountably aggressive after taking them. Their reaction was described as doctors, patients and families to monitor every depressed person prescribed SSRIs, child or adult, for suicidal inclinations. Monitoring was especially crucial at the beginning of treatment or when doses were changed.

The warning was followed by the publication in a July 2004 issue of the *Journal of the American Medical Association* (JAMA) of research that found the greatest risk of suicidal behaviour came in the first month after starting antidepressants, especially in the first nine days. But the same study found no greater risk of suicide among people on SSRIs than among those on two other popular antidepressants, amitriptyline (Elavil, Endep) and dothiepin (Prothiaden, Dolsulepin), older medications that belong to the tricyclic class of antidepressants.

All this leaves parents of depressed children – and adults struggling with depression – in a quandary about what is going on with this popular and effective class of drugs. No one, even the experts, is quite sure. 'It's very hard to tell what is a suicide attempt and what isn't,' says Scott Gottlieb, senior advisor for medical technology at the FDA. It is also difficult to tell if a drug is directly inducing suicide attempts.

When they are first diagnosed and start treatment, many people with the kind of severe depression that warrants medication are often too numb and lethargic to do anything – let alone commit suicide. As the treatment takes effect, they begin to regain some energy – just enough, in some cases, to try to kill themselves. The authors of the JAMA study suggest that one reason for the slightly higher risk of suicide early on is that patients are still very depressed. It generally takes about two weeks or more before people taking antidepressants start to feel better. 'Doctors should be more vigilant during this initial treatment time,' says Dr Gottlieb.

Hidden clinical trials

The issue took a legal turn in June 2004, when New York State sued GlaxoSmithKline, the British manufacturer of Seroxat, accusing the company of concealing clinical evidence that the drug could lead to suicidal thinking in children and adolescents and that it worked no better than a placebo. The controversy opened the public's eyes to what the *Wall Street Journal* called the 'black hole' in medical

Timeline: SSRIs under scrutiny

▶ **June 2003:** FDA advises against using paroxetine (Seroxat) to treat children or adolescents with depression because it may increase the likelihood of suicide.

▶ **October 2003:** FDA alerts doctors to reports of suicidal thinking and suicide attempts in studies of antidepressant drugs used in children with severe depression.

▶ **December 2003:** British drug regulators warn that SSRIs other than Prozac should not be prescribed to children.

▶ **January 2004:** American College of Neuropsycho-pharmacology issues a report stating that Zoloft and similar SSRIs do not increase children's suicide risk.

▶ **March 2004:** FDA issues another advisory, about the need to 'closely monitor both adults and children with depression, especially at the beginning of treatment or when the doses are changed'.

▶ **April 2004:** Researchers publish the results of their analysis of six trials of antidepressants in children, finding that the trials consistently exaggerated the benefits of the drugs and downplayed their side effects. Their conclusion, published in the *British Medical Journal*, was that antidepressant drugs could not be confidently recommended as a treatment for childhood depression.

▶ **June 2004:** New York State files a lawsuit accusing British drug maker GlaxoSmithKline of 'repeated and persistent' fraud for concealing data showing problems concerning the effectiveness and safety of its drug Seroxat when used by children and adolescents.

▶ **July 2004:** A study of 159,810 people who were taking antidepressants for the first time finds a slightly increased risk of suicide in the first month of drug treatment but notes that the risk is no greater with SSRIs than with drugs in the tricyclic class of antidepressants.

▶ **September 2004:** Dr David Healy warns that SSRIs could cause aggression and homicidal tendencies. FDA asks manufacturers to change drug labels to include strong warnings about possible dangers.

research, in which as many as half of all studies, particularly those with negative results, are never published or publicly presented.

The FDA has since started reviewing all reports of suicides or suicide attempts that are associated with antidepressants. It has also asked the manufacturers to change the labels on ten drugs to include stronger warnings about the need to monitor patients for worsening depression and the emergence of suicidal thoughts, regardless of the cause.

Doubts raised over increasing use of growth hormones

'Why does it matter if I'm small?' asked Libby Kershner. She was 9 years old and could not understand why her parents wanted her to take injections of human growth hormone. They explained that, without the hormone, she would never grow taller than 1.42m (4ft 8in). But Libby wasn't thinking about her adult height. She was thinking about the injections she would have to take every night.

Her parents prevailed, though, and for five years during the 1990s she had the injections. Today, a university student who has reached a height of 1.57m (5ft 2in), she is glad she did. 'I'm taller than some of my friends,' she says. 'I had low self-esteem. Growth hormone helped me grow mentally as well as physically.'

Since the 1980s, synthetic growth hormones have been helping abnormally short children, and there are thousands of families worldwide who are delighted with the results. But in the summer of 2004, the practice became a subject of controversy in Europe, as it had the previous year in the USA. That was when the European Union's Committee on Proprietary Medicinal Products changed the rules for who could receive somatropin or recombinant human growth hormone, a genetically engineered version of the body's own growth hormone.

In the past, somatropin injections had been available only to short children whose stature was the result of a medical problem, such as a growth hormone deficiency. In 2004, the EU committee allowed the treatment to be given to 'short normal children' – that is, those without actual growth hormone deficiency – as long as they had been small since birth. A similar ruling in 2003 by the US Food and Drug Administration (FDA)

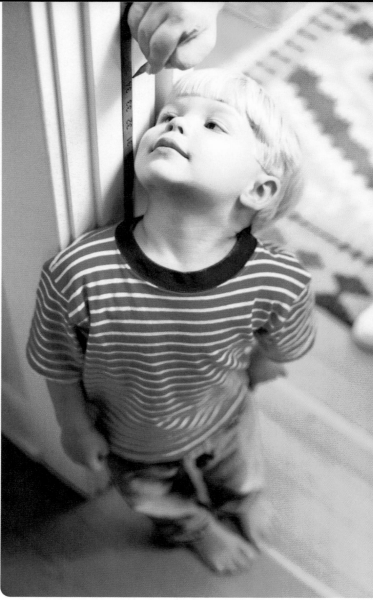

How does your child measure up? The European Union recently approved growth hormone treatment for 'short normal children'.

applied to children defined as 'exceptionally short' – that is, girls who, without treatment, would never grow taller than 1.5m (4ft 11in), and boys who would never get beyond 1.6m (5ft 3in).

The change raised eyebrows on both sides of the Atlantic among people who question the need to 'treat' short stature. Others welcomed the new rules. 'Don't trivialize what it means to be short,' says David Rothman, a co-author of *The Pursuit of*

Perfection: The Promise and Perils of Medical Enhancement. He points out that very short children often have low self-esteem. They are more likely to be picked on in school and passed over for sports teams. As teenagers, they often have more trouble getting girlfriends or boyfriends. Research shows that short men even get paid less than taller ones. But Rothman concedes that parents need to weigh up the pros and cons before seeking the treatment for their children.

Small gains In America, the FDA based its decision on the results of one major trial. After four and a half years of treatment, the participants in the trial had gained an average of 4cm (1½in). That may be enough to put a very short child in the bottom of the normal range, but it will not transform a natural jockey into a basketball player. In other studies, higher hormone doses gave greater gains. But is an extra few centimetres worth the extremely high cost of the treatment, the aggravation of nightly injections and the risk of side effects?

The pain factor Children are upset by the nightly injections. (Since most growth occurs at night, children take the injections before bed.) They can be given with fine needles that cause less pain than regular needles – but who wants to have injections for a condition that isn't a medical problem? The treatment often continues until late puberty, when the plates in the bones fuse, making further growth impossible. That is a lot of injections.

Safety concerns Any drug can have side effects. Even though growth hormone appears to be very safe, children sometimes develop complications, including swelling of the hands and occasionally of the brain. The swelling disappears when treatment is stopped, but doctors worry that the treatment could increase the risk of cancer in later years. Tall girls with a condition called acromegaly have excessive levels of growth hormone as youngsters – and higher rates of colon cancer as adults. 'But their levels of growth hormone are ten times those that

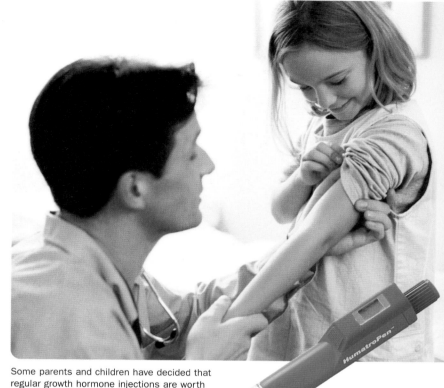

Some parents and children have decided that regular growth hormone injections are worth the discomfort and inconvenience. A 'pen' (right) can be used to inject somatropin, the synthetic human growth hormone.

we're giving these children,' says Pinchas Cohen, a professor of paediatrics at the University of California, Los Angeles, School of Medicine. He maintains that growth hormone is 'one of the safest drugs we have'.

A review by Great Ormond Street Hospital in London on the widespread use of prolonged growth hormone treatment highlighted questions about its 'tolerability, rationality and psychological effects' and called for more studies. The researchers pointed out that there was no evidence to determine final height outcomes in people receiving long-term treatment, and stressed that the treatment remained controversial in conditions where the response to it was only moderate. They said that it was difficult to justify the prolonged treatment of healthy children with short stature in that they had not been shown to suffer from a psychological disadvantage.

Innovative wound care tested on battlefield

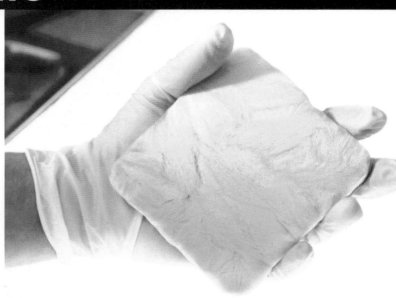

Stanching the flow: derived from the 'glue' that holds prawn shells together, this bandage encourages blood clotting and stops severe bleeding.

High-tech wound treatments made military headlines in 2004, as the coalition partners in Iraq tackled one of the most vexing challenges of battlefield medicine: out-of-control bleeding. The US military had launched an all-out attack on the problem (the leading cause of death from wartime injuries) following a horrific death in Somalia, immortalized in the film *Black Hawk Down*. The film depicted the real-life tragedy of an American soldier who died from loss of blood before he and his colleagues could be rescued.

'That soldier led a lot of people to say, "What can we put in a medic's hands, or in a soldier's hands, to help his buddy?"' explains US Army colonel David Burris, a spokesman for the department of surgery at the Uniformed Services University of the Health Sciences in Maryland. The answers range from a cheap product called QuikClot (available on the internet without a prescription) and a similar product called Chitosan, which is derived from shellfish. Both are under review by the British Army, as is recombinant factor V11a (NovoSeven), a product used to treat haemophilia and currently approved only for occasional emergency use in Iraq.

A low-tech but potentially very useful new item is a tourniquet that can be applied with one hand, allowing soldiers with arm wounds to stem bleeding on their own. The tourniquets are especially valuable because the body armour worn by today's soldiers means that most injuries occur in their arms or legs, through which major arteries and veins run, says Dr Burris. Eventually, he says, all military personnel in the field will carry them in their battle packs.

Then there is QuikClot. 'It literally looks like cat litter,' says Dr Burris. In fact, the two products are chemically related. Made of aluminium silicate, a type of volcanic rock, QuikClot is a powder that can be poured into a bleeding wound to encourage clotting; the wound is then covered with a bandage until the patient can be taken to hospital. 'We think it has saved at least a dozen marines and soldiers,' says Dr Burris. There are expectations that it will be used routinely by all sorts of emergency workers in the USA in the near future. Currently, all marines carry it in their first-aid kits and, according to Dr Burris, some soldiers took it to Iraq on their own initiative, ordering it either directly from the manufacturer, Z-Medica, or from its distributors.

Researchers have also discovered a high-tech clotting agent derived from the biological glue that holds prawn shells together. Called Chitosan, it is used in the form of a bandage 1.3cm (½in) thick and about the size of a coaster, with the consistency of a communion wafer. When pressed against a wound, the bandage sticks to the injury and absorbs liquid, thereby hastening clotting.

Such technology is not limited to the battlefield. Any medical product developed in the USA for the military must first be approved by the US Food and Drug Administration (FDA), so it becomes available to US civilians at the same time. Z-Medica has started marketing a trauma pack containing QuikClot to emergency workers, outdoor sports enthusiasts and motorists all over the country.

Food industry under fire over children's ads

A call for a ban on the television advertising of food and drink to children has been dismissed by the telecoms regulator, Ofcom. The ban was demanded by the British Medical Association (BMA) in response to soaring rates of childhood obesity in the UK – but the government favours voluntary action by the food and advertising industry.

'Children are being bombarded with adverts for products that are extremely bad for their health,' says Dr Peter Tiplady, chairman of the Public Health Committee of the BMA. 'Food manufacturers are targeting them by using sports personalities to send out the message that junk food and fizzy drinks will make them more popular.'

Meanwhile, a report by the International Obesity Task Force has concluded that sweetened soft drinks are as potentially as serious a problem in the UK as they are in the USA. 'We still have high sugar drinks being marketed to children in Britain as if the industry was unaware there was a problem,' says Neville Rigby, a spokesman for the task force.

The Food Standards Agency (FSA), a government watchdog, has now warned the food industry that it will face tough penalties if it fails to improve its record on food advertising for children. In July 2004 the FSA told the industry it had two years to get its house in order or face tougher measures. It said that voluntary action by manufacturers and caterers, such as clearer labelling and a reduction in advertising during children's television programmes, should be the first step to helping children and their parents make healthier eating choices.

Schools also have a major role to play in tackling the obesity epidemic, says Dr Tiplady. He points out that many schools have 'sold off their playing fields, installed junk food vending machines, and failed to provide healthy school meals'. The vast majority of secondary schools have machines selling sweets, crisps and fizzy drinks, which are valued as a source of extra income. Most parents dislike them. A *Times Educational Supplement* survey in April 2004 revealed that 79 per cent of parents in England and Wales – and 84 per cent of mothers – would like them to be removed from schools.

The FSA plans to issue guidelines on vending machines in schools and leisure centres, and to agree measures to improve school meals with the Department for Education. It has also called on supermarkets to remove sweets, snacks and soft drinks from checkouts and replace them with healthier options, such as fruit. The agency has advised the government to insist on mandatory labelling of energy, fat, saturated fat, sugar and salt content on all food products across the European Union. 'Parents want to give their children healthier diets and it's not always clear what the healthy choice may be at the supermarket, in a restaurant or at school,' says Sir John Krebs, chairman of the FSA. By June 2005 the agency intends to have published advice on a food labelling scheme which clearly states how healthy or unhealthy products are.

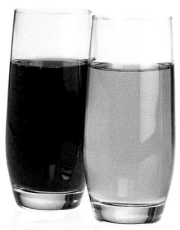
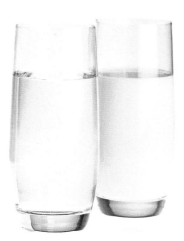

Many fruit drinks have as much sugar and as many calories as the most popular fizzy drinks. Nutritionists advise that water and milk are much healthier options.

PART 2

GENERAL HEALTH

DIGGING IN against the ravages of ageing? In the Ageing chapter, read about two common vitamins that can dramatically cut your risk of Alzheimer's disease and why taking a B-complex vitamin may be the best thing you can do to stay mentally sharp. Also discover which antibiotics appear to significantly slow the devastating effects of Alzheimer's disease.

In the Children's health chapter, learn why old standbys – including breastfeeding, exercise and watching less television – are looking better and better for improving your child's well-being. Parents will also want to read the shocking news about youngsters' diets, learn about a software program that benefits children with ADHD and find out why antibiotics may not be the answer to ear infections.

In the Wellness chapter, there are compelling new reasons to take vitamin D, cut back on salt, and buy wild – or canned – salmon instead of the farmed variety.

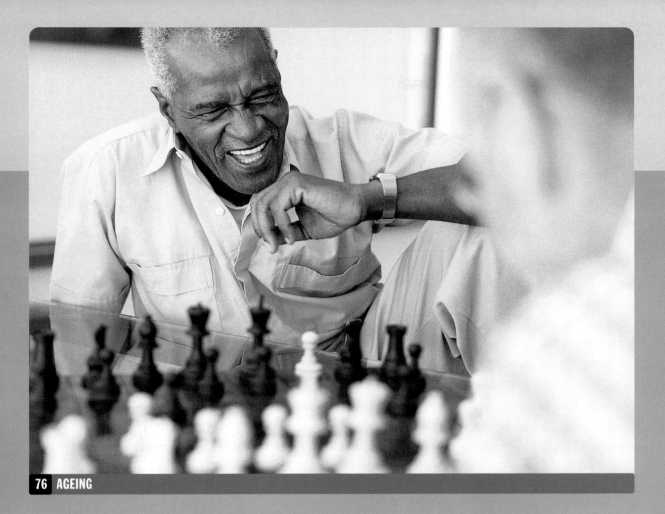

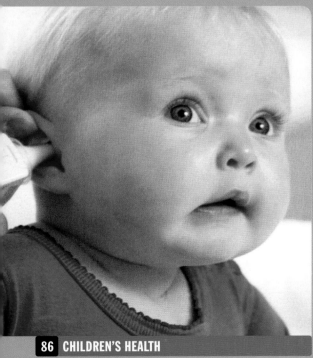

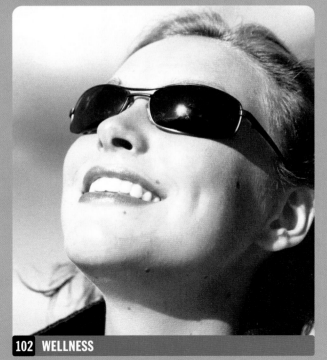

AGEING

In this section

Medical advancements offer more than a longer life – they promise a better life well into **old age**

On the high-tech front, vibrating insoles for your shoes may soon help you to keep your balance and avoid falls by subtly tickling nerve endings in your feet. And scientists have begun testing a system that uses artificial intelligence to help people with memory problems get through the day with a minimum of difficulty and a maximum of independence.

Alzheimer's disease, of course, is the cruellest memory thief, but a new way to peer into the brain promises a warning of the disease that would allow doctors to begin treatment sooner. That treatment may include antibiotics, as new discoveries have shed light on the role of infections in Alzheimer's as well as the ability of antibiotics to slow the disease's progress.

If you're hoping to avoid Alzheimer's, it turns out that a combination of two common vitamins could help you to do it. And there are more good reasons to take your vitamins, especially a B-complex supplement; they may help to sharpen your memory and protect your bones.

Alzheimer's disease
Coming soon: a snapshot of **early Alzheimer's**

Alzheimer's disease is the most common form of dementia, affecting around 500,000 people in the UK. There is currently no straightforward way to test for Alzheimer's in a living person and diagnosis is based on a process of eliminating other possible causes of dementia. However, that could be about to change. Imagine the following scenario: it's your 65th birthday and time for your first Alzheimer's check-up. A quick injection is followed by a painless positron emission tomography (PET) scan. If your brain is given the 'all clear' you can look forward to a future without serious memory loss. If the doctors see warning signs of Alzheimer's they put you on a drug regimen to keep you from developing the full-blown, memory-robbing disease.

As yet no part of that scenario is possible, but in the future it could be, thanks to a landmark discovery that enables the detection of the markers of Alzheimer's disease – clumps of protein deposits called amyloid plaques – in living brain tissue. Researchers at the University of Pittsburgh School of Medicine and their counterparts at Sweden's Uppsala University announced in a January 2004 issue of *Annals of Neurology* that a new imaging agent has been shown to make amyloid plaques visible during PET scans.

The dye, dubbed Pittsburgh Compound B, ushers in a new era of Alzheimer's research that is likely to speed up the development of plaque-reducing drugs and other treatments. Researchers already have several plaque-reducing drugs in the pipeline but now they will be able to monitor how the drugs work. They will be able to see the progression of the plaques visually and so decide whether a reduction in the clumps actually leads to a reduction in symptoms.

The new dye also provides a diagnostic tool that for the first time will allow Alzheimer's to be detected and treated well before mental decline sets in. People in their sixties may be able to fend off the

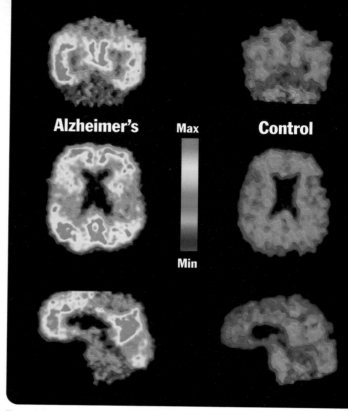

The column of three scans on the left shows amyloid plaque build-up (red and orange) in a brain with Alzheimer's disease. On the right, a healthy brain. A new dye has made the detection of the plaques possible in living tissue.

disease with drugs that reduce amyloids – the proteins that make up plaques – just as they fend off heart disease with cholesterol-lowering drugs.

How it works The Pittsburgh compound is an injectable radioactive dye, a variation on the dye used to detect plaques in autopsied tissue. The difference is that the new dye can safely enter the brains of living human beings through the bloodstream; prior to its invention, plaques could be imaged only after death. Once in the living brain, the new dye sticks only to amyloid deposits, making them easily detectable with a PET scan. Within two hours the dye is gone from the body.

Availability The dye's inventors are working with GE Health Care, a company that specializes in diagnostic tools, to fine-tune the new imaging agent for affordable, practical use in diagnosing Alzheimer's. It will require more laboratory work and then more tests on human volunteers. Therefore, even though researchers can move ahead with studies that use the new dye to find out more about the causes and treatment of the disease, the rest of us will have to wait several years before we can ask our GPs for an Alzheimer's test.

Alzheimer's disease
A new Alzheimer's treatment from old drugs

In the 20th century infection-fighting antibiotics tamed many afflictions. Now, two of these widely used drugs have been shown to slow the mental decline of Alzheimer's disease.

It's not just a token improvement that antibiotics are offering. Results of a carefully controlled study at five clinics across Canada revealed that the 43 Alzheimer's patients who took the antibiotics for six months experienced significantly less mental decline than the 39 who were given placebos (dummy tablets). The study authors, who presented their work to the Infectious Diseases Society of America in October 2003, rated the antibiotics' performance at least as effective as that of any of the three most common current drugs used in treating Alzheimer's – donepezil (Aricept), rivastigmine

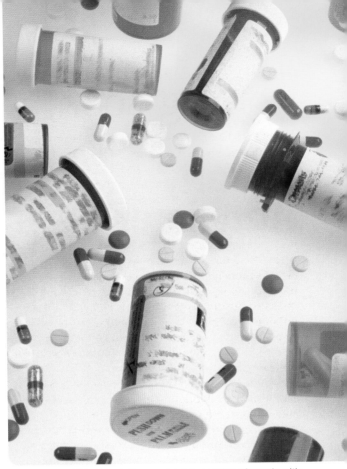

Antibiotics could hold back the mental deterioration of people with Alzheimer's disease, potentially giving them more good years.

[IS THERE AN INFECTION CONNECTION?]

If antibiotics work as a treatment for Alzheimer's, could the disease be caused by infection? Neurologists have known for some time that bacteria called *Chlamydia pneumoniae* – the ones responsible for several respiratory ailments – are found in the brains of most Alzheimer's patients. But just what these bacteria are doing has been hard to pin down. Even the researchers who discovered the antibiotic treatment for Alzheimer's don't think the drugs work by killing bacteria (see story above).

However, there's new evidence that *C. pneumoniae* does contribute to Alzheimer's. According to researchers from the Philadelphia College of Osteopathic Medicine,

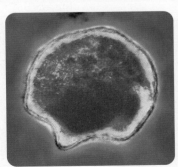

C. pneumoniae *bacteria cause respiratory infections. Could they be connected to Alzheimer's, too?*

healthy mice who had the bacteria sprayed into their noses soon developed amyloid plaques, the protein deposits in the brain that are the hallmark of Alzheimer's. That doesn't prove that the bacteria cause Alzheimer's, but the researchers think the bugs might act as a trigger for other causes.

Other recent British research has implicated the herpes simplex virus type 1 (the virus responsible for cold sores) as a strong risk factor for Alzheimer's as well as cytomegalovirus. Clearly more research is needed before the cause of Alzheimer's can be pinned on one particular infection, or several.

(Exelon), and galantamine (Reminyl) – all of which belong to the class of drugs known as cholinesterase inhibitors.

How they work The two antibiotics found to fight Alzheimer's – doxycycline (Vibramycin) and rifampicin (Rifadin, Rimactane) – are best known for their activity against *Chlamydia pneumoniae*, a bacterium that causes a number of respiratory illnesses, from sore throats to pneumonia. Although there's been some suspicion in the past that the chlamydia germ may be associated with Alzheimer's, the researchers don't think the antibiotics' effectiveness has anything to do with fighting infection. Doxycycline and rifampicin may instead slow the disease's progress by reducing inflammation in the brain, or perhaps by discouraging the accumulation of the protein clumps known as amyloid plaques that are a central feature of the disease.

Availability Doxycycline and rifampicin are established antibiotics with good safety records, and doctors could prescribe them for Alzheimer's treatment right now. Most GPs, however, will probably be reluctant to do so until a new, larger study duplicates the positive results of this one. Long-term treatment with any antibiotic increases the risk of bacteria developing resistance to that drug. However, the antibiotics may be useful in treating mild to moderate cases of Alzheimer's and it makes sense for people who've had no success with other treatments to discuss the possibility of an antibiotic regimen with their GPs.

RESEARCH ROUND-UP

How long will Mum or Dad live?

In a bid to help relatives plan future care, US researchers have followed the progress of 521 newly diagnosed Alzheimer's patients in Seattle aged 60 years and older over a period of nine years. The median survival period for the male patients surveyed was 4.2 years after diagnosis; for the women it was 5.7 years. But the formula devised requires expert evaluation of many factors, such as severity of symptoms and the patient's physical state. On average, Alzheimer's patients' life expectancy is half what it would be without the disease.

When blood pressure is too low

It is well known that high blood pressure increases the risk of developing Alzheimer's and middle-aged people are often advised to keep their blood pressure down to protect against heart disease and stroke as well. However, elderly people who are concerned about Alzheimer's would be well advised to make sure their blood pressure doesn't drop too low either. Several European studies have reported a higher prevalence of dementia in people with low blood pressure and a recent long-term study of more than 400 senior citizens aged 75 and over has come to the same conclusion.

After 21 years of monitoring the health of the study subjects (all of whom were dementia-free at the start), researchers at Albert Einstein College of Medicine in New York City found that those who had consistently low blood pressure in the early years of the study were twice as likely to develop dementia later on. In the study, any reading of 70 or lower for diastolic blood pressure (the second number in a blood pressure reading) was regarded as low. The study authors, writing in the December 2003 issue of the journal *Neurology*, suspect that the connection between low blood pressure and dementia is related to an inadequate supply of blood to the brain.

They also believe that the connection is age dependent – that is, the increased risk of dementia from low blood pressure applies only to people over 75. It seems that older people now have even more reason to keep a check on their blood pressure.

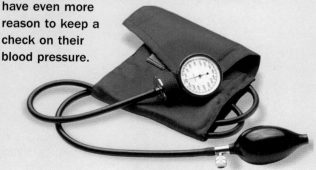

C plus E equals less risk of AD?

Could vitamins C and E help prevent Alzheimer's disease? In a recent study of 4,740 Utah residents aged 65 and over, the prevalence of Alzheimer's among those who took the vitamins daily for three years was 78 per cent lower than those who didn't. Just taking one, it seems, was not enough. According to results in the *Archives of Neurology* in January 2004, those who reported taking either vitamin C or vitamin E alone showed no decline in Alzheimer's risk.

So should older people start popping vitamin cocktails? The Alzheimer's Society advises caution. Although it is well established that antioxidants such as vitamins A and C have a preventive effect on cellular ageing by protecting the cells from free radicals, the doses of vitamins used in the Utah study were high: 500mg of vitamin C and 270mg (400 IU) of vitamin E.

Taken in high doses, some vitamins can have undesirable effects and more research is required before they can be recommended as a preventive measure. But you can boost your vitamin C and E intake naturally with a balanced diet including nuts, seeds, grains and at least five portions of fruit and vegetables each day.

Alzheimer's disease

Low testosterone linked with Alzheimer's

All men have less of the male sex hormone testosterone circulating in their bloodstreams as they get older. Now it appears that the less you have, the higher your risk of Alzheimer's disease.

Researchers who followed 574 men, aged 32 to 87, over two decades found that those who eventually developed Alzheimer's had, on average, half the amount of 'free' or unbound testosterone in their blood as those who stayed Alzheimer's-free. And the low free testosterone levels were detected as much as a decade before Alzheimer's could be diagnosed. This suggests that low testosterone could be a precursor, and perhaps even a cause, of Alzheimer's in men.

Only a small amount of a man's total testosterone circulates unbound in the blood. Previous studies have connected healthy free testosterone levels with a better ability to remember things. Now, the new study, published in a January 2004 issue of the journal *Neurology*, seems to show that the sex hormone also protects the brain against Alzheimer's.

A study by researchers at the University of Western Australia, published in September 2004, also implies that testosterone may have a protective effect. It found that men whose testosterone levels had been suppressed during chemotherapy for prostate cancer had raised blood levels of beta-amyloid – a protein associated with Alzheimer's.

The findings suggest that testosterone supplementation may make sense in men whose levels are low. But the researchers are unlikely to recommend this unless further studies confirm the link between testosterone levels and Alzheimer's, and safety concerns about testosterone replacement therapy are addressed. Testosterone supplementation is suspected of raising men's risk of prostate cancer and stroke.

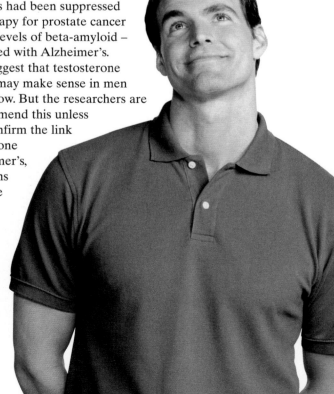

Balance
Tickling the feet for better balance

In a few years' time a lot of older adults may be walking around in shoes that gently 'tickle' their feet. New research shows that continuous vibrations on the soles of the feet dramatically improve balance control in elderly people while limiting sway in their standing posture. Most important, the steadying effect of these vibrations should cut down on serious falls, the number one cause of death due to injury in elderly people.

The breakthrough was announced in October 2003 in the *Lancet* after an unusual series of tests was conducted on adults both young and old. The volunteers were asked to stand on special gel-based vibrating insoles for about 30 seconds at a time. Since the vibration intensity was set at just below the lowest level that a human can feel, the participants had no idea when the vibrating mechanism was on or off. Special cameras aimed at reflector points on the volunteers' bodies clearly showed less side-to-side swaying when the insoles were vibrating, especially among the elderly subjects.

How it works Humans can stand and walk on two feet without tipping over only because nerve endings in the skin of our soles are constantly sensing pressure changes at the point where our feet meet the ground. The nerves fire off signals to the brain, which instructs the muscles to adjust accordingly. So, in reality, we're never 'standing still' – tiny muscle contractions are constantly taking place to keep us balanced and standing upright.

The problem for elderly people is that the nerve endings lose sensitivity over the years and fail to pick up many of the pressure changes. The vibrating insoles solve that problem because continuous exposure to uneven vibrations 'tickles' the nerve cells into heightened sensitivity. The nerve-brain-muscle performance thus improves, and better balance results.

Availability The Boston University researchers who ran the study have been working with a medical device manufacturer to design an affordable, battery-powered insole that can be inserted into shoes. But before they receive official approval they will need to conduct larger trials that overcome safety concerns such as the possibility of vibration damage. Therefore it may be some time before the insoles are on sale in the UK.

Fancy footwork

Video cameras aimed at reflectors on volunteers monitored their balance. When researchers activated subtly vibrating insoles, balance improved.

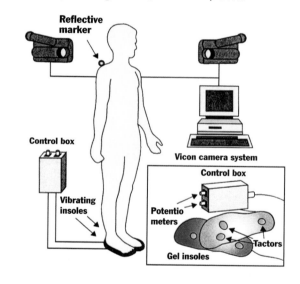

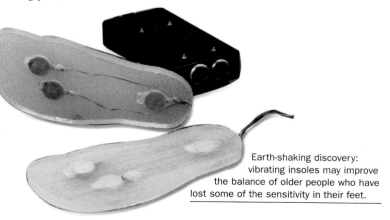

Earth-shaking discovery: vibrating insoles may improve the balance of older people who have lost some of the sensitivity in their feet.

Falls
Vitamin D keeps older adults firmly on their feet

Preventing falls is easier than you might think. Just by making sure you get enough vitamin D every day, you can cut your risk of falling in half. That means a simple multivitamin may be all that's needed to avoid the debilitating and often life-threatening consequences of fracturing a hip or other bone.

Swiss researchers gave a vitamin D supplement to half of 378 elderly residents of a retirement community. After about nine months, those who took their daily dose of D were 55 per cent less likely to fall than those who didn't, according to the study results, published in the February 2004 issue of the *Journal of the American Geriatrics Society*.

That's because vitamin D does more than team up with calcium to build bone strength. It helps muscles main-tain strength by regulating the release of parathyroid hormone (PTH). Too much PTH weakens muscles needed for balance. It also weakens bones, increasing the likelihood of a fracture resulting from a fall.

Vitamin D deficiency is common in Britain and other northern European countries, especially in winter. That's because light levels are low – and sunlight is essential for the body to be able to manufacture its own supply of vitamin D. Elderly people are particularly vulnerable since they tend to stay indoors, depriving their bodies of natural sunlight. However, the situation is easily remedied with supplements.

How much D do you need? Many multivitamins contain 10mcg (400 IU) of vitamin D, which is adequate for most people. However, if you're over 65, ask your GP about taking a heftier dose. Oily fish such as herring, salmon and tuna are naturally rich in vitamin D, so include them in your diet. Also make sure you're getting enough calcium: the Swiss study showed that the vitamin D is wasted if you're not. Most people need about 700mg of calcium per day.

General health
The B team makes the anti-ageing A-list

B vitamins are shaping up to be among the most valuable anti-ageing supplements on the market. A bevy of recent studies has shown that certain B vitamins protect older people against two of the most debilitating age-related maladies: failing memory and weakened bones. Add to this the well-known heart benefits of B vitamins, and you've got a virtual wonder drug sitting right there on the

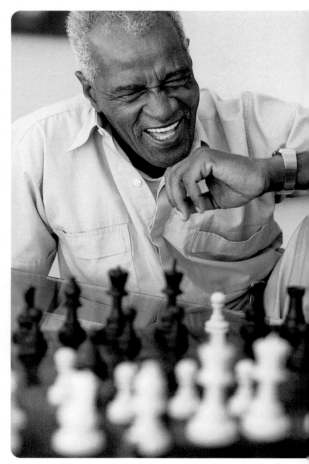

chemist's shelf. In fact, some researchers say that supplementing with a B-complex vitamin – or simply a daily multivitamin with a reasonable complement of B vitamins – could be the most important step you can take towards a sharp-minded and fracture-free old age.

B$_{12}$ for memory The anti-ageing superstar in the B family is vitamin B$_{12}$. New research from Goldsmiths College, London, and the Karolinska Institute in Stockholm, Sweden, confirms that getting enough B$_{12}$ makes you less likely to develop age-related memory loss. After taking blood samples and giving memory tests to 167 people with an average age of 83, researchers found that people with sufficient levels of vitamin B$_{12}$ in their bloodstreams scored much better on the memory tests than those with B$_{12}$ deficiencies.

The vitamin made the biggest difference for people who carried a gene variant known as APOE4 – the so-called Alzheimer's gene – but people without the APOE4 gene also benefited. Vitamin B$_{12}$ has also been shown to combat bone loss (see page 196).

The study, published in the April 2004 issue of *Neuropsychology*, recommends that people over the age of 50 should get their vitamin B$_{12}$ from supplements, since some older adults have trouble absorbing B vitamins from foods. Many nutritionists recommend that older adults take 100–400mcg per day, the amount found in many B-complex supplements. Good food sources of vitamin B$_{12}$ include brewer's yeast, eggs, meat and cheese.

Folate for bones Another B vitamin, known as folate or folic acid, helps to keep older bones strong by reducing levels of homocysteine, an amino acid. Experts already knew that an elevated level of homocysteine increases the risk of a heart attack, but now research has linked it to the brittle-bone disease osteoporosis.

In Dutch and American studies published in a May 2004 issue of the *New England Journal of Medicine*, the

Want to improve your chess game? Take a vitamin B-complex supplement. Older people who get enough vitamin B$_{12}$, found in the supplement, have sharper memories.

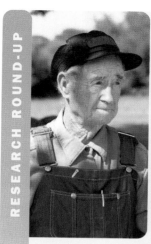

Long life is all about status

The question of why some people live longer than others has vexed scientists for decades. Theories put forward over the years include diet, lifestyle and adequate access to health care. But now a book by Sir Michael Marmot, professor of epidemiology and public health at University College London, has really put the cat among the pigeons. He proposes that a long life is related to a person's social status.

Sir Michael has studied life expectancy for over 30 years and his findings, detailed in *Status Syndrome: How your Social Standing Directly Affects your Health and Life Expectancy*, make fascinating reading. For example, an actor who has won an Oscar will live an average of three years longer than those who were nominated but missed out, and people with Ph.D.s live longer than people with only Master's degrees. Sir Michael thinks the phenomenon may have something to do with control. People who are higher up in the social pecking order tend to have more control over their lives.

25 per cent of people who were identified as having the most homocysteine in their blood had at least double the risk of an osteoporosis-related bone fracture compared with the rest of the participants.

High blood levels of homocysteine have also been linked with the risk of arterial disease, dementia and Alzheimer's disease.

Clearly, having too much homocysteine making the rounds in your system is something to avoid. But the study authors aren't recommending routine homocysteine tests. Rather, they say, a daily multivitamin that includes folic acid should be enough to keep your homocysteine levels in the healthy range. Most multivitamins contain around 200mcg of folic acid. Good food sources of folic acid include leafy green vegetables, beans and whole grains.

Memory loss
A **nicotine fix** for your memory

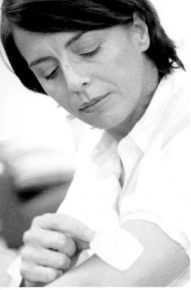

Patching up your memory: small doses of nicotine may give your brain a boost, making 'senior moments' less frequent.

Why would a non-smoker wear a nicotine patch? Because she's trying to quit – that is, trying to stop forgetting things. Researchers have discovered that small, steady doses of nicotine reduce the mild but annoying memory loss that accompanies ageing. This means that memory-boosting patches may one day become common.

By putting a group of elderly people 'on the patch' for a month and then testing their memories, a research team at Duke University in Durham, North Carolina, redeemed some of nicotine's dismal reputation. Nicotine, it was found, can alleviate symptoms of age-related memory loss by reducing the number of those forgetful 'senior moments', for instance. It may even prevent, or at least slow down, the decline of memory function in the first place.

How it works Most people think of nicotine only as the addictive ingredient in tobacco. But, as many a chain-smoking college student cramming for exams can testify, it can also enhance mental function. That's because nicotine duplicates the action of a natural brain chemical called acetylcholine, which is released at nerve endings to help with learning and memory. When nicotine is introduced into the brain, it's like boosting the workforce at a construction site. Beams are lifted and walls erected more easily.

Earlier research had suggested that nicotine's ability to mimic acetylcholine can help people with major brain disorders such as Alzheimer's disease. The new study, reported in October 2003 in the journal *Psychopharmacology*, unveiled nicotine's beneficial effects on age-associated memory impairment. Subjects who wore the nicotine patches noticed a marked improvement in their memories. Those who (without knowing it) had fake patches noticed no change at all.

An earlier British study demonstrated the memory-enhancing effects of nicotine in young men. Those who had been given an oral dose of nicotine were able to remember more words from a 32 item list than those who had been given a placebo.

Availability The study volunteers wore the same patches that are used for quitting smoking, which feed small doses of nicotine into the bloodstream through the skin. However, the researchers warn against using these patches for memory enhancement. For one thing, the study was very small, involving only 11 subjects. Its findings need to be duplicated in larger studies. Nicotine is a powerfully addictive drug, and using nicotine skin patches for the long term can be dangerous. The most likely next step will be the development of a nicotine-like drug that delivers nicotine's memory-enhancing benefits without its negative side effects.

Don't forget: it's never too late to quit

It's true that some researchers are exploring the possibility that nicotine may one day be used in a patch or drug to slow age-related memory loss. But don't turn to cigarettes for a mental boost in the meantime. The detrimental effect of smoking on mental function in old age is well established, and now there's more proof. Researchers from several European countries examined data on more than 9,000 elderly people and found that ageing smokers experienced mental decline at five times the rate of ageing nonsmokers. The more they smoked, the faster their memories failed.

Research looking at the smoking habits of 35,000 British doctors over 50 years found that men born between 1900-1930, who continued to smoke, shortened their lives by 10 years compared to nonsmokers. But the study, published in the June 2004 issue of the *British Medical Journal*, had some good news. Men who stopped at age 60 clawed back three years and stopping at 50 halved the hazard. So if you think that quitting later in life is pointless – think again.

Memory loss
A **high-tech friend** lends a helping hand

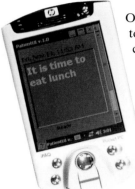

Older people with fraying memories can look forward to having a 24-hour friend around the house in the coming years. This particular friend will be made of computer circuits and motion sensors instead of flesh and blood, but it will still offer much of what's needed from a true companion: a helping hand, understanding and respect for your independence.

Autominder is a computerized creation of University of Michigan scientists that will help memory-impaired old-age pensioners manage their daily tasks – everything from using the bathroom and taking medication to finding their way around and even remembering to call their loved ones. It doesn't dole out reminders like an alarm clock. Instead, it uses artificial intelligence to interact with the user.

How it works All the information about the person's daily routine – mealtimes, medication, favourite TV programmes – is logged into a laptop computer that's set up in a safe place in the house. The computer communicates with a smaller unit that the user keeps on hand (either a handheld device or something that can be attached to clothes or body). This unit then issues reminders, either vocally or via a display in large type on a screen.

And that's just the bare bones of the operation. With strategically placed motion and contact sensors keeping track of the user's where-abouts and activities, the Autominder can use its intelligence to adjust its reminders to suit the situation. For example, if it knows that the user has just spent several minutes in the bathroom, it may delay a programmed bathroom reminder. If it senses that mealtime overlaps with a favourite weekly television programme, it may suggest an adjustment to avoid the conflict. It will even learn the best time to gently prod, 'Have you called your daughter lately?'

Availability Much fine-tuning and testing needs to be done before the Autominder (or similar technology under development at other research sites) will be ready to market. An early version, mounted on a small mobile robot, was recently field tested in a Pennsylvania retirement community. It was a hit with the users. 'They actually felt a sense of autonomy that they don't feel with a human caretaker,' says Martha E. Pollack Ph.D., lead researcher on the project. Dr Pollack expects Autominder to be available to the public around 2010 – just as the first wave of 'baby boomers' approaches age 65.

Meanwhile in Japan a robot called 'Wakamaru' is already becoming a household name. The robot is human-sized and its sophisticated programming enables it to be interactive in a 'human-like' way. It doesn't monitor its owner – it is more like a robotic 'friend'.

Paws to remember

Guide dogs for the blind are a time-tested blessing. So why not have guide dogs for the memory impaired? The idea makes sense, because Alzheimer's patients often lose their way outside their homes, wandering aimlessly until they someone helps them. Now, an Israeli dog trainer and a social worker have successfully trained and tested an 'Alzheimer's aid dog'.

They key to the project was finding the right dog, which turned out to be a female smooth collie from Finland named Polly (pictured below), who is able to stay calm when her master becomes confused and frustrated. Polly is her master's constant companion. She knows his routines as well as the neighbourhood around his home. When her master gets lost he simply tells Polly 'Home!' and she leads him there. Just as important, the dog relieves much of the loneliness that can afflict people with Alzheimer's. The UK charity Support Dogs also trains 'med-

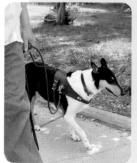

ical assistance' dogs to help people with Alzheimer's and other disabilities. The dogs selected by the charity often come from rescue homes.

CHILDREN'S
HEALTH

Top of the agenda in children's health is a campaign to stem the **obesity epidemic**

The evidence is mounting that dietary habits and weight problems become entrenched early in life. One study showed that toddlers' diets are shockingly deficient in fruit and vegetables and that young childen eat far too much junk food. In the 'good news' column, children of mothers who breastfeed are less likely to be overweight. Children who were breastfed even appear to have healthier cholesterol levels later in life.

Another way to safeguard your children's future health is to urge them to take more exercise. In addition to keeping kids slim, the right type of physical activity strengthens their bones, helping to prevent osteoporosis and fractures years later. Vigorous exercise can even ward off colds.

A major study found that the number of hours of television a toddler watches corresponds with how good – or bad – his attention span is at 7. For children already diagnosed with ADHD, research from Sweden shows that 'exercising' the brain can help to improve working memory.

Finally, find out why fevers can be beneficial and why the use of antibiotics for ear infections is increasingly losing favour.

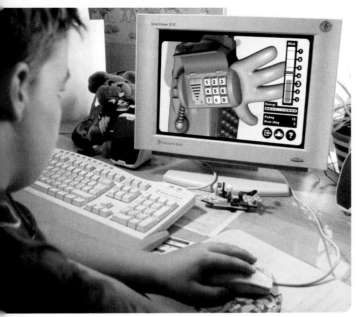

RoboMemo to the rescue: when children with ADHD performed increasingly difficult memory exercises using this computer program, their symptoms showed sustained improvement.

ADHD
Brain exercises make 'working memory' more efficient

As the number of children with attention deficit hyperactivity disorder (ADHD) continues to rise, researchers, doctors and parents are working to find treatments that offer an alternative to medication. The disorder is estimated to affect about 5 per cent of school-age children, with boys roughly three times more likely to be affected than girls.

Now, the results of a study in Sweden suggest that 'exercising' a particular part of the brain in children with ADHD can significantly improve the way they carry out cognitive tasks while reducing the symptoms of inattention and hyperactivity.

The problem Researchers have known for some time that certain regions of the brain that control 'working memory' are impaired in children with ADHD. Working memory involves tasks such as taking notes during a classroom lecture or trying to remember a phone number someone has just given

you while you continue to listen to that person talk. If you have problems with working memory, you have trouble remembering plans or instructions and solving problems.

Children and adults with attention deficit disorder have difficulty with working memory because it is dependent on the prefrontal cortex of the brain – a region that is smaller than usual in people with ADHD – and the neurotransmitter dopamine, which is not used effectively by those with the condition.

CANADA BANS BABY WALKERS

Safety campaigners in Canada achieved an important success in April 2004 with the introduction of a ban on the manufacture and sale of baby walkers. Baby walkers – plastic seats with wheels and oversize trays that babies use to propel themselves around a room – have long been recognized as a major cause of accidental injury. In some parts of Europe they have been banned since the early 1980s – but not in the UK or the USA. Despite implementation of new safety standards, in 1999 nearly 9,000 infants age 15 months and younger were injured in the USA as a result of baby walkers. In Britain, where no similar standards apply, there were 5,000 accidents in 1997.

Worried about the high accident rate and the risk posed by the devices to babies' natural development, the Chartered Society of Physiotherapists has repeatedly called for a ban in the UK – to no avail. But the Canadian health ministry has decided that infants lack 'the necessary skills, reflexes and cognitive abilities to safely make use of these products'. It has advised parents who have walkers to get rid of them.

RITALIN PRESCRIPTIONS SOAR

The number of children diagnosed with behavioural problems such as attention deficit hyperactivity disorder (ADHD) continues to rise – and with it the number of prescriptions issued for the controversial drug Ritalin. In 2003, more than 314,000 prescriptions were issued for Ritalin-type drugs (methylphenidates) in England and Wales – an increase of 24 per cent on the previous year. The annual cost to the NHS of the drugs now exceeds £10 million. Ritalin is a mild stimulant that works on the central nervous system to improve concentration. But its critics say it should be prescribed only in extreme cases. They claim that it can cause serious side-effects in some children, leaving them depressed, lethargic or withdrawn.

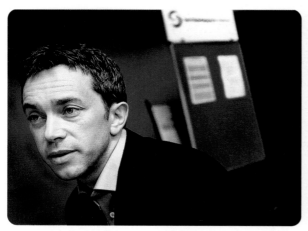

Brain researcher Torkel Klingberg uses software to strengthen the working memory of children with ADHD.

The solution To strengthen working memory in a group of children with ADHD, Dr Torkel Klingberg and his colleagues at the Karolinska Institute in Stockholm installed a specially designed software program on the children's home computers. For 30 minutes a day, five days a week, the children (aged from 7 to 12) completed various exercises on the computer, such as remembering the position of objects and recalling letters or digits. For one group, the exercises became steadily harder over the five-week study; for a second group, the level of difficulty remained low. The results were then uploaded to a mainframe computer and expertly analysed.

When the children were tested immediately after the experiment, those in the first group showed big improvements in their working memory compared with those in the second group. Ninety per cent of the improvements were still evident three months after the trial had ended, and parents and teachers also reported significant improvements in tasks requiring working memory, as well as less inattention.

Availability The software program used in the study, called RoboMemo, is manufactured and distributed by the Swedish company Cogmed Cognitive Medical Systems. The company began distributing its product in Sweden in late 2003 and hoped to start worldwide distribution in late 2004.

TOP trends

REPETITIVE STRAIN HITS CHILDREN

A disorder usually associated with office workers is becoming increasingly common among children who spend long hours at the keyboard. Repetitive strain injury (RSI) – which damages tendons, nerves, muscles and other soft body tissues – is often caused by the incorrect use of computers.

Peter Buckle, an expert in ergonomics at Surrey University, points out that many home computers are set up for adult use, and the standard keyboard, mouse and computer furniture do not take account of children's size: 'Most parents seem unaware of the possible dangers of children sitting for long periods unsupported, with necks twisted and wrists over-extended.' In a study of 2,000 young people aged 11–14, Buckle found that 36 per cent suffered serious ongoing back pain. He advocates more user-friendly equipment for children and urges parents to monitor their children's computer use at home, making sure that they take regular breaks and sit properly.

RESEARCH ROUND-UP

A clear picture of ADHD

For more than a decade, researchers have known that attention deficit hyperactivity disorder (ADHD) was a physical disorder of the brain. Then, in November 2003, scientists from the University of California at Los Angeles published images from MRI scans of the brains of children with ADHD. While earlier studies had suggested that the brains of children with ADHD differed from those of children without the disorder, the images

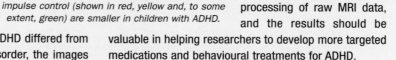

Areas of the brain associated with attention and impulse control (shown in red, yellow and, to some extent, green) are smaller in children with ADHD.

had never been clear enough to show exactly where the differences lay. The new images, published in the British medical journal *The Lancet*, clearly showed that the areas of the brain associated with attention and impulse control are smaller in children with the disorder. The clarity of the pictures was achieved by sophisticated computer processing of raw MRI data, and the results should be valuable in helping researchers to develop more targeted medications and behavioural treatments for ADHD.

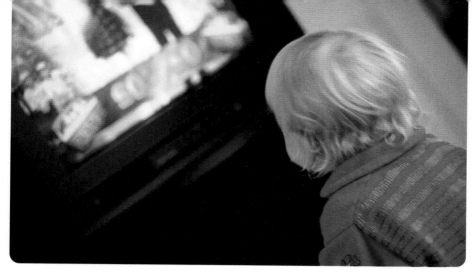

The fast-changing sounds and images provided by television may train young brains to expect the same stimulation in real life, thereby reducing toddlers' attention spans.

ADHD
Does television make children prone to ADHD?

Many a parent has wondered how older generations managed to bring up children without television for entertainment. But, for all its ability to keep children quiet and – sometimes – educate them, television is also gaining a reputation nearly as bad as that of smoking, with indications that it can contribute to weight problems and aggression. Now, a study by the University of Washington in Seattle suggests that regularly dumping your toddler in front of the box for long periods may predispose him or her to developing an attention deficit disorder.

What the study found Researchers compared the amount of television watched by 1 and 3 year-olds with their rate of attention problems at the age of 7. They discovered that every hour of television the toddlers watched daily increased their risk of later attention problems by 10 per cent. (Problems were assessed using a standard questionnaire that probes whether a child has difficulty concentrating, is easily confused, is impulsive, has trouble with obsessions or is restless.) The findings lend weight to a recommendation by the American Academy of Pediatrics' that children under 2 should watch no television at all.

On average, the toddlers in the study watched 2.2 hours a day at the age of 1 and 3.6 hours at the age of 3. Only a third of the 1 year-olds and just 7 per cent of the 3-year-olds watched no television. 'I was

RESEARCH ROUND-UP

New drug promises sounder sleep

A new drug licensed for use in the UK could mean more peaceful nights for some children with ADHD. Atomoxetine (Strattera) became available on prescription in July 2004, 18 months after it had been approved for use in the USA. It raises the levels of the natural chemical noradrenaline in the brain, but its effect on the symptoms of ADHD is not fully understood.

Unlike Ritalin and other methylphenidates – the only other drugs currently used to treat ADHD – atomoxetine is not a stimulant. Ritalin-type drugs, which contain amphetamines, cause insomnia; they cannot be taken in the evening, so symptoms are not controlled at night. A dose of atomoxetine, by contrast, works for 24 hours. 'Continuous relief from ADHD symptoms is new,' says Dr David Coghill, a psychiatry lecturer at Dundee University. 'It may allow children and their families to live a more normal life.'

Drug therapy for ADHD remains controversial. The National Institute of Clinical Excellence (NICE) advises that it should be given only to the most severely affected children. There are worries that Ritalin could cause depression or be abused because of its amphetamine content. But methylphenidates look set to remain the drug of choice for treating ADHD. 'We've been using them for 50 years, and we know how they work,' says Professor Peter Hill, a psychiatrist who has specialized in ADHD care: 'Atomoxetine will remain a second or third choice drug for the foreseeable future.'

shocked to incredulity by the amount of television these very young children are watching,' says Dr Dimitri Christakis, one of the authors of the study. Since children of that age are awake only about 12 hours a day, the data means that they are spending 20 to 30 per cent of their waking hours watching television, he notes.

Reshaping the brain Dr Christakis and his fellow researchers suspect that early and intense television-watching moulds children's brains in a way that later affects their ability to maintain concentration. Studies in newborn rats have shown that high levels of visual stimulation change the architecture of their brains.

With its rapidly changing images and scenes and its stimulating sounds and colours, television may condition the young brain to expect a similar high level of stimulation later in life. Obviously, real life moves at a much slower pace.

Although the Seattle researchers had no information about whether the children in the study had been diagnosed with ADHD, it is not the diagnosis that matters, says Dr Christakis. What is important is a child's attention span. 'We know that children who pay attention better do better at school. And those who achieve success early in school are more likely to do better later.' Other study results show that hyperactive children prefer the hyperstimulation of television to slower-paced activities, suggesting a potential vicious circle.

Since publishing the results of his study, Dr Christakis (who has young children of his own) has heard from numerous parents who say they rely on television to entertain their toddlers so that they can get things done, such as cooking dinner.

Dr Christakis has a ready answer: 'Television has only been around for about 50 years, but dinner has been around for ever. Obviously, there are other ways to get dinner on the table when you have young children.'

He agrees that dumping your child in front of the box can be convenient but points out that: 'Not everything that is convenient is necessarily good.'

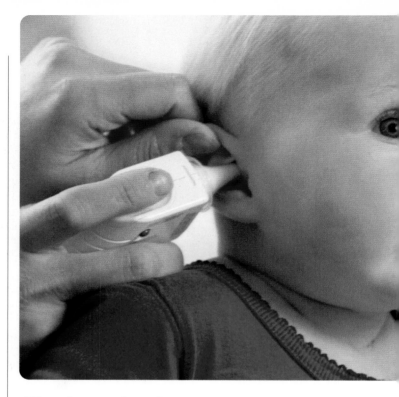

Allergies and asthma
Fevers effectively boost immunity

The next time your baby develops a fever, don't panic. It could mean that the infant will be less likely to develop allergies when he or she gets older. That was the conclusion of researchers at the Henry Ford Health System in Detroit, USA, who studied the medical records of 835 children from birth to their first birthday – and then followed the progress of the children until they reached the age of 7.

Earlier research had suggested that children who had had illnesses such as measles, tuberculosis and hepatitis A were less likely to develop allergies. The Detroit researchers looked at more common infections such as upper respiratory tract infections. 'And it appeared that having a fever in the first year was protective,' says Keoki Williams, a clinical epidemiologist at Henry Ford. The fever itself seemed to be the deciding factor, with fever-inducing infections involving the eyes, ears, nose or throat associated with a lower risk of allergies than similar infections that didn't result in fever. It didn't matter how high the fever was: the effect was the same for temperatures between 38°C (100.4°F) and 38.3°C (101°F), the cut-off point used in the study. But the number of fevers did matter. Among children who were fever-free in their first year, half were allergic to one or more irritants by

In the first year of life, repeated fevers caused by infection in the eyes, ears, nose or throat may train the immune system to tell the difference between germs and harmless intruders such as dust and pollen.

the age of 7. Among those who had one fever, 47 per cent were allergy-prone, but only about 33 per cent of children who had two or more fevers in infancy showed allergic sensitivity by the age of 7. The results were echoed in a separate German study which concluded that the risk of developing asthma by the age of 7 is reduced by about 50 per cent in those children who have had two or more episodes of common cold in their first year of life.

Stimulating immunity The findings back up the 'hygiene hypothesis', which holds that because people in Western industrialized countries are exposed to fewer germs than nature intended, their immune systems become overly sensitive, to the point where they react to harmless 'invaders' such as dust and pollen.

'There are important decisions in the first year of life going on at the level of the T-cell,' explains Dr Williams. T-cells act as ringleaders for the immune system, telling other immune cells how and when to react to a threat. 'If you have no exposure to early infections, it may be more likely that T-cells will respond to certain environmental challenges in an allergic way,' he says.

Infections significant enough to cause fevers probably stimulate the immune system enough to affect the development of T-cells. The findings may eventually help us to find a way to immunize children against allergies by manipulating their immune systems in early life. But in the meantime, says Dr Williams, 'I am not suggesting that you go out and expose your baby to other sick children.'

Are you rubbing allergens into your baby's skin?

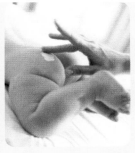

Peanut allergy may be caused by applying skin-care products containing traces of peanut protein to infants with eczema, says a report commissioned by the Food Standards Agency. In people with eczema the skin becomes broken or inflamed, leaving an abundance of immune cells potentially exposed to allergens.

In a separate study, researchers at the Children's Hospital in Chicago examined 293 paediatric skin-care products and found that more than a quarter of them contained common allergenic foods such as cow's milk, wheat, nuts and soya products, and 46 per cent contained other foods. Lotions, creams and baby oils were most likely to contain the foods. Even zinc and castor oil ointment, a preparation often used to treat nappy rash, is 30 per cent arachis oil (peanut oil).

Let Johnny play

There is no medical reason why a child with asthma should be a couch potato. But a study in Baltimore found that one in five children with asthma don't get enough exercise, even though running, swimming and other activities can help to control the disease. 'As long as your condition is well controlled and you consult your doctor regularly, asthma should not stop you doing any type of exercise,' says Asthma UK.

The Baltimore researchers interviewed the parents of 137 children aged 6 to 12 with asthma about their children's activity levels, and compared them with those of 106 children without asthma. They found that the healthy children were more active, spending an average of 146 minutes on physical activity daily, compared to 116 minutes for the kids with asthma. The absence of a place to 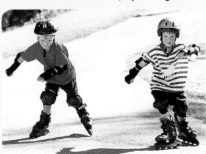 exercise was not part of the problem – but some of the parents were. A quarter of them were afraid that their children would have an attack if they exercised. The researchers noted that warm-up exercises and, if necessary, a change in medication should protect against any exercise-related asthma.

A little **pressure** prevents ear infections

Your daughter appears to be particularly vulnerable to ear infections. She has been prescribed several courses of antibiotics, but the problem continues to recur and your doctor has now suggested surgery to insert ear tubes, or grommets. You are reluctant, but what else can you do?

The answer may lie in a therapy called osteopathic manipulative treatment (OMT), which involves gentle stretching and pressure to move the muscles and joints.

During a six-month study of 57 children with frequent ear

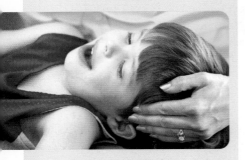

infections, the ones who had OMT in addition to routine care had fewer ear infections and surgical procedures.

Researchers at Oklahoma State University in Tulsa, who published their results in late 2003, say OMT helps partly by relieving compression of the bones surrounding the ear's Eustachian tube, allowing it to drain more freely.

Ear infections

Antibiotics are not much use in treating **infections of the ear**

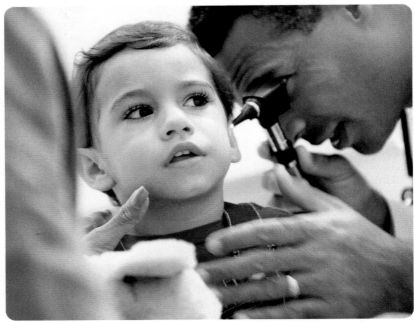

Your two-year-old wakes up in the night with a high temperature, crying inconsolably and evidently suffering from pain in the ear. The next day, you take the child to the local GP, knowing that this is probably an ear infection, but aware that your doctor may do no more than prescribe a painkiller such as paracetamol. Just a few years ago you would have been satisfied with nothing less than a course of antibiotics.

In response to recent European studies showing that antibiotics benefit only one in eight children with ear infections, attitudes to the drugs now vary widely in the developed world. Acute otitis media (AOM), or infection of the middle ear, is one of the most common diseases of early infancy and childhood – but antibiotic use for the condition ranges from 31 per cent in the Netherlands to 98 per cent in the USA and Australia. In the UK, the NHS guidance recommends that antibiotics 'should NOT be offered routinely' but could be used selectively in certain conditions such as for a child under 2 years of age.

In the USA, where half of all antibiotics prescribed for pre-school children are for the treatment of ear infections, new guidelines issued in March 2004 aim to cut antibiotic prescriptions by as much as 3 million a year. The concern is that they are ineffective for AOM and also that overprescribing has accelerated the rising rate of antibiotic-resistant bacteria, particularly those that cause ear infections.

In Britain, it is estimated that a typical GP will see about 20 children with AOM each year. With some 37,000 practising UK GPs, that means an annual incidence of some 740,000 cases. But government guidelines, revised in June 2004, make it clear that in many cases antibiotic treatment is not effective.

What the guidelines say The guidelines point out that AOM is usually a self-limiting illness and some 80 per cent of cases resolve within three days without treatment. The use of antibiotics has also not been shown to reduce the risk of complications.

Antibiotics can, however, be used selectively in children under 2 years of age, if children have the infection in both ears, if they have a temperature above 38.5°C (101.3°F) or are vomiting, or if there is swelling suggesting a particularly severe infection. Amoxicillin is the recommended first-line antibiotic in most cases as it is usually effective and has few adverse effects.

In the majority of cases, they say, simple analgesia (painkillers) is the mainstay of treatment. Both paracetamol and ibuprofen are appropriate but aspirin should be avoided in children under 16. Treatment with antihistamines or decongestants is not recommended.

Drop the drops for ear infections

If your doctor writes a prescription for antibiotic eardrops when your baby has an ear infection, you may want to think twice before using it. A study presented at a meeting of ear, nose and throat doctors in January 2004 found that the commonly used eardrops loxacin (Floxin) and ciprofloxacin (Cipro) can lead to an increase in drug-resistant bacteria and fungi in the ear.

Two doctors at the Temple University School of Medicine in Philadelphia found a link between eardrops and fungus in children who had had ear-tube surgery, prompting them to examine samples from children's ears taken before and after they received eardrops. They found a notable increase in drug-resistant bacteria and fungi in children who used the drops. (Antibiotics kill off all bacteria – even beneficial ones – leaving a disrupted chemical environment that allows fungi to grow.) They advise parents to avoid antibiotic eardrops in young children and for minor infections. In older children, the drops should be used with care, along with ear suctioning to remove excess fluid.

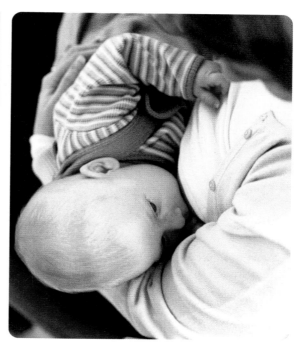

General health

More reasons to **breastfeed**

The idea that breastfeeding is better for babies than bottle-feeding is not new, but the evidence continues to accumulate. Now it appears that infants who are breastfed rather than bottle-fed are less likely to become overweight later in life. They may even be less prone to getting diseases such as heart disease or diabetes.

Signs of a healthy heart In a groundbreaking study published in the medical journal *The Lancet* in May 2004, researchers from the Institute of Child Health in London looked at more than 200 Scottish teenagers whom they had studied as babies. The babies – all premature – had been randomly assigned either breast milk or formula.

Compared with teenagers who had been bottle-fed as babies, those young people who had been breastfed had significantly lower levels of LDL, or 'bad' cholesterol, in their bodies, as well as lower levels of C-reactive protein – a indicator of inflammation that is now thought to play a major role in heart disease and other serious illnesses, including diabetes and cancer. The differences were so substantial that they translated into a 25 per cent reduction in the risk of heart disease.

Researchers suspect that the reason for the differences is that the bottle-fed babies grew faster than the breastfed ones, spurred on by their consumption of the nutrient-rich formula. This in turn led to the permanent metabolic changes that the researchers noticed in the teenagers, including increased resistance to insulin and changes in the cells lining their blood vessels – both of which are among the risk factors for early cardiovascular disease.

Breastfed children are slimmer
These findings fit like a jigsaw puzzle with those of another recent study, published in February 2004 in the US journal *Pediatrics,* which concluded that the longer a mother breastfeeds the less likely it is that her baby will grow into an overweight child. The American study was one of the largest ever conducted into the link between breastfeeding and weight later in life.

Researchers found that 4-year-old children who were never breastfed and those who were breastfed for less than a month were much more likely to be overweight than those who had been nursed for longer. The protective effect of nursing seems to kick in at about the age of 3 months and increase from then on. The longer the children had been breastfed the less likely they were to become overweight.

One theory is that breastfeeding reduces the risk of weight problems because breastfed babies learn of their own accord to regulate the amount they eat – for example, they fall asleep or turn their heads away when they have had enough, as opposed to bottle-fed babies, who continue to have nipples placed in their mouths.

Many experts say that, ideally, women should try to continue breastfeeding for at least one year after birth, while gradually introducing other nutritional elements into their babies' diet.

Let children go to the bathroom when they need to go

If your 6 year-old suddenly starts wetting his pants in the classroom, don't blame it on stress or changes in routine. Instead, ask what the teacher's bathroom policy is. A survey of 1,000 primary-school teachers by the University of Iowa found that about 80 per cent set specific times for lavatory breaks (a policy not unknown in Britain) which contributes to incontinence and can lead to bladder and kidney infections.

Between 5 and 15 per cent of school-age children have daytime incontinence, says the study's main author, Christopher Cooper, associate professor of urology at the university. According to Dr Cooper, children in the early years of primary school are simply not old enough to hold their urine or bowel movements until a particular time.

Resisting the urge can result in accidents or urinary problems. (Children in one study named accidents as the third most stressful thing that could happen to them, after the death of a parent and going blind.) Children who learn to 'hold it in' continually tighten the muscles that prevent leakage of urine or faeces. 'They can become very good at this,' says Dr Cooper, 'but then they have trouble learning to relax the muscles when they are allowed to go to the bathroom.' This in turn leads to incomplete emptying of the bladder, which can contribute to infections. In another unhealthy trend, some children may try to restrict their fluid intake to avoid frequent visits to the bathroom.

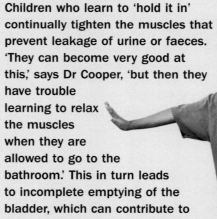
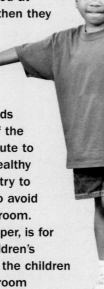

The answer, says Dr Cooper, is for parents to talk to their children's teachers and request that the children be allowed to go the bathroom whenever they feel the need to.

General health

Sports keep the doctor away

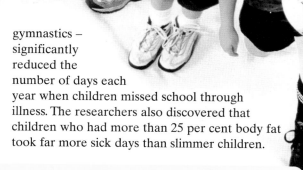

Children who participate regularly in sporting activities apparently have stronger immune systems and are less likely to come down with colds or flu.

We all know that exercise is good for us – but there is now another reason to encourage children to take regular exercise rather than spending long hours in front of a television or computer screen. Not only does exercise keep off excess weight and strengthen muscles and bones but, according to the results of a study at Brock University in Ontario, it can also fend off colds and flu.

The Canadian researchers found that the more children participated in high-energy sports such as football or basketball – any activity that significantly increased their heart rates – the less likely they were to be ill enough to miss school. Earlier studies on adults had shown that moderate exercise could strengthen the immune system, says Panagiota Klentrou, associate professor in the department of physical education at Brock.

But no one had ever examined the effects of exercise on children's immunity – even though, as Dr Klentrou points out, they are the ones most likely to suffer from viral infections throughout the year. It turned out that 8 hours or more a week of vigorous activity – such as football, swimming or gymnastics – significantly reduced the number of days each year when children missed school through illness. The researchers also discovered that children who had more than 25 per cent body fat took far more sick days than slimmer children.

RESEARCH ROUND-UP

Stopping nosebleeds faster

Have you ever tried to stop a young child's nosebleed and wondered how it was possible for a nose to bleed so copiously? The next time it happens, you will have a solution at your disposal that doctors in casualty have been using for more than 40 years.

The device is a nasal plug impregnated with a substance called micro-dispersed oxidized cellulose (m-doc, for short), derived from cotton, which aids coagulation. The tiny fibres – each nine times thinner than a human hair – act as a 'scaffold' on which the blood can clot. The plugs also form a protective gel-like covering over the wound – but they won't stick to the wall of the nose or cause further bleeding when removed. Over-the-counter plugs containing m-doc are now available from pharmacies under the name Seal-On.

Designed to stop bleeding from everyday cuts and scrapes as well as nosebleeds, Seal-On is also available in the form of spray powder, adhesive pads, sterile pads and sheer bandages.

Fast food world

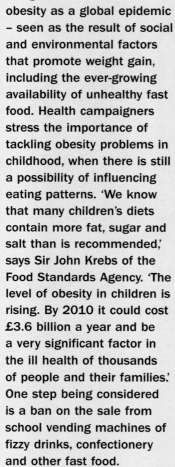

In 1998 the World Health Organization designated obesity as a global epidemic – seen as the result of social and environmental factors that promote weight gain, including the ever-growing availability of unhealthy fast food. Health campaigners stress the importance of tackling obesity problems in childhood, when there is still a possibility of influencing eating patterns. 'We know that many children's diets contain more fat, sugar and salt than is recommended,' says Sir John Krebs of the Food Standards Agency. 'The level of obesity in children is rising. By 2010 it could cost £3.6 billion a year and be a very significant factor in the ill health of thousands of people and their families.' One step being considered is a ban on the sale from school vending machines of fizzy drinks, confectionery and other fast food.

A study published in the journal *Pediatrics* in January 2004 found that in the USA today fast food makes up more than 10 per cent of children's overall calories – a fivefold increase since the late 1970s. Similar trends are seen all over the world.

Obesity
Early dieting is doomed to failure

If your preschool-age daughter is rather plump and you are thinking about putting her on a diet, think again. A recent American study found that girls who are at risk of being overweight at the age of 5 and begin dieting often end up putting on extra weight by the time they are 9. The plain truth is that diets don't work. University of Pennsylvania researchers followed 153 5-year-old girls for four years, evaluating their weight, attitudes about their weight, eating patterns and satisfaction with their bodies.

The researchers identified 32 girls who had begun to gain excess weight by the age of 5. By the time they reached the age of 7, those girls were eating significantly more than girls who weighed less, munching snacks even when they weren't hungry. They were also more dissatisfied with their bodies, more concerned about their weight, and more likely to diet. These patterns were still prevalent by the age of 9.

The theory is that the girls' attempts to diet backfired in much the same way as dieting does for adults – namely, depriving yourself of the food you want results in binge eating and encourages you to eat whenever food is available, whether you are hungry or not.

The study's message is clear, says Dr Matt Longjohn, executive director of a campaign to reduce childhood obesity in Chicago. 'Diet is a four-letter word. You have to make lifestyle changes,' he says. 'If a child is overweight, I'm not saying look the other way, but focus more on creating positive opportunities in her daily life for physical activity rather than focusing on diet and weight.'

Teenage dieting also fails
Another recent study found that dieting doesn't work for teenagers, either. After following more than 15,000 boys and girls between the ages of 9 and 14 for three years, researchers at Harvard Medical School found that the children who dieted gained more weight on average – around 1kg (2lb) more a year – than those who weren't dieting, possibly because the dieting teenagers were more likely to binge.

Obesity
Weight-loss drug for US teenagers

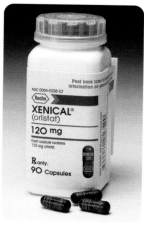

Xenical prevents some of the fat contained in food from being absorbed by the body.

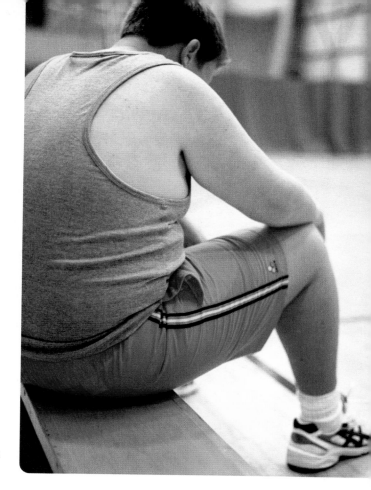

Seriously overweight American teenagers can now be prescribed a drug to help them get rid of unwanted pounds. In December 2003, the US drugs-monitoring authority approved orlistat (Xenical) for children between the ages of 12 and 16. The drug had already been sanctioned for adults.

The approval comes amid a huge growth in obesity among American children. The problem is particularly worrying for adolescents because studies show that overweight teenagers are likely to become overweight adults. Between 1994 and 2000, the number of overweight adolescents in the USA grew from 5 to 11 per cent. Today, about 30 per cent of American teenagers are overweight, and 15 per cent of those are obese.

A similar problem exists in the UK. Government figures show a 25 per cent increase in the number of overweight and obese children since 1995, with almost 17 per cent of children now estimated to be obese. But British health advisers shun the idea of using drugs in the treatment of childhood obesity, stressing instead the importance of diet, activity and behaviour change as the vital components in the management of the problem.

How it works Xenical blocks the action of the enzyme lipase, which usually breaks down the fat we eat so that the body can absorb it. When lipase is blocked, about 30 per cent of the fat in food is never absorbed and is excreted in faeces.

People taking the drug still have to follow a low-fat diet and exercise regularly if they want to lose weight, says Dr Marc Jacobson of the Schneider Children's Hospital in New York, who directed a clinical trial on the use of Xenical. Adolescents taking the drug should also take a daily multivitamin supplement, since Xenical can reduce absorption of fat-soluble vitamins such as vitamins E and A.

Who should take it? Xenical isn't for the slightly overweight teenager who wants to slim. It is for the young person whose weight problem is so serious that it affects his or her health. That means someone with a body mass index (a measurement that takes into account height and weight) of more than 30, or more than 27 if the person also has Type 2 diabetes, high blood pressure or abnormal cholesterol levels.

Side effects include increased bowel movements and cramps, but none of the 16 teenagers who used it in Dr Jacobson's study dropped out because of side effects, and all lost weight. 'Some of the kids who lost significant amounts of weight had dramatic changes in their social life and their ability to play sports and go out with other kids,' he says.

Availability Xenical is available in the USA with a doctor's prescription but it has not been approved for use in adolescents in Europe.

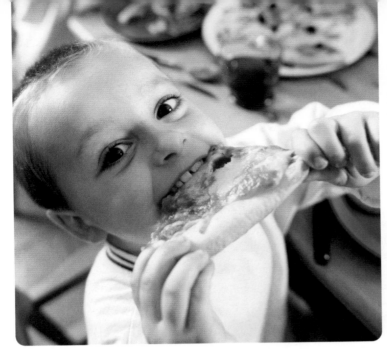

Young children are consuming fatty foods at an alarming rate, often to the exclusion of fruit and vegetables.

Obesity

Babies' diets are 'shocking'

When you think of finger foods for toddlers, you might picture sliced apples and bananas and little cubes of cheddar cheese. In fact, an image of chips, pizza, hot dogs and similar fare would be more accurate, according to a new American survey. The survey evaluated the eating habits of 3,000 randomly selected children between the ages of 4 months and 2 years and noted that they were eating the same kind of unhealthy food as their parents. It found that a third of children under 2 ate no fruit or vegetables on any given day.

An investigation for BBC's Six O'Clock News backed up these findings. It revealed that parents were putting junk food such as burgers into the blender to feed to their babies – some mothers said they had been told to blend up whatever they were eating to wean their children. Health visitors from all over the country reported seeing regular incidences of babies and children being given mashed-up fried chicken, Chinese takeaway or other fast food rather than home-cooked foods or fresh produce. The salt and fat content of these foods can result in obesity and even more serious effects.

The American survey also found that the toddlers were eating far more calories than they needed at their age, setting them up for weight problems later on. The results were 'shocking', says Kathleen Reidy, director of nutrition sciences at the baby-food maker Gerber, which sponsored the study. 'We are seeing problematic eating habits we associated with older children – few fruits and vegetables, too many sweetened drinks, too much fat – in children as young as 9 months.'

Most worrying is the fact that the foundation of a child's diet is established in the first two years of life, says Dr Reidy. Studies show that what a child likes and eats at age 2 is what he will like and eat at age 8. 'The issue we saw screaming out at us was that we're not developing these healthy eating habits early,' she says.

Obesity

The wrong breakfast may make kids fat

If your child's typical breakfast is a bowl of sugar masquerading as cereal or a couple of pieces of toasted white bread with jam, it may be contributing to overeating later in the day – and, potentially, to weight gain. That was the conclusion of a study conducted by Oxford Brookes University to test the effects in children of high and low-GI foods.

The glycaemic index and what it means

What most sugary cereals and white bread have in common is a high glycaemic index (GI), a measure of how much a food increases the level of sugar in the blood within two to three hours after eating it. High-GI foods include refined grains, such as cornflakes, and simple sugars, such as sugary jams.

Since they are quickly digested and absorbed into the bloodstream, high-GI foods send the level of sugar in the blood skyrocketing. In response, the body mass-produces the hormone insulin, which escorts blood sugar out of the bloodstream and into cells. As a result, blood sugar levels plummet, leaving us hungry again in no time – or so the thinking goes.

The popular theory is that eating low-GI foods such as wholegrain breads and cereals helps to keep the appetite in check, facilitating weight loss. Several recent studies have supported this notion, but few of them have involved children.

'Test' breakfasts and lunch observations

In the Oxford Brookes study, a group of 37 children (some overweight, some not) were given one of three breakfasts for three consecutive days: a low-GI breakfast, a low-GI breakfast with added sugar, and a high-GI breakfast. All the meals included fruit juice, cereal and milk, with or without bread and butter or margarine, and all contained exactly the same number of calories. All the children who took part in the investigation reported feeling full after eating the meals.

The second part of the experiment involved the unobtrusive recording by the researchers of how much food the children consumed at lunchtime (lunch was served buffet-style). They concluded that the breakfast a child ate had a 'statistically significant' effect on how much he or she ate at lunch. Children who ate high-GI breakfasts were more likely to eat more at lunchtime than children who ate either of the low-GI breakfasts.

'This is the first study to observe such an effect in a group of normal and overweight children, and it adds to the growing body of evidence that low-GI foods may have an important role in weight control and obesity management,' commented the authors of the investigation.

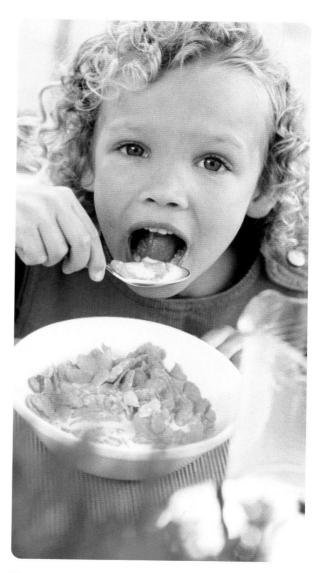

When children eat high-GI foods, such as cornflakes, for breakfast, they are more likely to overeat later in the day.

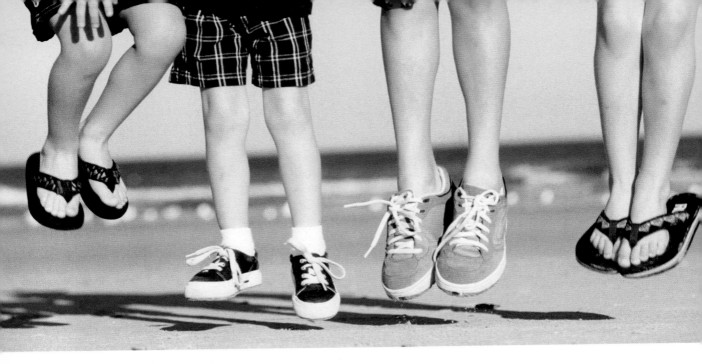

Osteoporosis
Jumping to build up young bones

Who would have thought that simply jumping up and down for a few minutes a day, interspersed with some skipping, could make a major difference to a child's bones later in life? That was the conclusion of researchers in British Columbia who studied the effects of a two-year exercise programme on pre-pubescent boys and girls.

Persuading 9-year-old children to start thinking about osteoporosis may seem like overkill, but it's important, says study author Kerry MacKelvie of British Columbia Children's Hospital in Vancouver. Today, one in every three women and one in 12 men over 50 in the UK will have an osteoporosis-related fracture in his or her lifetime. 'Banking' bone during childhood and adolescence is crucial to ensure that the skeleton is in good shape to withstand the inevitable bone loss that occurs in everyone from about 40 onwards. In some people, problems start to occur much earlier.

'In the last few years, people who work with kids and think about health started to realize that the lack of physical activity in children was behind a lot of the problems we see emerging in teens and adults,' Dr MacKelvie says.

The exercise programme The study involved 383 children at 14 schools. For the children at 50 per cent of the schools, it was business as usual. At the

other schools, the children participated in 12-minute circuit training programmes three times a week during two seven-month sessions (with a summer break in between). The programme included nine stations at which the kids did simple activities such as jumping up and down off a step or jumping over hoops set into the ground. The action of jumping puts weight on the femur (the large thighbone) and the hip, both common sites of fractures.

The key was to provide diversity of movement, says Dr MacKelvie, since research shows that doing activities to which you are not accustomed (such as running or walking) has a greater effect on bone.

The results After two years, Dr MacKelvie and her colleagues found that the children who had completed the programme had gained about 4 per cent more bone mass in the hip and lower spine than children who had not followed the programme.

The boys exhibited no significant change in the lower spine – which was possibly due in part to the different ways in which boys and girls jump and land – but their bone strength increased 7.5 per cent more than that of the boys who hadn't participated in the exercises.

'We consider these changes to be substantial,' says Dr MacKelvie. 'If you looked up the drug studies for older women, you would see that bisphosphonates

Will more milk reduce breakages?

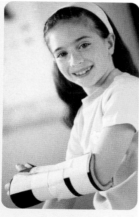

A decline in the consumption of milk may be to blame for a rise in bone breaks among children around the time of puberty, say researchers at the Mayo Clinic in Rochester, Minnesota. Comparing recent data with information recorded in 1971, they found that the incidence of forearm fracture had risen by 42 per cent over the period. Most fractures occurred around the time of the growth spurt during puberty – perhaps because bones become more porous at that time.

'Our study does not explain why fracture rates increased,' says Dr Sundeep Khosla of the Mayo Clinic. 'But the data raises concern about whether development of bone mass in today's children is impaired by lifestyle and dietary factors.' Decreased milk consumption, increased consumption of soft drinks and changing patterns of physical activity have all been mentioned as possible causes.

and other therapies for osteoporosis can hope to increase bone mass by only about 1 to 2 per cent per year. There is greater potential for exercise in the prevention of osteoporotic-related fractures.'

The issue of bone strength is important, she says, since it is the combination of strength and bone mass that offers the ultimate protection from fracture.

What it means The study demonstrates that short bursts of physical activity can have a significant impact on bone mass and strength. The National Osteoporosis Society in Britain comments that the results highlight 'the benefits of longer-term exercise in children whose bones are growing in strength'.

IN*Brief*

▶ Pollutants impair lung growth

According to the World Health Organization (WHO), there is now 'substantial' evidence about the harmful effects of air pollution on pregnancy and infant health, Recent research confirms findings that pollutants can impair the lung growth of a baby in the womb. The pollutants responsible are particulates, tiny fragments of soot emitted from vehicle exhausts. The WHO report says that the evidence is compelling enough to infer a link between particulate pollution and respiratory deaths in infants in the first year of life.

▶ Jabs against addiction on the way

A nationwide scheme to vaccinate children against drug addiction is being considered by the government. Childhood immunization would give adults protection from the euphoria experienced by drug users, making it pointless to take heroin or cocaine, for example. Professor David Nutt of Bristol University, a leading government adviser on drugs, says, 'People could be vaccinated against drugs as you are against measles. You could say that cocaine is more dangerous than measles, for example.' Appropriate vaccines are expected to come on the market within two years.

▶ Fish oils linked to prevention of allergies

An Australian study found that fish-oil supplements taken during pregnancy may help prevent allergies in children who have a high risk of developing them. Fish oils contain omega-3 fatty acids, which reduce inflammation and play an important role in a range of vital bodily processes, from regulating blood pressure and blood clotting to boosting immunity. Researchers speculate that fish oils may affect some part of the foetus's developing immune system, lowering the risk of future allergies.

▶ Be positive about potty training

If you are potty-training your toddler, for best results keep thinking positive. Researchers at the University of Pennsylvania at Philadelphia found that parents who were told to praise their children and avoid negative terms ('stinky nappy', for example) during potty training had children who became toilet trained sooner than parents who received only basic instructions.

WELLNESS

Imagine going into your doctor's surgery and puffing into a tube to find out whether you have a major illness, such as

cancer

Or consider never having to have another painful injection, instead receiving medications through needles so small you can't feel them. Both these developments were in the works in the past year and could become a reality in the near future.

Among the here-and-now developments: Experts are urging people to consume less salt and more potassium, and to maintain healthy levels of the 'sunshine' vitamin D. The weight-loss supplement ephedra was banned in the USA because of the health risks it posed, spurring manufacturers to promote new alternatives. And one researcher who tested 2 tonnes of salmon discovered that there were sufficient contaminants in the farm-raised variety to pose a real health risk. (UK experts disagree.)

Heart health may be linked to being happily married, caring for grandchildren and even drinking hard water. Finally, don't take the 'drink 8 glasses of water a day' advice too literally. It turns out that when it comes to staying properly hydrated, you should use common sense and urine colour as guides.

Anxiety

Do-it-yourself acupuncture for **anxiety**

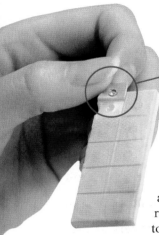

Watching their child being wheeled into an operating theatre is one of the most stressful things parents ever experience. But a simple acupuncture device could help reduce such anxiety, according to a US anaesthetist.

Dr Shu-Ming Wang, who works at at Yale University School of Medicine divided the mothers of children who were about to have surgery into two groups. In one, she inserted tiny acupuncture needles known as press needles into each mother's ear at a specific point that is known to produce relaxing effects. (A press needle is a short, fine needle attached to a wire loop covered with sterile skin tape – it resembles a drawing-pin.) In the other group, Dr Wang inserted needles into places that aren't known to produce a calming effect.

The mothers then spent 30 minutes with their children before the children were anaesthetized for surgery. When the women were surveyed about their anxiety levels, those who had the 'real' acupuncture treatment were found to be significantly less upset than mothers in the other group. The children of the less anxious mums were also significantly less anxious as they went into the operating room.

Dr Wang, who has taught the technique, says that most hospital doctors who are familiar with acupuncture should be able to offer the treatment.

In the UK, acupuncture has BMA approval and is available in NHS pain clinics and increasingly from GPs to treat a range of ailments. Pyonex, a press needle designed for self-care home use, is now available in the UK.

TOP Trends

THE HIGH COST OF OBESITY

The obesity epidemic is hitting us where it hurts: in our wallets. In the UK around 22 per cent of men and 24 per cent of women are obese. Life insurance companies are all too conscious of the health risks associated with obesity and, increasingly, insurance policyholders are seeing their premiums grow in proportion to their waistlines.

The UK National Audit Office estimated the cost of obesity to the NHS at £480 million for 1998 (the latest year for which figures are available) while the indirect cost to the economy, according to Liam Donaldson, England's chief medical officer, is £2 billion a year and predicted to reach 3.6 billion by the year 2010.

HEALTHIER EATING UNDER THE GOLDEN ARCHES

The fast-food chain McDonald's made several moves in 2004 to promote healthy heating. Innovations included the biggest menu change in 30 years – the launch of Salads Plus, with cherry tomatoes and rocket among the 21 fresh new ingredients; a new low-calorie 'Go Active' salad; and lower-fat chicken nuggets with reduced salt content. Its series of 2-minute educational films featuring the YumChums, developed with the leading nutritionist Anita Bean, aims to inform children in a fun way about how to keep fit, healthy and happy by eating a balanced diet.

The food chain's decision to phase out its 'supersized' French fries and drinks came on the heels of the film *Super Size Me,* which generated considerable publicity. The film charts a man's 11kg (25lb) weight gain as he follows a 30-day diet of McDonald's food and drinks including super-sized items. McDonald's denied that phasing out super sizes had anything to do with the film.

EGGS FOR A HEALTHY HEART

Eggs are an important source of protein, vitamins and minerals but their high cholesterol content has been a cause for concern. Not only are earlier fat warnings proving unfounded, but now some egg types contain significant amounts of omega-3 fatty acids (typically found in fish oil) which help to reduce blood cholesterol and blood pressure levels. Laid by free-range hens who have been fed a diet rich in essential fats, the eggs are on sale in most supermarkets. Look for the 'omega-3 enriched' label on the carton.

In the USA, some hens are now fed lutein-rich marigold extract so that they lay eggs whose yolks are rich in the yellow eye-protecting nutrient.

Diagnostic tests

New breath test will diagnose diseases

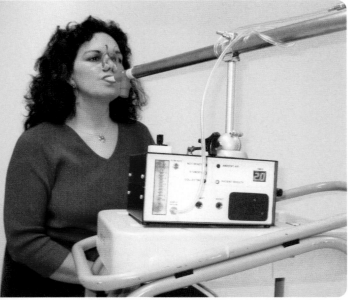

An ill wind? Patients simply have to exhale into a breath collection apparatus for two minutes in order to capture compounds that provide a 'fingerprint' of diseases.

Finding out if you have developed cancer or another serious condition may soon be as easy as whistling or blowing out a candle.

Each breath you exhale carries chemical hints about processes going on in your body, and a new device can store your breath so it can be analysed for subtle signs of disease. The device – the breath-collecting apparatus (BCA) – features a tube into which a person exhales for several minutes and a special trap that collects chemicals from the exhaled breath, says Dr Michael Phillips, professor of clinical medicine at New York Medical College in Valhalla, who developed the BCA.

Analysing breath to help track down a diagnosis isn't new. In the UK breath tests are used to detect single conditions, such as *Helicobacter pylori* in dyspepsia. And doctors can test for lactose intolerance – a problem that keeps some people from properly digesting dairy foods – by measuring hydrogen in a person's breath. Police officers routinely 'diagnose' excessive alcohol consumption with breath tests. However, the new technology analyses much tinier amounts of breath components than any other test has been able to do.

A new clue to disease In the early 1970s, says Dr Phillips, Nobel prize winner Linus Pauling froze exhaled breath in a tube and discovered that the air contained traces of volatile organic compounds (VOCs), carbon-based chemicals evaporated in the air. Dr Phillips has since measured many Americans' and Europeans' breath with his device and discovered that healthy people generally exhale the same 200 or so VOCs, in tiny concentrations. When people have diseases, however, they exhale some *different* VOCs. By comparing the breath of healthy people with that of people who are ill, he has been able to create three-dimensional 'fingerprints' of various diseases.

Testing for cancer and diabetes In early 2004, the US Food and Drug Administration (FDA) approved the device to test for organ rejection in people with recent heart transplants. Additional studies were evaluating its usefulness for detecting diabetes, breast cancer and lung cancer. Breath testing may also eliminate the injections that many people with diabetes face daily or several times a day – in order to obtain blood samples from which to check their blood sugar levels. Researcher Dr Pietro Galessetti Ph.D. and his colleagues at the University of California, Irvine, recently conducted tests on 10 volunteers to see if they could use VOCs in the subjects' breath to measure their blood sugar levels. The method appeared to work, and the researchers plan to test it on more people.

Before this method becomes useful on a large scale, patients will need access to breath-analysing equipment that is small and cheap. Currently, Dr Phillips' apparatus is relatively simple, but the technology used to examine the trapped breath is expensive and cumbersome, so researchers must send breath samples to a central laboratory for analysis. Dr Phillips envisages a future in which doctors will have their own equipment loaded with different disease 'fingerprints', providing a rapid diagnosis in the surgery. Patients will no longer have to endure blood sampling or invasive diagnostic procedures to know what is going on in their bodies.

'All they'll have to do is sit down and breathe for a couple of minutes,' he says.

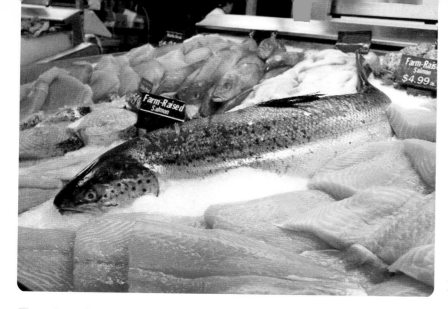

A US study found high levels of dioxins and PCBs in farm-raised salmon, but the UK Food Standards Agency says they are within the WHO safety levels.

Food safety

Is your salmon swimming in contaminants?

'Eat plenty of fish' has been the advice of doctors and nutritionists for years, especially to prevent heart problems. But an analysis by US scientists of 2 tonnes of salmon, including farmed salmon from Scotland, revealed that many fish, particularly the farm-raised variety, contained enough contaminants to pose a potential health risk.

Farm-raised versus wild Dr David Carpenter, director of the Institute for Health and the Environment at the University at Albany in New York and his team bought whole salmon and fillets from vendors in Europe and North America for testing and also analysed samples of feed given to farm-raised salmon in Europe, North America and South America. As reported in a January 2004 issue of the journal *Science*, the researchers found that levels of dioxins and PCBs in farm-raised salmon were more than 10 times higher than in wild salmon. Dioxins, formed by burning oil and coal, can persist in the environment for many years. PCBs are industrial chemicals. Concentrations of the pesticide DDT, were also higher in farm-raised salmon.

The differing levels of contaminants are probably due to the different diets of the fish. The researchers found contaminants in the food given to farmed

salmon, which is rich in fish oil and fish meal. The food samples from Europe were more contaminated than those from North or South America. And the levels of contaminants were higher in salmon farmed in Scotland and the Faroe Islands than in farmed fish raised in North or South America.

What's the risk? The contaminants detected are fat soluble. This means that they are stored in the fat of the fish that are processed into food for farmed

[FISH TO AVOID WHEN YOU'RE PREGNANT]

Pickles and ice cream started sounding even better to expectant mothers in December 2003. That's when the Food Standard Authority's Committee on Toxicity of chemicals in food, consumer products and the environment produced an updated statement on a survey of mercury in fish and shellfish, and advised pregnant and nursing women, as well as those considering becoming pregnant, to limit their intake of certain fish.

Some types of seafood contain unacceptably high levels of mercury, which can be harmful to a foetus or a breast-fed infant. The survey concludes that eating more than a 140g portion of either shark, swordfish or marlin each week might be verging on dangerous for pregnant women, but two 140g portions of fresh tuna or four 140g portions of canned tuna should not damage a developing foetus.

Mercury concentrations in UK-farmed salmon and trout were found to be reassuringly low in a Bristol University study published in 2003.

salmon, and in turn, in the fat of salmon that eat the food then in the fat of people who eat the fish.

That's a problem, Dr Carpenter says. Some of these contaminants are known to cause cancer, and some can lower the IQs of babies born to mothers who have the toxins in their bodies. DDT can cause liver cancer and damage humans' nervous and reproductive systems. The chemical was banned in the USA in 1972 (in the UK in 1984) but takes more than a decade to break down in the environment, and is still used in other parts of the world.

In light of his findings, Dr Carpenter suggests that only people who stand to gain from salmon should eat the farm-raised fish. Middle-aged people with heart disease can benefit from the omega-3 fatty acids in the fish, which help to protect against heart problems. On the other hand, he says, the risks of eating farm-raised fish outweigh the benefits for children and young adults, who are less likely to have heart problems and have more decades of life in which to develop cancer from the contaminants.

Other research studies Dr Carpenter's findings are in line with recent British research. A 2002 study by the School of Biomedical and Life Sciences at the University of Surrey, Guildford, confirmed previous reports of relatively high concentrations of PCBs in farmed Scottish salmon. Another study, published the same year, suggests that the average consumer could be at risk of exceeding tolerable limits of dioxins and PCBs by increasing their intake of farmed salmon by as little as one portion a week. The authors of the report called for further research.

UK government guidelines The Food Standards Agency (FSA) states that Dr Carpenter's study does not present any new safety concerns, and that the levels of dioxins found in farmed salmon are within the safety levels set by the World Health Organization (WHO), the European Union (EU) and the US Food and Drug Administration (FDA). It states that any possible risks of eating oily fish are outweighed by the benefits to heart health.

The FSA advises people in the UK to eat at least two portions of fish a week, one of which should be 'oily' fish such as salmon. Although the FSA's own research has shown no significant difference in levels of contaminants between farmed and wild salmon from the UK, it is carrying out further research. Meanwhile, it says, there is no reason to avoid eating Scottish or any other farmed salmon.

Poultry:
how to avoid spreading
tummy bug
bacteria

Next time you make a chicken casserole, don't rinse the meat first. A 2004 survey by the Food and Drink Federation revealed that four out of five Britons who cook poultry meals at home could be increasing the risk of food poisoning by rinsing raw poultry under the tap. Food safety scientists have found that this seemingly sensible action can splash any invisible bacteria on the bird onto nearby taps, surfaces and foods.

Poultry is a source of salmonella and campylobacter bacteria, both potential food poisoning culprits. The majority of campylobacter infections arise from cross-contamination, such as blood from raw poultry dripping onto cooked foods or salad. Salmonella infection is commonly linked to undercooked poultry and to raw and lightly cooked eggs: thorough cooking at the right temperature removes the risk.

'Spreading germs when preparing food is easily done, but easily prevented,' says Martin Paterson, deputy director general of the Food and Drink Federation. The survey showed that many food safety messages are hitting home. Of those interviewed, 9 out of 10 always wash their hands after touching raw meat and before handling salads and cooked foods; more than 50 per cent store meat on the bottom shelf of the fridge to avoid juices dropping onto other foods; and about 6 out of 10 use separate chopping boards and knives for cutting raw meat and vegetables.

Heart health

Ulcer bug is also a cholesterol suspect

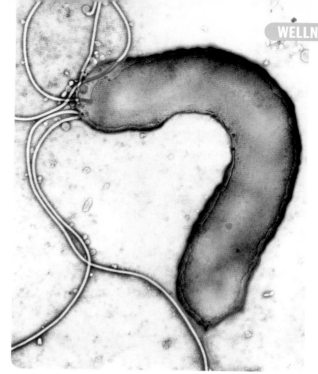

The curved (or sometimes spiral) *Helicobacter pylori* bacterium is involved in peptic ulcer formation. It may also have an adverse effect on your cholesterol profile.

Helicobacter pylori, a bacterium that lives in the stomach, is best known for causing peptic ulcers, but the organism may also play a role in unhealthy cholesterol levels, researchers from Austria and Germany have discovered. On the positive side, getting rid of the bug may be a quick and easy way to improve your cholesterol profile and thereby help to reduce the risk of heart disease.

In a study published in a January 2004 issue of the *American Journal of Cardiology*, researchers looked at 87 people with ulcers who tested positive for *H. pylori* and took drugs, including two antibiotics, to eradicate the bacteria. The patients' cholesterol levels were tested before they began taking the drugs and again a year later.

Once the *H. pylori* bacteria had been eliminated, the participants' total cholesterol increased significantly, but the increase was mostly in their levels of high-density lipoprotein (HDL, or 'good') cholesterol – the kind that gobbles up low-density lipoprotein (LDL, or 'bad') cholesterol and helps to prevent the formation of artery-clogging plaque. The participants' HDL levels were seen to have increased by almost 25 per cent.

It is still unclear why *H. pylori* would affect cholesterol, says lead researcher Hubert Scharnagl Ph.D., of the University of Graz Clinical Institute of Medical and Chemical Laboratory Diagnostics in Austria. One theory is that the bacteria trigger inflammation in the body that affects cholesterol balance. When the bugs are eradicated, the inflammation subsides, and the ratio of good to bad cholesterol improves.

Although additional studies are needed to establish the connection between *H. pylori* and cholesterol, people whose cholesterol tests show that they have low levels of HDL should consider being tested for the bacteria, Dr Scharnagl says.

RESEARCH ROUND-UP

Hard water may be soft on your heart

Hard water leaves crusty limescale deposits on taps and 'furs up' kettles, but the benefits it may offer to your heart could be a consolation.

A recent Finnish study found that increased water hardness – the concentration of minerals such as calcium and magnesium – was linked to a reduced risk of heart attack. Rates of heart attack vary widely in Finland, which has relatively soft water. Researchers looked at data on nearly 19,000 men ranging in age from 35 to 74 and compared it with data on water hardness throughout the country. They found that for each increased unit of water hardness, risk of heart attack fell by 1 per cent.

The magnesium present in hard water may be responsible for the beneficial effect. Earlier research linked higher magnesium intake or higher blood levels of the mineral with reduced risk of high blood pressure and heart disease.

Heart health

Chest pain? Make the **right call**

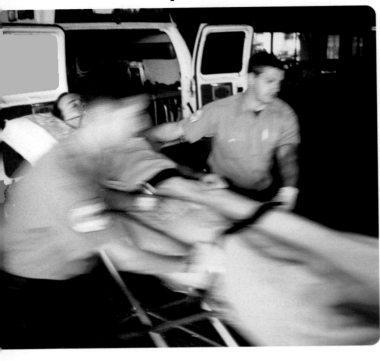

You're having chest pain. Could it be a heart attack? Should you dial 999?

Although two-thirds of emergency hospital admissions have a non-cardiac cause for their chest pain, the advice from NHS Direct is unequivocal: if you think you may be having a heart attack call an ambulance immediately. While you are waiting for help, take an aspirin. Delay in seeking treatment is a major cause of heart attack fatalities. Women, for instance, tend to think heart attacks are a male problem.

So how would you know if your chest pain signals a heart attack? The usual sign is a crushing pain in the centre of the chest which often wraps around the body like a vice and may spread to the arms, throat, jaw, back or abdomen. You may also be short of breath and feel weak, sick or sweaty.

British Heart Foundation advice is: never ignore chest pain, especially if you have coronorary heart disease. If you suspect a heart attack, call 999 and phone your doctor.

Hale and hearty grandparents?

Being with your grandchildren may gladden your heart, but does it put you at risk? A Harvard study of 54,000 middle-aged and older women in the *American Journal of Public Health* in November 2003, showed that grandmothers who cared for grandchildren, even part time, had a higher risk of heart disease than those who were't carers.

If true for the UK the finding could challenge both family links and our system of childcare. 'Six out of 10 families turn to grandparents as carers, saving a possible £5 billion a year in childcare costs', says Gordon Lishman, Director-General of Age Concern. 'Modern grandparents are central to family life in Britain and a constant source of support to their own children and grandchildren.'

It would also be a new phenomenon. A review of women in the 18th and 19th centuries, reported in *Nature* in March 2004, showed that grandchildren enhanced grandmothers' longevity and fitness.

Living happily – and longer – ever after

Men derive more health benefits from being married than women do – something researchers already knew. Now, a new study shows that women, too, are healthier when married, but only when they're happy in the relationship.

The 13-year study assessed the marital status and cardiovascular disease risk of 493 women. Researchers measured the women's physical risk factors, including blood pressure and glucose and cholesterol levels; lifestyle risk factors, such as smoking and exercise; and their psychological risk factors, such as stress, anxiety and depression. Women who were highly satisfied with their relationships showed lower cholesterol, less weight gain and less depression than those women who were unhappy in their relationships or were single, widowed or divorced, says Linda Gallo Ph.D., head researcher at the University of California, San Diego.

Another US study, published in the annals of *Behavioral Medicine* in 2003, shows that hugging your partner is good for your cardiovascular system.

Nutrition

Vitamin D takes centre stage

You probably know that your body needs calcium for healthy, strong bones. Many calcium supplements also contain vitamin D because the two work as a team to protect your skeleton, but now it turns out that vitamin D may be important in its own right in more ways than we knew.

Recent research shows that the 'sunshine vitamin' may play a key role in preventing certain cancers as well as multiple sclerosis (MS). In one study vitamin D was also shown to be an effective treatment for widespread musculoskeletal pain. And it appears that some researchers fear that too many of us have woefully low levels of the nutrient.

The body makes vitamin D when the skin is exposed to sunlight. People who live far from the equator, though, and those who rarely venture out of doors or always wear sun-block are at risk of deficiency. Most of us could apparently do with more vitamin D in the winter, and older people may need supplements because, with age, the skin becomes less able to convert sunlight into vitamin D.

Protection from colon polyps For four years, researchers coordinated through Dartmouth Medical School in New Hampshire followed people who'd had precancerous colon polyps removed. Half were given calcium supplements, and the other half placebos (dummy pills). The vitamin D levels of 803 subjects were also assessed twice with blood tests.

The people who took calcium supplements were less likely to develop more polyps – provided they also had higher-than-average vitamin D levels. Vitamin D was also associated with a reduced risk of recurrent polyps, but only in the people who received the calcium supplements. The combination of calcium and vitamin D is also thought to help protect against cancers of the breast and prostate.

Multiple sclerosis prevention Researchers have long known that people who live near the equator have lower rates of multiple sclerosis than those who live farther away. Vitamin D may be the reason, says Kassandra Munger M.Sc., a Harvard researcher who led the first prospective study exploring the relationship between vitamin D and MS. This type of study follows a group people without a disease to see who develops it and how they differ from people who don't develop it. The study evaluated data from nearly 200,000 women. Those who took at least 400 IU of supplemental vitamin D daily had a 40 per cent less chance of developing MS than those who didn't take it.

The researchers' next step is to examine samples of blood from millions of individuals, which are stored in a military repository, to see if people with low levels of vitamin D in their blood are more likely to develop MS. In MS, the immune system attacks the protective insulating sheath around nerves, and vitamin D may protect against the disease by preventing that kind of assault.

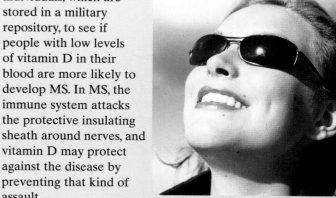

The pain connection A study published in the December 2003 issue of the journal *Mayo Clinic Proceedings* uncovered a surprising link between persistent pain and low levels of vitamin D. Dr Greg Plotnikoff noticed that many patients he saw at a University of Minnesota community health clinic suffered unexplained pain despite having otherwise normal checkups. He had read European studies that connected pain with vitamin D deficiency and decided to test for the deficiency in his patients.

Nearly all the 150 patients whom Dr Plotnikoff studied turned out to be low in vitamin D, including all those under the age of 30. The people who were severely deficient required prescription-strength doses of the vitamin to restore normal levels.

Vitamin D deficiency is believed to lead to changes in the inner bone that cause it to become rubbery and press outwards on the outer layer of bone, probably causing aches and pains. If you have unexplained pain, ask your doctor for a blood test that measures vitamin D, suggests Dr Plotnikoff, .

How much is enough? In the USA the Recommended Dietary Allowance (RDA) daily for vitamin D is 5mcg (200 IU) for adults under 50, 10mcg (400 IU) for people aged 51 to 70, and 15mcg (600 IU) for people over 70. But in the UK there is no recommendation for adults exposed to sunlight although the Food Standards Agency advises 10 mcg (400 IU) a day for people confined indoors.

Nutrition

Vitamin E
is better from
a box than from
a bottle

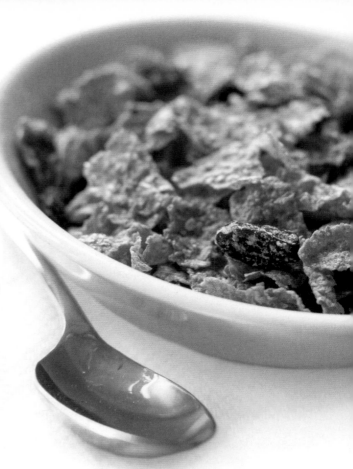

To get the most benefit from vitamin E, it may be better to take it *in* rather than *with* your breakfast. That's the finding of a small study that compared the vitamin's 'bioavailability' – how well the body can use it – when it is consumed in pill form versus in a cereal with added vitamin E.

Three women and two men participated in the trial, conducted at the Linus Pauling Institute at Oregon State University in Corvallis. They first took vitamin E in a 270mg (400 IU) capsule – typical for a vitamin E supplement – with a glass of fat-free milk. Later, they ate cereal containing 20mg (30 IU) of the vitamin with fat-free milk. Next, they ate cereal containing 270mg (400 IU) of the vitamin with fat-free milk. Finally, they consumed a 270mg (400 IU) vitamin E capsule with cereal that had no vitamin E, with fat-free milk. The vitamin E in the capsules and cereal was specially tagged with deuterium – an isotope of hydrogen – so that the researchers could measure it in the subjects' bloodstreams. The cereal company General Mills sponsored the research.

The subjects' bodies were able to absorb the 270mg (400 IU) in the cereal far more readily than the same amount in capsule form. And their bodies derived more of the vitamin from eating the 20mg (30 IU) cereal than taking the 270mg (400 IU) capsule, according to the January 2004 issue of the *American Journal of Clinical Nutrition*.

What it means Vitamin E is an antioxidant that may help reduce the risk of heart disease. The study findings support previous studies which found fewer protective results from supplements than from vitamin-rich diets. Sara Stanner, Senior Nutrition scientist at the British Nutrition Foundation, says: 'You can't replace the benefits of a varied, balanced diet by taking any supplement. Eating fortified cereals is a good way to boost a number of vitamins and minerals.' Wheatgerm, nuts and vegetable oils

are other good sources of vitamin E . In the UK no recommended daily intake of vitamin E has been set but some experts suggest that those at high risk of heart disease should take up to 800mg (1200 IU).

Nutrition

Government bid to shake that salt habit

The UK government has called on food firms and supermarkets to produce rigorous strategies that will reduce the level of salt in processed foods. Last autumn, the Food Standards Agency launched a £4m post and TV advertising campaign to highlight the excessive salt in everyday diets which they contend poses a significant health risk as many studies have linked high salt intake to high blood pressure. The Department of

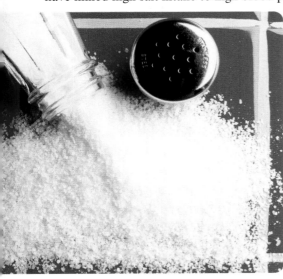

Health and the Food Standards Agency want to cut total daily salt intake to no more than 6g for an adult and 4g for a child. Most of us eat far more than that – and much of our intake is currently 'hidden' within processed foods. Manufacturers are not yet legally required to list the salt or sodium in their products, but many do and claim they are working closely with the FSA to 'produce both plans for and actual substantial salt reductions.'

Salt is also an issue in the USA where the Institute of Medicine, a private organization which advises the US government on nutritional guidelines and other scientific matters, published its report on salt and potassium in 2004, recommending even lower salt consumption levels.

The current US recommendation is 2.4g sodium (6g salt) daily, as in the UK. (As salt is composed of 40 per cent sodium and 60 per cent chloride, 2.5g salt contains 1g sodium.) The institute recommended no more than 1.5g sodium (3.75g salt) a day for adults under 50, 1.3g sodium (3.25g salt) daily for adults aged between 50 and 70, and only 1.2g sodium (3g salt) a day for people aged over 70.

The body needs some sodium to regulate its fluid levels, maintain healthy blood pressure and to generate electrical impulses in nerves and muscles. But excessive intake increases the risk of high blood pressure, stroke and coronary heart disease.

While you're cutting back on salt, you may want to boost your intake of another mineral – potassium – according to the same US report. People need 4.7g daily, which is roughly twice the amount that young adults generally consume. Potassium helps to maintain proper fluid levels in your body and may help to prevent high blood pressure. Sources include bananas, spinach, citrus fruits, tomatoes and potatoes.

FUTURE BREAKTHROUGHS

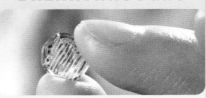

MICRONEEDLES: Too tiny to hurt

Pioneering work in the USA means that by 2010, doctors may be able to put medications into your body with devices that combine the efficiency of a hypodermic needle with the painlessness of a patch.

The devices are microneedles, that are so small that they are invisible to the naked eye. In fact, their length is measured in millionths of a metre – too short to cause any pain when they pierce your skin. They may be hollow or solid and made of silicon, metal, glass or polymer.

Microneedles could be affixed to a medicinal patch that is applied to the skin, allowing the medication to seep into your body through the tiny holes made by the needles, according to Dr Mark Prausnitz Ph.D., associate professor of chemical and biomedical engineering at the Georgia Institute of Technology in Atlanta.

The tiny needles offer an option for delivering drugs that can't be taken by mouth or supplied via conventional patches. Dr Prausnitz is particularly interested in using microneedles to administer vaccines, thereby saving infants and children from the pain of receiving multiple injections.

The BioValve company has licensed Georgia Tech's microneedles and is developing drug-delivery methods that use them.

Nutrition
Super foods
to protect against
free radicals

Your body is constantly under assault from tiny trouble-makers called free radicals, but two studies published in the summer of 2004 show which foods offer you the best protection against their vandalism.

Free radicals are unstable oxygen molecules that can damage your cells' DNA. Although your body generates some free radicals during normal metabolism, as part of its defence against disease, sometimes it goes into over-production, triggered by factors such as cigarette smoke and pollution. Damage from free radicals – a process called oxidation – is thought to play a role in ailments such as heart disease, cancer and Alzheimer's disease, as well as in premature ageing.

To combat oxidation you need antioxidants, compounds that neutralize free radicals. Many brightly coloured fruits and vegetables are rich dietary sources of antioxidants, which include vitamins E and C and beta carotene (the plant form of vitamin A), among other compounds.

The strongest antioxidant foods The new studies, conducted by the US Department of Agriculture (USDA), tested the antioxidant capacity of 100 different foods.

Among the fruits studied, the highest in antioxidants per serving are blueberries, cranberries, blackberries and prunes. Top scorers among vegetables are red beans, red kidney beans and pinto beans, followed by artichokes. Some nuts are rich in antioxidants, with pecans scoring higher than many fruits and vegetables. Among spices that the researchers tested, ground cloves, ground cinnamon, dried oregano and turmeric top the list of those with antioxidant power. And there's also one powerful antioxidant food that will appeal to chocoholics: cooking chocolate.

Eat your vegetables Whether a food is fresh, frozen or cooked can affect its antioxidant potency, but the bottom line of this research is that 'individuals should eat more fruits and vegetables. I am coming to the conclusion that there needs to be at least one food with high antioxidant capacity included in each meal,' says Ronald Prior, PhD, a research chemist with the USDA and one of the study authors.

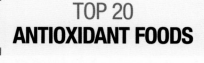

[TOP 20 ANTIOXIDANT FOODS]

The following foods are ranked according to their antioxidant power per serving (strongest first), using portion sizes set by the USDA. Some spices and cooking chocolate are also high in antioxidants but weren't measured per serving and aren't included in the list.

SMALL RED BEANS
WILD BLUEBERRIES
RED KIDNEY BEANS
PINTO BEANS
CULTIVATED BLUEBERRIES
CRANBERRIES
ARTICHOKES
BLACKBERRIES
PRUNES
RASPBERRIES
STRAWBERRIES
RED DELICIOUS APPLES
GRANNY SMITH APPLES
PECANS
CHERRIES
BLACK PLUMS
RUSSET POTATOES (COOKED)
PLUMS
GALA APPLES
WALNUTS

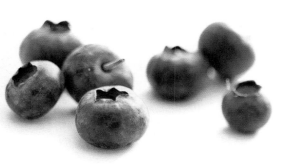

Nutrition
Fructose comes under suspicion

Fructose, a sugar found in fruit and honey, may not be naturally good for you – particularly if you're concerned about your weight. A can of soft drink contains roughly the same amount as two apples, but while it may may quench your thirst, the type of sugar it contains may also trigger your hunger.

A US study in the June 2004 issue of the *Journal of Clinical Endocrinology & Metabolism* investigated the different ways that common types of sugar affect the hormones in the body that tell us when we're full or hungry.

Soft drinks – particularly in the USA – are sweetened with high-fructose corn syrup (HFCS), a thick liquid made from cornstarch, which contains fructose and glucose (another form of sugar) in similar proportions to those that occur in table sugar (sucrose). Increasingly, food and beverage manufacturers are using HFCS instead of sucrose as it's cheaper, and the liquid is easier to mix into soft drinks.

What the study showed The researchers looked at 12 healthy, normal-weight young women who ate three meals in a laboratory, each one accompanied by a specially prepared beverage sweetened with either fructose or glucose. After a month, the experiment was repeated, but this time, the volunteers drank the beverage they hadn't had the first time. In each instance, frequent blood samples were taken for analysis.

The researchers found that when the women drank the fructose drinks – which contained as much fructose as two cans of soft drink – their bodies produced less of a hormone called leptin, which makes you feel full, thus encouraging you to stop eating. The volunteers also had higher levels of a hormone called ghrelin after eating the meals accompanied by fructose. Ghrelin stimulates the appetite, making you want to eat more.

According to the study, Americans are consuming at least 26 per cent more fructose than they were three decades ago, primarily because they are drinking more soft drinks. This increase in fructose consumption may be playing a role in the national increase in obesity – possibly by making people eat more because of their altered hormone levels.

How relevant is the research? The American Corn Refiners' Association points out that the study examines exaggerated use of either fructose or glucose, whereas they occur together in almost equal proportions in both table sugar and HCFS. In Britain there is greater awareness of fructose since regulations now require it to be listed on food labels. Much less corn syrup is used in soft drinks although some is used in food. The UK Food Standards Agency says that more evidence is needed before it will be able to single out HFCS from its general advice to consume sugary foods more sparingly.

Lowering your total sugar consumption is a wise move, and burning more calories through exercise is a sure way to lose weight or keep it off.

Nutrition
Old hydration advice doesn't hold water

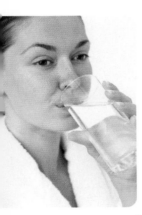

Guidelines about how much water to drink a day appear to be changing. Americans have been told to drink when thirsty and in the UK the message is ' look at your urine'.

The Institute of Medicine (IOM), a private group that sets guidelines for nutrients that Americans need, released its recommendations for water intake in the spring of 2004. Its report stated that the average sedentary man, should take in 3.7 litres (nearly 7 pints). For women, a daily intake of 2.7 litres (about 5 pints) is deemed adequate. But those amounts include the fluids found in foods. The report also said that healthy people can manage with less; drinking when you're thirsty will keep you properly hydrated. Of course, if out in the heat or taking part in exercise, you should drink more – to compensate for the extra water lost through breathing rapidly or sweating. Interestingly the report also said that caffeinated drinks could be included in your daily fluid intake as their diuretic effect was minimal unless you drank them to excess.

A spokeswoman for the British Nutrition Foundation said that the best indicator of whether you're drinking enough is the colour of your urine. UK health professionals recommend an intake of 1.5 to 2 litres (2½-3½ pints) a day as liquids in our temperate climate, and more when taking vigorous exercise or in the heat. We should also derive about a third of our total daily adult water intake from food. Fruit and vegetables are the main providers; canteloupe melon for instance is 95 per cent water. But wholewheat bread is 38 per cent water by weight and roast turkey is 62 per cent.

Another 2004 report challenged age-old advice to drink more fluids during illness. This can be harmful researchers from the University of Queensland in Australia reported in a February issue of the *British Medical Journal*. A hormone produced when people have pneumonia or bronchitis causes them to store water rather than passing it in urine. Drinking too much can cause excessively low sodium in people with these conditions as the excess water can dilute the blood and upset the normal water-sodium ratio – a condition called hyponatremia – leading to confusion, lethargy and even coma.

Supplements
Herbal supplement banned

As 2004 dawned, fans of the herb ephedra – a key ingredient in weight-loss products that were widely sold on the internet – descended on health food stores in the United States, emptying shelves of the popular supplement. The spree followed news that the FDA would soon ban sales of the herb because it posed 'unreasonable risk of illness or injury'. In February 2004, the FDA did just that, prohibiting the sale of any supplement containing ephedrine alkaloids, components found in ephedra.

Widely promoted as a way to help you lose weight and enjoy better athletic performance, ephedra was found in a variety of US products. The stimulants purportedly stoked users' metabolisms, helping them to burn calories faster. The side effects, however, included higher blood pressure, irregular heart rate and jitters.

A risky herb The ban followed years of contemplation by the FDA as reports of harm linked to the herb accumulated. A February 2003 study commissioned by the National Institutes of Health looked at 16,000 'adverse events' reported after ephedra use, which included several heart attacks, strokes and deaths that may have been attributable to the supplement. The study found some evidence that ephedra could be useful for short-term weight loss, but there was little to support its use for improved athletic performance.

Despite the popularity of ephedra in the USA, before the ban it accounted for less that 1 per cent of all herbal preparations sold in the USA (but 64 per cent of adverse reactions). In the

THE NEXT **EPHEDRA?**

For a year or two before the FDA ban on ephedra, a number of companies producing ephedra supplements started marketing other products for weight loss; an internet search reveals thousands of products now described as 'ephedra-free'. You're likely to see more of the following in the near future say US medical herbal experts. But these are not devoid of controversies of their own.

- **Bitter orange.** Also known as citrus aurantium, this supplement contains synephrine, a mild stimulant. Some research has shown that it helps to promote weight loss, but it is chemically similar to ephedrine and can raise blood pressure. The same week that the ephedra ban was announced, a US senator urged the FDA to ban bitter orange, too, and the agency is reportedly monitoring the supplement closely.
- **Garcinia cambogia (tamarind).** This supplement, extracted from an Asian fruit, contains a chemical called hydroxycitric acid. It is said to facilitate weight loss, but a study published in the *Journal of the American Medical Association* in 1998 found that dieters who took it lost no more weight than dieters who took placebos.
- **Green tea extract.** The internet is filled with claims for this supplement, but evidence supporting those claims is scant. A small Swiss study in 1999 found that people who took green tea extract burned more energy – thus calories – over a 24-hour period than those who took a placebo. The researchers claimed that the results weren't attributable simply to the caffeine in the tea.

UK, where its use has always been more restricted, a small number of adverse reactions and one death have been reported.

The legal status of ephedra varies from country to country. In the United Kingdom, where its safety is under scrutiny by the Medicines and Healthcare products Regulatory Agency (MHRA), ephedra remains legal, although it is restricted to a maximum dose of 600mg and a maximum daily dose of 1800mg. In addition, any herbal medicines containing ephedra may only be supplied following one-to-one consultations and must be obtained from a pharmacist, registered medical herbalist or doctor.

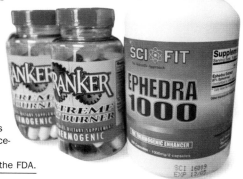

Bottles of ephedra were pulled from store shelves in the United States. Popular as a weight-loss and performance-enhancing supplement, the stimulant scored poorly with the FDA.

IN*Brief*

▶ New moves to make hospitals safer places

No-one looks forward to going into hospital – and there's always the fear that you might come out feeling worse than when you went in.

New independent research, based on four years of hospital statistics, concludes that hospitals must improve recording of medical errors and of hospital-acquired infections such as the MRSA superbug. The National Patient Safety Agency (NPSA), which estimates that one in 10 patients is harmed to some degree as a result of their care in NHS hospitals, is now developing systems to improve reporting of medical errors and maximize patient safety. 'Encouraging staff to be open about their mistakes, with the aim of ensuring that they are not repeated, should help reduce hospital deaths and make the NHS a safer place for everyone that uses it,' says a spokeswoman for the NPSA.

To reduce the risk of medication errors, London's Charing Cross hospital has introduced a new barcoding system which links patients to a computerized drugs trolley, or Smart Cart, on the ward.

A *British Medical Journal* report in August welcomed the publication later in the year of surgeons' performance, following the inquiry into cardiac deaths at Bristol Royal Infirmary as 'a first step towards transparent public accountability'.

▶ Door-slammers live longer

According to a US study of nuns and priests, showing your anger when you're upset may help you to enjoy more years of life. The study, which followed 851 Catholic clergy members in their seventies for about five years, found that those most likely to be depressed and direct their anger inward were almost twice as likely to die earlier than those who expressed anger openly with actions such as slamming doors.

PART 3

YOUR BODY
HEAD TO TOE

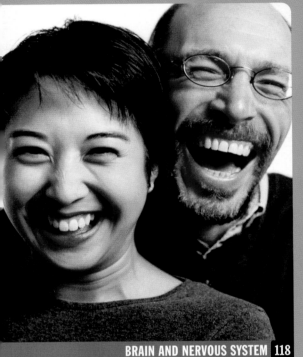

BRAIN AND NERVOUS SYSTEM 118

RESEARCHERS are leaving no stone unturned in the search for medical breakthroughs. Their discoveries include anti-cancer compounds from the deep sea, a miraculous clot buster for stroke patients modelled on the saliva of vampire bats, and a hormone derived from the saliva of Gila monsters that could be the next major weapon against Type 2 diabetes. Old thinking is being turned on its head as scientists put forward revolutionary theories about the origins of cancer and osteoarthritis – theories that could lead to new and better treatments. And doctors are pulling out the big guns – or rather, tiny new instruments – to grab artery-blocking clots and remove them before they cause permanent damage.

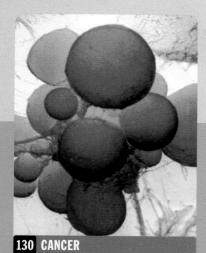

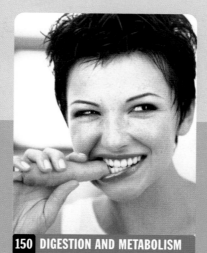

150 DIGESTION AND METABOLISM

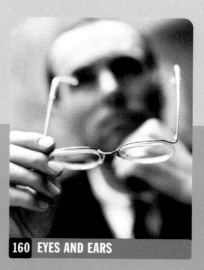

160 EYES AND EARS

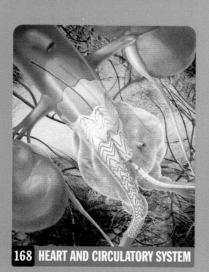

168 HEART AND CIRCULATORY SYSTEM

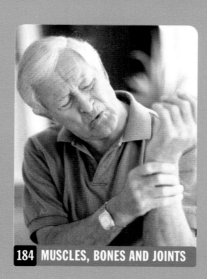

184 MUSCLES, BONES AND JOINTS

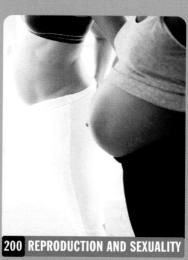

200 REPRODUCTION AND SEXUALITY

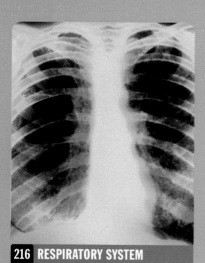

216 RESPIRATORY SYSTEM

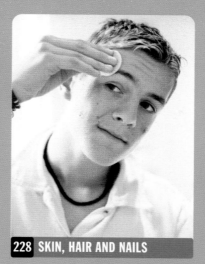

228 SKIN, HAIR AND NAILS

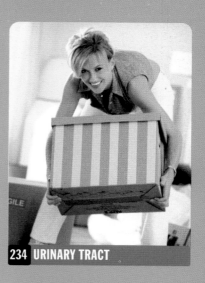

234 URINARY TRACT

BRAIN
AND NERVOUS SYSTEM

Some of the latest approaches to treating stroke sound like the work of **mad scientists**

But the scientists are sane and their methods are sound. To save lives and reduce disability, they are experimenting with a clot-dissolving drug derived from the saliva of vampire bats and a tiny, corkscrew-shaped device that doctors can use to reach into the brain and retrieve a clot before it can cause further damage. In some stroke patients, the corkscrew device has reversed paralysis and speech loss.

What sort of mood are you in? If you are a woman over 50 and you are depressed, studies show that you have an increased risk of dying of a heart attack or stroke. On a lighter note, one researcher decided to find out why having a good laugh makes us feel good.

Laughing till it hurts is one thing; chronic headaches are another. People who suffer from them may soon benefit from drugs used to treat epilepsy. Acupuncture is also proving effective for headaches, including migraine. And there is a particularly good reason to get migraines under control: research has confirmed that they can damage the brain.

Cerebral palsy

Increased limb control for children with cerebral palsy

Children with cerebral palsy, a disease that impairs areas of the brain governing movement and muscle tone, often have weak or stiff muscles in their limbs and poor control over them. When one side of the body is more seriously affected than the other, the children tend to favour the stronger side, sometimes to the point of ignoring the weaker side altogether. So what can we do to help those children use both sides of their bodies and learn to perform daily tasks such as dressing and feeding themselves with more confidence and more success?

Traditional physiotherapy can bring some benefit, but a technique called constraint-induced movement therapy (CIT) may be more effective. CIT is a well-established method of helping adults to regain body function after strokes or brain injuries. Researchers at the University of Alabama at Birmingham are now using it to treat children with cerebral palsy. And two mechanisms are thought to underlie its effectiveness. First, CIT treatment allows the patient

to overcome a strong tendency to avoid using the affected arm. Second, the treatment is thought to exploit the human brain's ability to adjust itself to special demands, such as learning new skills.

How it works Dr Edward Taub and colleagues at Birmingham tested CIT against conventional physiotherapy in 18 children aged from seven months to eight years who had more impairment in one arm than in the other. In the CIT group, each child's stronger arm was restrained for 90 per cent of waking hours in a cast – the same type as that used on a broken bone but split down the middle and taped so that it could be removed if necessary.

For 6 hours a day, the children 'played' with a therapist, performing activities designed to improve their motor skills in the weaker arm. Each time they succeeded in a task, they were encouraged to strive for the next level. For example, a child might start by removing and replacing a large piece of

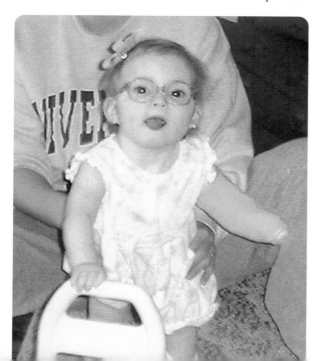

A child with cerebral palsy wears a cast on her stronger arm to help develop motor skills in the weaker one. The cast can be opened to check for any skin problems.

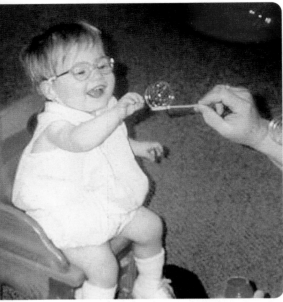

A 15-month-old child with cerebral palsy uses her weaker hand to pop bubbles. Before treatment, she had almost no use of her left arm and hand.

jigsaw puzzle with a knob on it. As he progressed, the puzzle pieces would be replaced by smaller ones. In another activity, the child would reach for a soap bubble, with the ultimate goal of popping it with the tip of one finger.

After three weeks, children in the CIT group had gained an average of nine new motor skills and functions in their affected arms, while those given conventional therapy had gained two new skills. 'In some cases, children start from zero use of the affected arm,' says Dr Taub, 'and at the end of three weeks, they may be pushing up to a sitting position or crawling for the first time in their lives.'

In the UK, Anetta Sterr, professor of cognitive neuroscience at Surrey University, and her team have developed a repetitive training programme using CIT for children and young adults with restricted arm control. According to Dr Sterr, initial evidence shows that 'the intervention improves upper-limb movements in patients with traumatic brain injury, stroke and cerebral palsy'.

Depression

Depression can seriously affect your heart

Feelings of sadness, hopelessness, lack of worth: there is no question that depression can break the spirit. It now seems increasingly likely that it may also break the heart.

Results of a recent American study provide strong evidence that depression significantly increases a woman's chances of dying from a heart attack or stroke. The conclusions were based on information collected as part of the Women's Health Initiative, the largest study of post-menopausal women ever undertaken, with more than 90,000 participants aged 50 and older. They reinforce the findings of researchers at the Queen's Medical Centre in Nottingham, who concluded in 1998 that men with a recorded diagnosis of depression were three times more likely to develop heart disease than men of the same age who were not depressed.

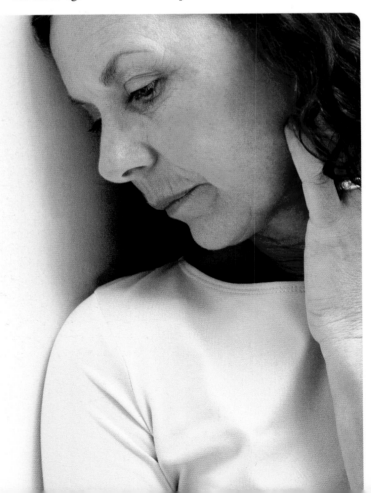

What the study shows The US study looked at symptoms of depression, such as feelings of sadness, bouts of crying and restless sleep, and at cardiovascular disease risk factors, including age, high blood pressure, high cholesterol, smoking, overweight, diabetes and physical inactivity. 'After accounting for all of the other established factors, depression was still a risk factor for cardiovascular death,' says Sylvia Wassertheil-Smoller, a leader of the study. Women with depression were 12 per cent more likely to have high blood pressure and 60 per cent more likely to have experienced stroke or angina. Women who had depression but none of the classic risk factors for heart disease were 50 per cent more likely to die of heart disease in the four years of the study than women who were not depressed.

What is the connection? It is not clear what links depression to heart disease, but there is some evidence that depression lowers oestrogen levels – and the loss of oestrogen that occurs after the menopause is known to increase the risk of cardiovascular disease. Another possibility is that stress hormones released during depression contribute to heart disease. No one yet knows whether treating depression reduces the risk of heart disease. But the other effects of depression are significant enough to indicate that women with depressive symptoms should be monitored and treated.

Restless legs and a restless mind

It attacks at night: an odd sensation in your legs that won't go away unless you move or rub them. Lie still, try to sleep … and back it comes. For people with restless legs syndrome (RLS), insomnia comes with the territory – and so, it seems, can mental distress. Researchers in Turkey found that people with RLS have higher anxiety and depression levels than people with well-behaved legs, and the more severe the syndrome the more severe the anxiety and depression. No one knows for sure, but it is thought that the mental distress results from the RLS, rather than the other way around.

RESEARCH ROUND-UP

Brain is different in depressed teenagers

Adolescent depression is not a character flaw or the result of bad parenting but a genuine illness, says Frank MacMaster of Canada's National Research Council. And he should know, because he has done something that countless parents have sometimes wished they could do: he has peered inside the brains of adolescents.

In MacMaster's study, 34 adolescents, half of whom were suffering from clinical depression, underwent MRI scans. The scans revealed that an area of the brain called the hippocampus was 17 per cent smaller on average in the depressed teenagers than in those teenagers who were not depressed. The hippocampus plays a critical role in memory, and a disruption of this function may help to explain why depression has a negative impact on academic performance. One objective of the research is to aid doctors in the diagnosis of teenage depression.

Depression linked to low testosterone

Research at the University of Washington in Seattle, has shown that 30 per cent of men over 55 have low testosterone, which can lead to diminished appetite and libido, fatigue, irritability and decreased muscle mass. Now depression has been added to the list. The researchers looked at the medical records of 278 men aged 45 and older with no signs of depression. Over a two-year period, nearly 22 per cent of the men with low testosterone became depressed, compared with just 7 per cent of men with a normal level.

A blood test can reveal your testosterone level. But, if it is low, testosterone supplementation may not be the answer, since it may raise the risk of prostate cancer and stroke.

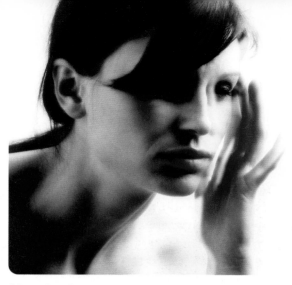

Headache

Epilepsy drugs work to subdue headaches

There are plenty of drugs that can be used to treat headaches, from over-the-counter pills for dull aches to powerful prescription medicines for migraines. But people who experience frequent headaches are much better off if they can prevent the pain in the first place rather than trying to control it once it starts. Help may now be at hand from an apparently unlikely source: anti-seizure drugs.

In clinical trials, two drugs approved to prevent seizures in people with epilepsy are showing that they can also keep headaches at bay. How these drugs – topiramate (Topamax) and gabapentin (Neurontin) – work against headaches is not totally understood. Stephen D. Silberstein, professor of neurology at Thomas Jefferson University in Philadelphia, says Topamax – and probably other drugs for epilepsy – may work by calming an over-active brain. During a migraine, nerve cells that respond to pain become activated. They release a chemical that causes inflammation of the nerve endings. 'It's the same thing that happens to the skin in hives,' says Dr Silberstein. 'This is a very new way of thinking about migraine.'

What the studies show. In the latest study of Topamax, nearly half the patients taking the drug had at least a 50 per cent reduction in migraines after six months, with about 6 per cent of patients

becoming completely migraine-free. In an Australian study of Neurontin, 36 per cent of people with chronic headaches stopped having them entirely after three months. 'Some say that gabapentin is far better for the management of pain than it is for the management of epilepsy,' says Roy G. Beran, an author of the study who works as a neurologist at Liverpool Hospital in New South Wales.

While all medications have potential side effects, Topamax and Neurontin appear not to cause the weight gain common with many other drugs used to prevent headaches, such as the antidepressant amitriptyline (Elavil), beta blockers and valproate (Depacon), another anti-seizure drug. In fact, people taking Topamax tend to lose weight, at least initially, which may encourage them not to stop taking it.

Availability Neurontin is not currently approved for treating headaches, but some doctors prescribe it for patients who are not experiencing relief from other preventive medications. In the USA, the Food and Drug Administration approved Topamax for migraine prevention in adults in August 2004.

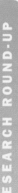

RESEARCH ROUND-UP

Sticking it to headaches

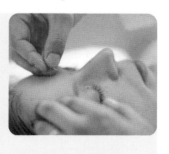

Acupuncture has been successfully used as a medical therapy for some 2,000 years, but convincing the Western medical establishment of its value has not been easy. Critics have poked holes in several small studies that showed that the ancient healing method eases the pain of headache. Now, a large British study should help to persuade persistent sceptics that acupuncture is a useful treatment for chronic headaches.

Most of the study's 401 participants in England and Wales suffered from migraines, and a few had chronic tension headaches. Half received standard care, including drugs, while the other half got standard care plus acupuncture – up to 12 treatments over three months. At the end of the year-long study, people in the acupuncture group had significantly fewer and less severe headaches than people in the standard care group. They also used less medication, had fewer visits to a doctor and took fewer sick days.

Headache

Migraine: brain threat confirmed

The pain and other disturbing symptoms of migraines can be intense enough to make some sufferers suspect that the headaches could cause damage to their brains – and they are right. Research in the Netherlands has confirmed that migraines increase the risk of brain infarcts, or areas of dead brain tissue.

In the Dutch investigation, more than 400 randomly selected people had MRI scans. The risk of brain infarcts turned out to be 13 times higher in people who had a history of migraine with visual disturbance (an 'aura', such as sparkling lights) than in those who had never had a migraine. People who had experienced migraines with or without an aura had higher risks of infarcts in the cerebellum, the region of the brain that is responsible for controlling voluntary movement, posture and balance.

Several earlier studies have revealed that migraine is a risk factor for stroke, which clearly leads to brain damage and infarcted tissue. What is new about the Dutch research is that it demonstrates the presence in migraine patients of previously unsuspected infarcts.

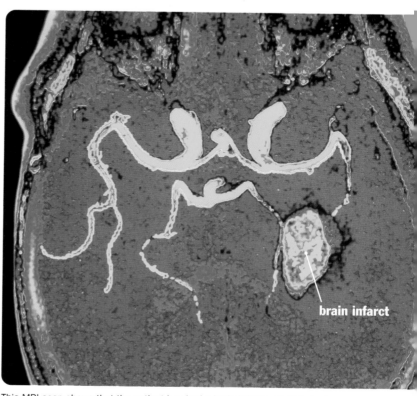

brain infarct

This MRI scan shows that the patient has had a brain infarct – that is, brain tissue has died. The link between infarcts and migraines is being studied, and that research may lead to new methods for managing the debilitating headaches.

Waking up with headaches? You may have anxiety and depression

Morning headaches were once believed to be the exclusive problem of people with sleep disorders such as insomnia, snoring and sleep apnoea. While it is true that sleep disorders are associated with morning headaches, a large study of people in several European countries has discovered that waking up with headaches is more likely to be caused by anxiety and depression.

Of the nearly 19,000 people surveyed in five countries, 7.6 per cent reported waking up with a headache at least sometimes. People who suffered from anxiety or depression were at least twice as likely to wake up with headaches as were happier, calmer individuals. The researcher notes that the relationship between headaches and depression can work both ways: the headaches may be a symptom of depression, but if they are severe enough they can also be the cause.

Humour
Laughter brings its own rewards

Have you ever wondered why we are drawn to humour – why we are content to watch endless *Fawlty Towers* repeats or endure an unreliable friend who has a rapier wit? For Dr Allan Reiss of Stanford University in California, such rumination led to a discovery. Using MRI scans, Dr Reiss established that humour makes us feel good because it activates the brain's reward centres – the areas also activated by amphetamines, financial gain and even the sight of an attractive

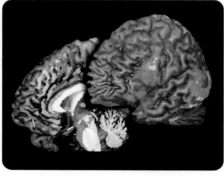

The brain's reward centres 'light up' when you have a laugh, induced in this case by a cartoon.

face. His finding confirms the results of research carried out in 2001 in Toronto and at London's Institute of Neurology. The earlier study, published in the journal *Nature Neuroscience*, threw light on the biological nature of humour and suggested an explanation for the fact that some types of brain damage destroy a person's sense of humour.

What the new study shows Dr Reiss and his colleagues at Stanford used MRI scans to monitor volunteers' brain activity while they read cartoons. When participants thought a cartoon was funny, they pushed a button.

The scans revealed that the funnier a person found a cartoon, the more intense the activity in the brain's reward centres. The study was published in the December 2003 issue of the journal *Neuron*. Its findings could increase our understanding of the normal variations in personality and behaviour. For example, some individuals use humour as a coping mechanism and stress reducer, but we all know people who don't. It is possible that people who rely less on humour simply find it less rewarding.

Comprehending the brain mechanisms that underlie humour may one day help scientists to identify people who are at risk of depression, in that the loss of the ability to appreciate humour is a common symptom of depression. The Stanford team's findings also support the theory that humour can be used to fight depression and other ailments.

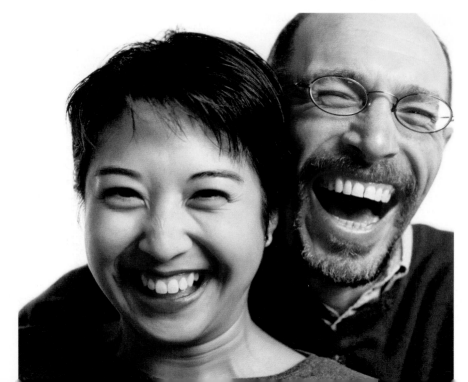

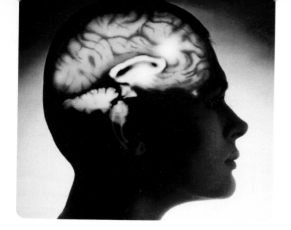

Memory
Bad memories?
Forget them

Victims of post-traumatic stress disorder (PTSD) are frequently afflicted by disturbing flashbacks. But, according to Dr Michael Anderson of the University of Oregon, 'People who suffer PTSD represent only a very small fraction of the people who experience trauma. The great majority of people who experience trauma never develop PTSD and eventually are able to adapt in the face of these events.' He believes that they do so by suppressing their unpleasant memories – and that the process of suppression gradually erases them.

Dr Anderson and his team persuaded a group of volunteers to memorize pairs of words, then asked them to remember some pairs and forget others. When the volunteers attempted to forget some of the word matches, MRI scans revealed that certain areas of their brains – in particular the frontal cortex – became extremely active. This region 'manages' other areas of the brain, including the hippocampus, which controls conscious memory.

The amount of forgetting that occurred in the participants was directly related to how activated the frontal cortex was – and that forgetting could become permanent.

The Oregon researchers presented their findings to the US Society for Neuroscience in December 2003. They hope their conclusions will enhance the scientific understanding of a number of conditions, including PTSD. 'Now that we know which areas of the brain are activated when things are working normally,' says Dr Anderson, 'we can take this knowledge and ask whether people with PTSD have damage in this network.'

FUTURE BREAKTHROUGHS

Patches for pain

If you have ever had major surgery, you know what a nuisance pain control can be. With your arm attached to a morphine drip, it is difficult to move around in bed, let alone do something complicated such as making your way to the bathroom. In the near future, patients who need pain relief could be swapping drips, pumps and needles for skin patches the size of credit cards. Worn on the upper arm or chest, the patch has a button that the patient pushes to deliver small doses of the pain medication fentanyl (Duragesic). It has been tested at 33 North American hospitals, where post-operative patients found that it worked just as well as standard self-administered pain control. And the patches need far less attention from nursing staff than drips and pumps. The new pain control method is currently under review by the Food and Drug Administration.

Stroke helmet: cooler heads may prevail

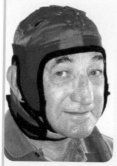

Stroke patients may one day arrive in hospital with cool heads, thanks to special helmets with liquid cooling technology, which were originally developed by the American space agency NASA. Researchers say that the soft, aviator-style helmets are a safe and effective way to lower brain temperature, which may reduce stroke damage and allow more time for other treatments to be administered.

In animal studies, cooling the brain after a stroke has reduced damage to brain tissue by up to 70 per cent. The tricky part is cooling the brain without cooling the entire body, which would interfere with the heart and the immune system. In a recent study, the special helmet cooled brains by an average 3.4°C (6°F) in the first hour without much effect on body temperature. Researchers could use the helmets for an average of 6 to 8 hours before body temperature fell too low. They envisage the helmets being used in ambulances to keep brain tissue alive while stroke patients are transported to hospital.

Stroke

A corkscrew for blood clots

If a blood clot lodges in a brain artery, can a corkscrew save your life? Some researchers think so.

A clot in the brain is a time bomb. Because blood cannot get past it, the parts of the brain fed by the artery are starved of oxygen and begin to die. That is what happens in an ischaemic stroke, by far the most common type. In the UK, a third of people who suffer a stroke die within 10 days and many of those who survive are severely impaired. In one study, after six months 83 per cent still required assistance with daily tasks and 47 per cent remained physically dependent on others long term, suffering from a variety of physical and mental problems.

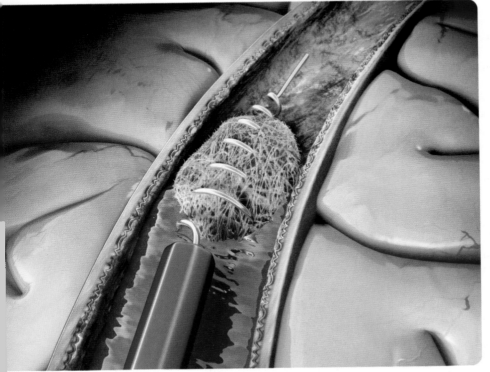

At the tip of a catheter, a tiny clot-grabbing corkscrew.

Once an ischaemic stroke has occurred, there is a very narrow window in which to administer an emergency clot-dissolving drug, called a tissue plasminogen activator (TPA), to minimize damage. After 3 hours, it is too late – and most people arrive in hospital too late. TPA also takes time to work, and in the meantime brain cells in the affected area continue to die.

Imagine that, instead of waiting for a drug to dissolve the clot, doctors could reach in and remove it. This has become possible with the advent of a new corkscrew-shaped wire designed to grab blood clots and pull them out. Called the MERCI Retrieval System, the device can be used effectively up to 8 hours after a stroke has occurred. (MERCI is the acronym for 'mechanical embolus removal in cerebral ischaemia'. An 'embolus' is a clot.)

How it works The device is inserted through a catheter into an artery in the groin and then guided by angiography, a

The MERCI Retrieval System pulls a blood clot out of a vessel in the brain of a stroke patient. The device can be used up to 8 hours after a stroke has occurred. By contrast, the clot-dissolving drug TPA must be used within 3 hours.

special X-ray that involves a dye, to the blood clot in the brain. The retriever itself is a thin metal wire with a 'memory'. When it is threaded through the catheter the wire is straight, but after it has been sent into the artery it takes on its unique corkscrew shape. Once the clot has been captured in the corkscrew, a balloon inflates to stop blood flow temporarily, and both the clot and the corkscrew are retracted into the catheter, which is then pulled out of the body.

Success stories The MERCI system was tested on 114 patients who had suffered severe strokes but could not receive TPA. (Some people cannot be given the drug, including those who have recently had surgery, because it can cause bleeding in the brain.) 'These were the most severe stroke patients, and without the procedure, they were likely to be dead or severely disabled,' says Sidney Starkman, a leader of the study who is co-director of the stroke centre at the University of California, Los Angeles.

In 54 per cent of the patients the blocked vessels were successfully opened and the clot was retrieved, dislodged or broken into pieces. Three-quarters of them survived, and about 40 per cent had little or no lasting disability. In some cases, the procedure immediately reversed paralysis and loss of speech.

'If the blood vessel was opened and the brain had not yet suffered severe irreversible damage, then the patients had a very good to excellent chance of recovery,' says Dr Starkman. 'What was remarkable in these patients was that some were made nearly normal the moment that the vessel was opened with the MERCI retriever.'

Availability The MERCI Retrieval System is at present in the testing stage. The manufacturer, Concentric Medical of Mountain View, California, is seeking approval from the Food and Drug Administration, but it is too early to tell when the device may be available.

The MERCI procedure is not an option for everyone who suffers a stroke. In order for the system to be used, the blockage must occur in a major brain artery, and the clot must be visible on an angiograph. Furthermore, the procedure can be performed only by doctors specially trained in neurology and radiology (and even they require extra training).

INBrief

▶ Injury to the brain may have psychiatric consequences

People who experience traumatic brain injuries often also have to contend with long-term psychiatric problems. In 2004 researchers at the University of Warwick investigated the outcomes of 526 children between the ages of 5 and 15 who had suffered severe, moderate or mild head injury. They found frequent behavioural, emotional, memory and attention problems in one third of the severe group, one quarter of the moderate group and 10–18 per cent of the mild group. Personality change since the injury was reported in 148 of the children. A recent US study of adults who had experienced brain injury produced similarly startling results. It found mental illness in 49 per cent of people with moderate to severe injuries and in 34 per cent of people with mild injuries. By comparison, in a group of randomly selected people with no brain injury, 18 per cent had some form of mental illness (including depression).

▶ Legacy of lead is mental Illness

In the 1960s, lead was still commonly added to petrol on both sides of the Atlantic. Following several studies showing the toxic effects of leaded petrol, especially on children, it was been gradually phased out in the UK, and has been virtually unavailable in this country since 2000. In the USA, leaded petrol has been banned for more than two decades now, but some people may still be living with its effects. Scientists from Columbia University in New York City found that adults whose mothers had high levels of lead exposure during pregnancy in the 1960s had double the risk of schizophrenia compared with those whose mothers had less exposure.

▶ Stress a factor in MS

Some experts believe that stress can contribute to the development of multiple sclerosis (MS), a neurological disorder. To test this belief, Danish researchers conducted a large study of people who had experienced the most stressful event of all – the death of a child. Sure enough, parents who had lost children had a 50 per cent higher risk of developing MS than parents who had not. The risk was doubled in parents whose children died unexpectedly.

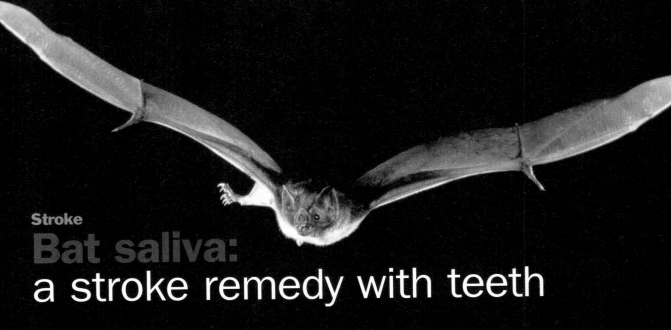

Bat saliva:
a stroke remedy with teeth

Doctors who treat stroke patients have something in common with vampire bats: they are both keenly interested in keeping blood flowing. Scientists have struggled for a long time to devise ways of dissolving clots that block blood flow to the brain and cause strokes. Meanwhile, vampire bats have been happily feeding on their victims while a natural enzyme in their saliva keeps the victims' blood coming. So, the scientists reasoned, why not put the enzyme to work in humans?

As a consequence, an experimental drug named desmoteplase (after the vampire bat, *Desmodus rotundus*) – a synthetic version of the bat saliva enzyme – could become the second clot-busting drug approved to treat strokes.

The first, tissue plasminogen activator (TPA), revolutionized stroke treatment when it was introduced in 1996. Suddenly there was a drug that increased by 50 per cent the number of stroke patients who could return to work and lead normal lives. But TPA has a major drawback: unless it is given within 3 hours of the stroke, it can do more damage than good, degrading the body's clotting system and causing bleeding in the brain. Because the window of opportunity is so small, only about 5 per cent of people who have an ischaemic stroke (the most common type, which involves a clot) receive the drug. Left untreated, a clot may dissolve on its own but is more likely to continue obstructing blood flow, leading to disability or death.

Researchers are optimistic that the newer drug will prove to be a kinder, gentler clot-buster because it has the almost magical ability to home in on a clot without disrupting the rest of the body's clotting mechanism. That means that it can be administered safely many hours after a stroke occurs.

Teaming up with MRI scans The bat-saliva drug is only part of the story. Researchers have begun using it in conjunction with ultra-sophisticated MRI machines that can identify with great accuracy which patients will benefit from the drug. With ECHO-Planar MRI, 'you can image the whole brain every second,' says George C. Newman, director of the stroke programme at the University of Wisconsin in Madison. It is used to measure the portion of the brain that has already been injured and areas where there are injured but salvageable brain cells.

During an international study, the high-tech MRIs allowed researchers to administer desmoteplase up to 9 hours after a stroke. 'A lot of people have potentially salvageable tissue at 6, 9, 12 – up to 24 hours' after a stroke,' says Steven Warach, chief of the stroke diagnostics and therapeutics section at the National Institute of Neurological Disorders and Stroke. 'There's individual variability,' he explains. 'The MRI can tell us which patients have salvageable tissue.'

The impact of desmoteplase combined with the advanced MRIs could be enormous. 'We're potentially moving 50,000 people a year from disability and dependence into the back-to-work range,' says Dr Newman.

Availability Desmoteplase is still in the early phase of clinical trials. More studies will be needed before the drug can gain official approval, which is still several years away.

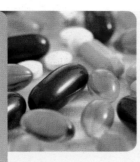

Smokers need to dose up on vitamins

If you smoke, giving up is the best way to prevent a stroke. Short of giving up, eating foods with plenty of vitamins may reduce your risk. A study in Rotterdam found that smokers who consumed plenty of vitamin C were 70 per cent less likely to have strokes than those who received less of the vitamin. Study participants whose diets were highest in vitamin C took in more than 133mg a day, while people consuming the lowest amounts received less than 95mg daily. How do you know you are getting enough? A red pepper contains 226mg of vitamin C and a glass of fresh orange juice 124mg. You will get about 100mg from130g (4½oz) strawberries or a 225g (8oz) of cooked broccoli.

Smokers also saw a benefit, although not as dramatic, from vitamin E. Eating a diet rich in vitamin E resulted in a 20 per cent reduction in stroke risk. Good food sources of vitamin E include vegetable oils, margarine and nuts.

The better way to treat aneurysms

Aneurysms are weakened parts of blood vessels that bulge out and can rupture, causing a brain haemorrhage. Typically, they are treated with a surgical procedure called clipping, in which a piece of the skull is removed to gain access to the blood vessel, then the aneurysm is 'clipped' at its base to prevent further blood flow. A better option, according to Dr Andrew Molyneux and Richard Kerr at Oxford's Radcliffe Infirmary, is a procedure called coiling. Coiling, also known as endovascular treatment, involves threading a catheter through a major artery from the groin or leg to the brain. There, tiny metal coils are packed into the aneurysm, slowing blood flow and causing a clot to form at the base of the bulge. The clot prevents blood from reaching the aneurysm and causing a rupture. While there are some patients for whom surgery is still the best treatment, coiling should be suitable for eight out of ten people who suffer haemorrhage from an aneurysm.

The researchers looked at data for more than 2,000 patients in neurosurgical centres in Europe, Australia and North America. They concluded that out of every 100 patients treated around seven could expect to be better off one year after treatment if they had the endovascular procedure rather that conventional surgery.

IN*Brief*

▶ Patching up Parkinson's

The drug rotigotine, which can control involuntary movements in Parkinson's patients, may soon be added to the list of medications available in patch form. The patches, applied once a day, deliver the drug continuously, thereby smoothing out the symptom fluctuations that are common with pills. And the fact that no swallowing is involved is a boon to some Parkinson's patients. The drug manufacturers were expected to seek approval in Europe and the USA by the end of 2004. The patches could be available by the end of 2005.

▶ Taking the edge off a Parkinson's treatment

At high doses, levodopa (Larodopa) – a drug commonly used to treat Parkinson's disease – can cause twitching and jerking. Lowering the dose stops the side effects, but it usually makes the Parkinson's symptoms reappear. A French study of 50 patients with severe Parkinson's showed that low doses of the antipsychotic drug clozapine (Clozaril) control involuntary movements in patients taking levodopa better than placebos (dummy pills).

▶ Stifling saliva in Parkinson's patients

Drooling is an embarrassing problem and potential choking hazard for many people with Parkinson's, a disease that interferes with the ability to swallow saliva. Help may now be at hand from an unlikely source: botulinum toxin B, a relative of Botox. The toxin interrupts the nerve messages to the salivary glands telling them to secrete. When injected into the glands of 16 people with Parkinson's, the toxin substantially decreased drooling. Relief from excessive salivation can in some cases last up to three months, and the injections can be repeated at any time. The treatment is still at the experimental stage.

CANCER

Scientists are busy trying to find out how to use stem cells to cure **major diseases**

Meanwhile, a radical theory rapidly gaining acceptance holds that 'bad seed' stem cells are the root of all cancers. If true, the theory could completely change the way cancer is treated.

For people who have cancer now, major drug developments are big news. The first cancer drug that works by starving a tumour of its blood supply has been approved for colon cancer and may soon be approved for other cancers as well. And, instead of tamoxifen, women who have survived breast cancer may soon be prescribed drugs called aromatase inhibitors to stop breast cancer from recurring, as three new major studies have found these to be more effective. Researchers are also mining the sea for cancer cures and have discovered at least one sea sponge that may be many times more powerful than today's cancer drugs.

Finally, experts have identified several factors that increase a person's chances of surviving cancer. Exercise is one. There's also new evidence that cancer patients need their sleep – their lives may depend on it.

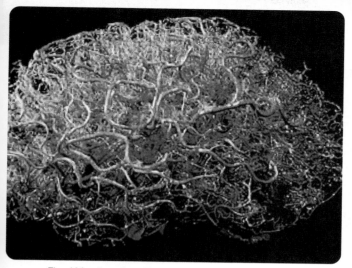

The 400 miles of capillaries in your brain have a surface area of about 9m² (100sq ft.). Only tiny molecules can slip through the tightly knit cells lining these blood vessels.

Brain cancer
Sneaking cancer drugs into the brain

Despite breakthrough after breakthrough for nearly every kind of cancer in recent years, one part of the body has remained cut off from most advances: the brain. Finally, that seems to be changing, as doctors are discovering how to sneak chemotherapy drugs past the gates that bar access to the body's all-important command centre.

'We spend untold millions and billions on drugs to treat disease in the nervous system, including brain tumours, but most drugs won't ever get to the tumour,' says Dr Edward A. Neuwelt, professor of neurology and neurosurgery at Oregon Health and Science University in Portland. That's because of the blood-brain barrier, or BBB.

The barrier – really a single layer of cells that line blood vessels throughout the brain – is designed to protect the brain from toxins and keep its environment as stable as possible. That means it lets in only certain molecules, usually very small ones and only those that are fat soluble. Most chemotherapy drugs are made up of large, water-soluble molecules.

Dr Neuwelt first succeeded in slipping standard chemotherapy treatments past the BBB nearly 20 years ago, but those drugs were often ineffective

TOP Trends

MARROW TRANSPLANTS FOR OLDER PATIENTS, TOO

Bone marrow transplants can save the lives of some cancer patients, but older patients typically don't receive them because the treatment is so physically debilitating. That's changing as more doctors turn to kinder, gentler 'mini' bone marrow transplants.

In a traditional transplant, doctors remove a quantity of bone marrow, then deliver massive doses of chemotherapy to kill any cancer cells and the patient's remaining bone marrow. Finally, they replace the marrow by infusing either the patient's own marrow or a donor's to restore blood-making stem cells. Intense chemotherapy is responsible for most of the hardships inherent in the transplants. But the mini-transplant uses lower doses of chemotherapy and thus leaves some of the patient's original bone marrow intact. Patients who receive mini-transplants appear to do just as well and are much less likely to develop acute graft-versus-host disease, in which the infused cells attack the patient's organs.

STOMACH CANCER – CASES HALVE

Deaths from gastric cancer in the European Union fell by half between 1980 and 1999, from 18.6 per 100,000 down to 9.8 per 100,000, according to a study in the Annals of Oncology, February 2004. Over the same period they dropped by 45 per cent in Eastern Europe and by 40 per cent in Russia. And the steady decline in mortality was observed in the middle-aged and young population, suggesting that the trend will continue, according to the study authors from the Cancer Epidemiology Unit at the Institut Universitaire de Médecine Social et Préventive in Lausanne, Switzerland. Explanations may include a better, more varied diet; better food conservation; reduced smoking and better control of Helicobacter pylori infection, a bacterium linked to stomach cancer.

against brain cancer. In the past few years, he's been able to use a unique procedure to sneak through new targeted treatments called monoclonal antibodies. These drugs attach to specific proteins on cancer cells and can be up to 100,000 times as large as the standard molecules the BBB allows in.

How it works Getting the drugs to a brain tumour isn't easy. Patients have to be hospitalized for the procedure, and it requires careful cooperation among medical specialists. A catheter is snaked through a patient's groin into a main artery that

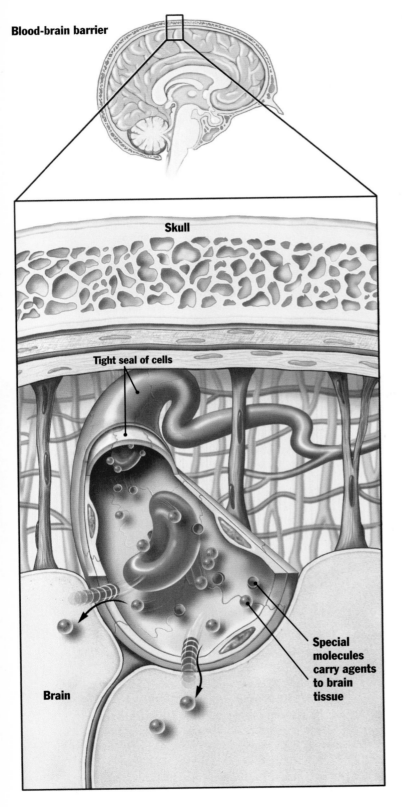

Blood-brain barrier

Skull

Tight seal of cells

Brain

Special molecules carry agents to brain tissue

supplies the brain, then a concentrated sugar solution is fed through the catheter. The solution sucks the water out of the barrier cells lining the blood vessels. This makes the barrier 'gappy' so that the cancer drug can squeeze through. The effect lasts about 30 minutes before the cells rehydrate and the barrier closes again. Once the barrier closes, the patient receives a different drug to neutralize the cancer treatment in the rest of the body, so that it does not harm healthy cells.

Other approaches Dr Neuwelt's work is the most advanced but it isn't the only effort to breach the BBB. In May 2004, the British biotech company Xenova Group began late-stage clinical trials in Europe and the USA of a chemotherapy drug called TransMID. The drug is a combination of a protein called transferrin and a poison called diphtheria toxin. The diphtheria toxin gains entry into a cancer cell when the transferrin is taken up by transferrin receptors on the surface of the cancer cell. Transferrin receptors are particularly prevalent on rapidly dividing cells (such as cancer cells). Once inside, the diphtheria toxin kills the cancer cell. To overcome the BBB, TransMID is pumped directly into the tumour via two catheters implanted in the brain.

Another drug that is causing a lot of interest is called clomipramine. This is normally prescribed as an antidepressant, but it is able to cross the BBB and has potential as a brain cancer treatment. It is thought that the drug acts on mitochondria within the cancer cells, effectively blocking the cells' breathing mechanism. A UK trial, coordinated by the University of Portsmouth, is under way to fully test the efficacy of the drug.

Availability Any weapon in the fight against cancer is always welcome and the above mentioned treatments are on a fast track to receive approval for use in the USA and Europe.

The blood-brain barrier keeps out not only toxins but medicines, too. One approach to sneaking medicine past the barrier: identify molecules that are already able to pass through, then attach drugs to them.

Breast cancer

Better drugs
may replace
tamoxifen

For more than 25 years, women who have survived breast cancer have taken a drug called tamoxifen to prevent the cancer from returning. Some women who are at high risk of breast cancer also take tamoxifen to avoid developing it. But now, thanks to the results of three major studies – two unveiled in late 2003 and the other in March 2004 – drugs called aromatase inhibitors may be set to topple tamoxifen from its perch as the pre-eminent weapon against breast cancer.

Aromatase inhibitors include anastrozole (Arimidex), exemestane (Aromasin) and letrozole (Femara). Taken after menopause, they work by reducing the amount of oestrogen women make. Tamoxifen, on the other hand, prevents oestrogen from doing its job in cells. Either way, reducing oestrogen's effects slows down or stops the growth of breast cancers that depend on the hormone.

The studies compared either Arimidex, Aromasin, or Femara to tamoxifen in breast cancer survivors. In all three trials, researchers found that the aromatase inhibitors did a better job of preventing breast cancer recurrences than tamoxifen. In the Femara trial, in fact, the drug worked so much better than tamoxifen that the study was stopped early to enable the women who weren't taking Femara to receive it.

Potential for prevention Dr Larry Norton, deputy physician in chief and director of breast cancer programmes at Memorial Sloan-Kettering Cancer Center in New York City and a lead researcher in the Femara trial, envisages a day when postmenopausal women might take an aromatase inhibitor every day to prevent breast cancer in the same way that they brush their teeth every day to prevent cavities.

That probably won't happen with the current line of aromatase inhibitors, however. Arimidex and Femara, nearly identical compounds that work by suppressing the enzyme that contributes to oestrogen production, seem to increase a woman's risk of osteoporosis. No one knows for sure yet if Aromasin, which also destroys the oestrogen-producing enzyme, has the same effect, but researchers think it doesn't. All three drugs also cause hot flushes. Drug companies are working hard to find new versions that have fewer side effects.

Making the switch Dr Norton and other cancer specialists have already begun switching patients to aromatase inhibitors after they have been on tamoxifen for a couple of years. 'There are only two things left to figure out,' he says. 'Do the benefits last, and is it better to use an aromatase inhibitor right off the bat or after two to three years of tamoxifen?' Large international studies are under way to answer both of these questions.

According to Cancer Research UK, although the benefits of aromatase inhibitors have been shown in the short term, 'we don't know about the long term risks or benefits'. An ongoing UK trial will look at the long-term effects. In 2000, 9,000 postmenopausal women who had had breast surgery began a five-year treatment with tamoxifen alone, anastrozole alone or a combination of the two drugs. They will be followed for a further five years to allow time for differences between the treatments to become apparent. The results will be available in 2010.

Heading off cancer

When oestrogen binds to receptors on certain cancer cells, the cells divide, and the tumour gets larger. Aromatase inhibitors prevent oestrogen production.

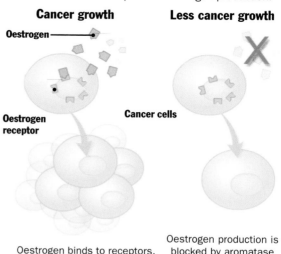

Cancer growth

Oestrogen

Oestrogen receptor

Less cancer growth

Cancer cells

Oestrogen binds to receptors, causing cancer growth.

Oestrogen production is blocked by aromatase inhibitor.

Breast cancer

Antibiotic use linked to breast cancer

Long-term use of antibiotics, some of the world's most commonly used medications, may join the list of factors that cause breast cancer. That's the finding from the second study ever designed to look at a possible connection between the drugs and the cancer.

After reading a 2000 Finnish study that suggested antibiotic use might contribute to breast cancer risk, Christine Velicer Ph.D., a research associate at the Group Health Cooperative Center for Health Studies in Seattle, USA, decided to conduct her own study. Because Group Health has a pharmacy database going back to 1977, is located within an area that requires that all cancers be tracked, and is part of the USA's National Cancer Institute's Breast Cancer Surveillance Program, she and her colleagues had access to all the data they needed to explore the connection in more detail.

They compared medical information and history of antibiotic use for more than 10,000 women who have been enrolled in the health insurance organization for an average of 17 years. About 2,000 of the women had developed breast cancer.

What the study found The researchers discovered that women who took antibiotics for more than 500 days (or more than 25 individual prescriptions) over an average period of 17 years had double the risk of breast cancer of women who took none. The more antibiotics the women took, the greater their risk of the disease. The risk remained the same across all classes of antibiotics, a finding that surprised the researchers.

'We thought we'd see that some types increased the risk and others decreased the risk', says Dr Velicer. 'We were very surprised at the consistency of our findings.'

Understanding the link Dr Velicer emphasizes that this study and the Finnish study before it do not mean that antibiotics cause breast cancer.

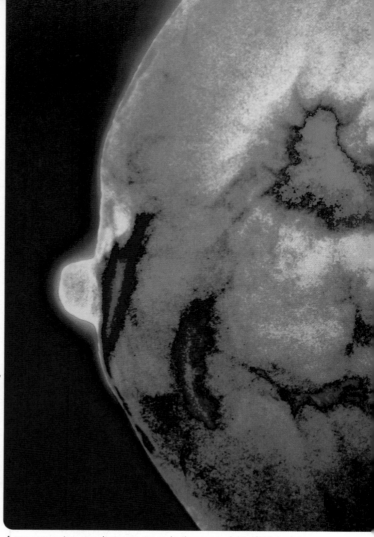

A cancerous tumour shows up green in the upper right of this colour mammogram. Being overweight is one risk factor for breast cancer. Now it appears that heavy use of antibiotics may be another.

There are several possible reasons for the link the research has revealed.

- Antibiotics may affect various immune functions that in turn affect the production of oestrogen, the hormone that plays a role in the development of breast cancer.
- Antibiotics disrupt the 'good' bacteria in the gut, the kind that aid digestion. This in turn may affect a woman's ability to absorb important chemicals that are found in plant foods and known to protect against breast cancer.
- Antibiotics affect certain chemicals that contribute to inflammation in the body, such as prostaglandins, cytokines, and COX 1 and 2 enzymes, all of which may also be involved in the development of cancer.

'As the research develops, we'll be able to see what's going on,' says Dr Velicer. For instance, it may not be the antibiotics themselves that are responsible for the increase in breast cancer risk but rather the fact that women who need to use antibiotics frequently have weaker immune systems that make them more susceptible to cancer.

Overall, she says, the possible increased risk to women who often take antibiotics is about the same as for any other common risk factor for breast cancer, including early menstruation, having children later in life or never having children, taking hormone therapy and being overweight.

The bottom line, says Dr Velicer, is that women should still take antibiotics when they need them. 'Antibiotics have a huge benefit in our society, and they need to be used wisely, and that's not going to change,' she says. But she emphasizes the phrase 'used wisely', because antibiotics are often overused – for instance, to treat viral infections such as colds, even though the drugs have no effect on viruses. The results of Dr Velicer's study were published in a February 2004 issue of the *Journal of the American Medical Association*.

Antidepressants may interfere with cancer treatment

About 1 in 12 cancer patients suffers from depression. Now, a small study suggests that the medications most commonly used to treat depression – selective serotonin reuptake inhibitors (SSRIs) such as paroxetine (Seroxat) and fluoxetine (Prozac) – could interfere with the action of tamoxifen, a drug commonly used to prevent a breast cancer recurrence.

The study followed 12 women with breast cancer who were given paroxetine for four weeks during their standard course of tamoxifen therapy. Blood tests before and after taking paroxetine revealed significantly lower amounts of a chemical related to the breakdown of tamoxifen after taking the drug, indicating that their bodies were less effective at breaking down and absorbing tamoxifen.

The researchers emphasize that this is a very preliminary study and that more studies are required before recommending any changes in current treatments for depression.

Exercise
improves breast cancer
survival

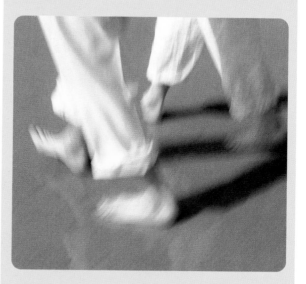

Everyone knows by now that exercise is good for you. Now, a Harvard study has found that exercise also significantly improves a woman's chance of surviving a battle with breast cancer.

Earlier studies had shown that exercise improved a woman's quality of life after a breast cancer diagnosis. This study, however, found that just one to three hours of walking a week cut a woman's risk of dying from breast cancer by 19 per cent, while women who walked three to five hours a week slashed their risk by 54 per cent.

What's the connection? 'Exercise may lower the levels of hormones that stimulate cancer to grow,' says lead researcher Dr Michelle D. Holmes, who presented the study at a major cancer meeting in March 2004.

Studies have also shown that regular physical activity prevents breast cancer developing in the first place. Cancer Research UK says that being active may lower your risk by about a third.

Breast cancer

Virtual reality
makes chemo-therapy a walk in the park

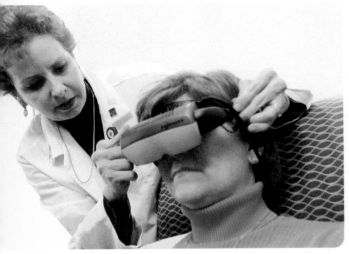

Susan M. Schneider R.N., Ph.D., fits a chemotherapy patient with virtual reality goggles at Duke University Medical Center. The 'mental holiday' reduces the ill-effects of the treatment.

Which would you rather do while undergoing chemotherapy for breast cancer: sit in a room filled with other sick people who are also getting infusions of toxic chemicals, or walk on a beach? How about deep-sea diving or touring an art gallery?

Chemotherapy patients can't actually do any of these activities while in the hospital, of course, but soon they may be able to put on a pair of goggles and experience them through computer-generated virtual reality.

A small study recently found that women with breast cancer who used virtual reality during their chemotherapy sessions experienced less fatigue, nausea, vomiting and inability to concentrate immediately after chemotherapy than women who didn't use the technique. Such symptoms affect about 60 per cent of chemotherapy patients. Additionally, the women who 'escaped' via virtual reality thought the chemotherapy sessions – which

averaged 67 minutes – lasted an average of only 42 minutes. The results were published in the January 2004 issue of *Oncology Nursing Forum*.

'Just the process of receiving chemotherapy can be stressful,' says Susan M. Schneider, R.N., Ph.D., director of the graduate oncology nursing programme at Duke University School of Nursing in Durham, North Carolina, and lead researcher in the study. 'Deciding with the physician which chemo-therapeutic agents are best, completing lab work and waiting for appointments can wear someone down. By the time a woman gets to the clinic for her treatment, she is often emotionally exhausted. The virtual reality provides a mental vacation.'

In 2004, Dr Schneider was completing larger studies of patients who have colon, lung and breast cancer to better understand who might benefit most from virtual reality and how to achieve more lasting reductions in post-chemo symptoms and fatigue.

Availability Currently, virtual reality is in use at just a couple of hospitals that are evaluating it, says Dr Schneider. But this could soon change if more studies like this one demonstrate its benefits.

FUTURE
BREAKTHROUGHS

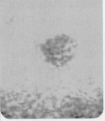

Low-frequency vibrations show up tumours in a special ultrasound scan.

Cancer screening without radiation

One day a doctor or nurse may be able to screen you for breast cancer simply by waving a handheld device over your skin – no uncomfortable mammogram required. A group of surgeons, computer specialists and physical scientists at the University of Dundee in Scotland have invented just such a device, dubbed Sonoelastographic Breast Imaging. The device can detect the tiniest of breast lesions because the lesions are stiffer than surrounding breast tissue, so they move differently when the imaging tool hits them with sound waves. Instead of waiting days for your results, you'd get them immediately. Researchers are now gearing up for large-scale clinical studies to test the device's effectiveness.

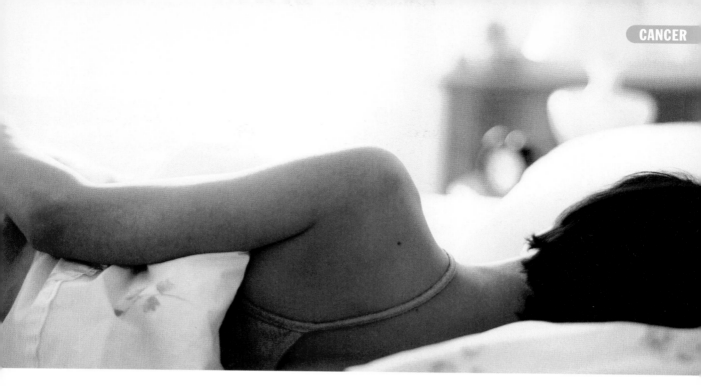

Breast cancer

Fight cancer with your eyes closed

Most people don't appreciate the value of a good night's sleep until it eludes them. The next day they feel grumpy and generally less able to cope. Now, a study from researchers at Stanford University suggests that poor sleeping patterns, often the result of stress, can affect the course of breast cancer.

What the study found Dr David Spiegel, associate chair of psychiatry and behavioural sciences at Stanford, has conducted groundbreaking work showing that women with breast cancer who participate in support groups or psychotherapy live longer than women who don't. In searching for the reason behind this finding, Dr Spiegel tested levels of the so-called stress hormone cortisol throughout the day in 17 women whose breast cancer had spread, then compared those numbers with cortisol levels in 31 healthy women.

Normally, he says, cortisol levels are highest in the morning and lowest at night. Two-thirds of the breast cancer patients tested, however, had altered cortisol levels: they rose throughout the day, a sign of a disrupted circadian rhythm (the normal cycle of sleep and waking). When questioned, the women with disrupted hormone levels admitted they had trouble falling asleep and sleeping through the night. As it turned out, they also died sooner than women with more normal cortisol cycles did. The results of that study were published in the online version of the journal *Psychoneuroendocrinology* in January 2004.

The link between cortisol, cancer and sleep is complex, and much remains to be understood, notes Dr Spiegel. A possible explanation for the link is that high levels of cortisol, which belongs to a class of chemicals that suppress the immune system, might prevent the immune system from effectively fighting the cancer. Additionally, cortisol may trigger a response similar to that of oestrogen or progesterone, hormones that stimulate growth in many breast cancer tumours.

What it means One way to control cortisol levels is to get enough uninterrupted sleep, says Dr Spiegel. Many of the women he sees don't get enough sleep because they're trying to do too much during a time when they should be taking it easier, he says. Additionally, women with breast cancer should try to manage stress as best they can. Creative visualisation and meditation can help to reduce stress as can regular physical exercise.

Breast cancer
MRI screenings
help women
at high risk

Say your mother and aunt had died of breast cancer. And an older sister had it. And, when you went for genetic counselling and testing, you learned that you carry a genetic mutation that dramatically increases your risk of the disease. How can you ensure that if you do get breast cancer, you detect it early?

Until recently, the answer might have been to have regular mammograms. But a major Dutch study published in a July 2004 issue of the *New England Journal of Medicine* found that for women at high risk magnetic resonance imaging (MRI) scans are a more precise tool. The study, involving nearly 2,000 high-risk women, found that MRIs identified breast cancers that mammograms missed, particularly more deadly, invasive types.

Beyond mammograms In Britain women aged between 50 and 74 are offered a mammogram every three years (older women can ask for the test). But women with family histories of breast cancer or those who carry genetic mutations that substantially increase their risks are usually advised to have earlier, more frequent screening.

The problem is that younger women have denser breasts, and mammograms aren't very good at telling the difference between a mammary gland, which shows up white on a mammogram, and cancer, which also shows up white. 'It's like trying to find a polar bear in a snowstorm,' explains

Dr Marissa Weiss, a Philadelphia-based radiation oncologist who is also president of a consumer website for breast cancer (www.breastcancer.org).

MRI screening, on the other hand, 'allows you to separate the appearance of regular gland tissue from the appearance of cancer, and that's powerful,' she says.

There are drawbacks to MRIs, however, which is why the tests aren't used for screening on all women. Firstly, they're much more expensive than mammograms. Secondly, MRIs are more likely to produce false positives, that is, suspicious readings that result in biopsies that turn out to be negative. In fact, in the study, MRI screening led to three times as many unneeded biopsies as mammography.

Still worth doing Nonetheless, notes Dr Weiss, 'if a woman is at high risk because she has a gene abnormality or because breast cancer is prevalent through her family, absolutely she should consider having regular MRIs'. That doesn't mean she should give up on mammograms, though. The two should be used in conjunction, she says, because 'they provide different pieces of information'. For instance, the study found that mammography is better than an MRI at identifying ductal carcinoma in situ, the most common type of noninvasive breast cancer.

In Britain the chances of being referred for an MRI scan depends on where you live since the equipment is not evenly distributed throughout the country. MRI is not routinely used to screen for breast cancer, but may be recommended after suspicious findings revealed on mammography. A multi-centre study is currently under way in the UK which aims to determine whether MRI is an effective way of screening women with a high risk of breast cancer. If successful it may lead to MRI scans being available for high risk women in future.

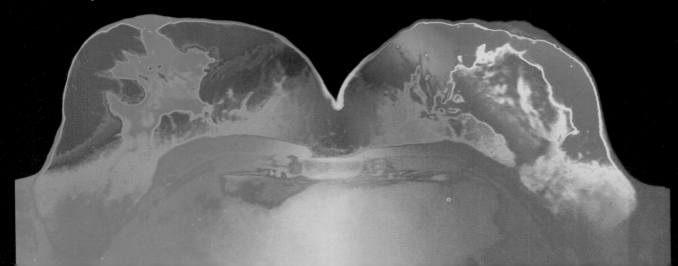

Colon cancer
Tumour-starving drug approved

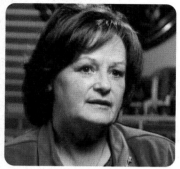

Grace Vanhoose

Grace Vanhoose received her death sentence in February 2002. That's when the colon cancer she thought she'd beaten three years earlier returned with a vengeance, showing up in her spine and neck. She had Stage IV cancer, the worst and final stage, and was told she had just a few months to live.

But Vanhoose didn't give up. She found a doctor who enrolled her in a clinical trial to test a new idea in cancer treatment – that a tumour could be killed by choking off its blood supply. Today, Vanhoose, 57, of Everett, Washington, is back at work as an administrative assistant, feeling great and looking forward to living for many more years, not months. The drug she credits with saving her life is called bevacizumab (Avastin).

Avastin is the first of a new class of cancer drugs, called angiogenesis inhibitors, to be approved in the USA. The drugs were the subject of an article in the *New York Times* in the late 1990s, which declared they would be the long-awaited cure for cancer. While it's doubtful the drugs will ever justify that early hype, researchers remain hopeful that Avastin and other angiogenesis inhibitors currently in the pipeline will radically change cancer treatment for the better.

How they work The drugs work on the theory that to survive, tumours form a network of blood vessels – a process called angiogenesis – and that shutting down that network leads to a tumour's ultimate demise. Avastin works in conjunction with chemotherapy; in addition to shutting down a tumour's blood supply, it decreases the pressure between cancer cells, allowing more chemotherapy drugs into the tumour.

In clinical trials, late-stage colon cancer patients taking Avastin lived an average of five months longer. That may not seem like a lot, but to oncologists like Dr Deborah Lindquist of Northern Arizona Hematology and Oncology Associates in Flagstaff, who had five patients enrolled in the trial, it's tremendous. All five had cancers that had spread to the liver, a certain death sentence, yet three are still alive nearly three years after starting the drug. That, says Dr Lindquist, gives patients the time they need to enrol in other trials and try other treatments.

Availability Avastin, produced by the biotech company Genentech, is not licensed in the UK and is only available to a small number of people who are taking part in clinical trials. It can be prescribed on a 'named patient basis' – when a specialist thinks it may help a particular patient.

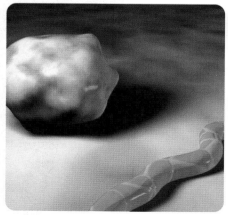

A tumour is an abnormal mass of cells that divide without control. To grow, these cells need nutrients from surrounding blood vessels.

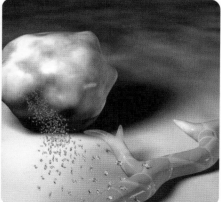

When a tumour needs a bigger food supply, it secretes a protein that appears to stimulate blood vessels to grow towards the tumour.

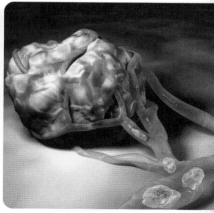

The new blood vessels reach the tumour, feeding it nutrients and allowing it to grow even more.

General cancer
What causes cancer?
A new theory

When you hear 'stem cells', what comes to mind? Probably those highly sought-after cells that have the power to transform themselves into any other kind of cell – heart, lung, muscle, brain – and may have the potential to repair damaged tissue and cure terrible diseases such as Alzheimer's, Parkinson's, and even paralysing spinal injuries. These cells are so highly valued not only because they can turn into other types of cells but also because they can replicate, or divide, indefinitely, creating an infinite supply.

But what if stem cells had evil twins, 'bad seeds' whose powers of limitless regeneration were used not to heal but to spread disease – specifically cancer – throughout the body?

This theory is called the cancer stem cell hypothesis, and it's getting further from hypothesis and closer to fact. If it proves to be true, everything we've ever thought about what cancers are, how they grow, and how to treat them may be only about 10 per cent right.

'It gives us a new framework to think of in studying cancer and targeting treatments,' says Dr Peter Dirks, a neuro-surgeon, assistant professor at the University of Toronto, and a leader in cancer stem cell research.

The worst of the worst Put simply, the cancer stem cell hypothesis theorizes that aberrant stem cells, a kind of 'black sheep' of stem cells, are to blame for the rapidly dividing cells that become cancer. If this theory is true, instead of hitting cancer with the big guns of chemotherapy and radiation, which take their toll on patients, it would be better to target just those stem cells – and treating cancer would be almost as simple as treating strep throat.

The theory is an old one, dating to the 1960s. Back then, however, scientists didn't have the tools to prove it. The explosion of research into stem cells in the past decade, along with techniques to fish out stem cells from organs, has reinvigorated scientific interest.

'Essentially, the theory says that in a cancer, not every cell in the tumour has the ability to regrow the tumour,' says John E. Dick, Ph.D., who directs the Program in Stem Cell Biology at the University of Toronto. This in turn goes against all we've ever thought about cancers.

Dr Dick, Dr Dirks and others have found that in leukaemia and brain and breast cancers at least, there are several different types of cancer cells in the same tumour. In leukaemia, which is Dr Dick's area of specialty and in which the bulk of the cancer stem cell work has been conducted, a tiny minority of rogue stem cells creates other cells called progenitor cells, which rapidly divide and produce billions of abnormal cells that overwhelm the blood.

Stem cells divide quite slowly, and sometimes they hibernate, hiding out in the body (exactly where is unknown) for months or even years before 'turning on' again. Thus, the traditional approach to cancer treatment – attacking rapidly dividing cells with chemotherapy drugs or radiation – is likely to miss them, leaving them to revitalize and start producing more cancer cells down the road. This helps to

'Bad seed' cancer theory

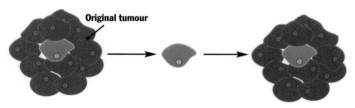

Traditional cancer therapies kill rapidly dividing tumour cells (red) but may spare the slowly dividing stem cells (blue), allowing the tumour to regrow.

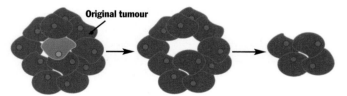

In theory, killing the cancer stem cell should halt the tumour's growth and perhaps lead to its disappearance.

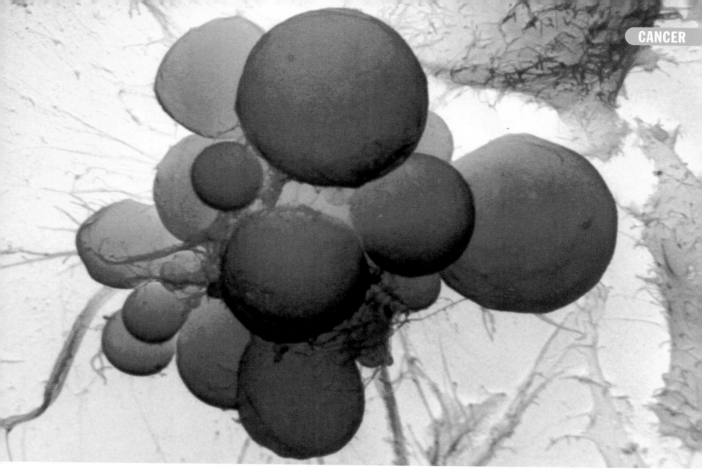

Tumour cells, magnified here 7,500 times, grow and divide without restraint. If cancer stem cells indeed spawn them, destroying those stem cells is vital to killing the cancer.

explain why Dr Dirks might remove a brain tumour, think he got it all, and then have the patient relapse a few months or years later. 'The whole stem cell cancer hypothesis suggests that we might wipe out 99 out of 100 cells. But if we don't get the key cell, the cancer is just going to regrow,' he says.

The future of cancer treatment Although so far stem cells have been identified only in leukaemia and in brain and breast cancers, researchers suspect they're at the root of all cancers. The question, of course, is how to stop them.

There are several potential approaches. Drugs could be designed to attack the mechanism within the stem cells that makes them self-renewing or to turn on a signal that makes them die. Antibodies could be developed that target proteins on the surface of the stem cells, delivering a poison directly to the cells. Or, in a kind of counterintuitive process, treatments may involve getting stem cells to mature into cancer cells; once mature, they stop regenerating and die off.

Researchers will have to tread carefully, however. Dr Dick and Dr Dirks suspect that cancer stem cells are actually normal stem cells gone bad. It will be vitally important that treatments targeting the black sheep cells don't inadvertently hit normal stem cells, they say.

The idea of stem cells as the root of all cancers also suggests new ways of determining how deadly a cancer might be. In the brain cancers he's studied so far, for instance, Dr Dirks has found that the higher the ratio of stem cells to other cancer cells, the more aggressive the tumour.

The next steps The whole field of stem cell cancer research is barely a decade old. It will take many more years of basic research before the findings bear fruit, but that doesn't keep scientists such as Dr Dick and Dr Dirks from being very excited.

Says Dr Dirks, 'Finding this culprit gives us hope that further research on these key cells will yield further breakthroughs about how cancer grows so we can more effectively treat it.'

General cancer
Fishing for cancer cures

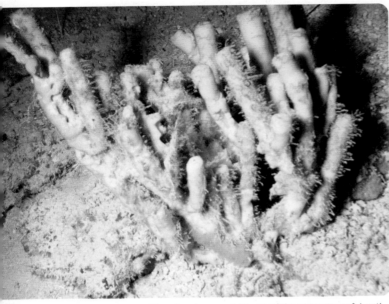

The deep-sea sponge Discodermia may yield one of the most powerful anti-cancer compounds ever discovered.

Creatures that spend their lives anchored in one place on the ocean floor have evolved powerful chemical defences to keep their enemies at bay. Now, scientists have discovered that those same unique compounds can apparently protect your body, too – against a broad range of cancers.

Researchers from Harbor Branch Oceanographic Institution in Fort Pierce, Florida, are leading the quest to find breakthrough medicines in the cells of organisms such as sponges, sea squirts and molluscs. They're probing the depths of the Earth's oceans with state-of-the-art, deep-diving, manned submersibles equipped with sophisticated robotic equipment to collect marine organisms 1,000m (3,000 ft) beneath the surface.

Nature's defences The sea creatures garnering so much attention are 'sessile', meaning that once they become adults they remain firmly attached to one spot. This makes them ideal for research, says Amy Wright Ph.D., director of Harbor Branch's division of biomedical marine research. 'Because they're stuck in one place, they make chemical

compounds to protect themselves from predators and keep other organisms from crowding their space,' she explains. As it turns out, those compounds may be powerful weapons against human diseases.

Back in 1984, Harbor Branch scientists exploring the deep waters off the Bahamas found a small piece of sponge that contained a chemical with remarkable cancer-killing ability. But it took 20 more years before scientists were able to find the sponge again, says Dr Wright, who has spent much of her career searching for it. In October 2003, she and her colleagues located it in water 300m (1,000ft) deep in the Bahamas, in an area known as the dead zone because it has so little animal or plant life. Dr Wright and her colleagues are testing chemicals in the sponge for anti-cancer properties. (The chemical that first attracted their attention has also been identified by a second marine research team – in a different sponge in a different part of the world.)

Pancreatic cancer cure? Meanwhile, laboratory tests suggest that a compound called discodermolide, isolated by the Harbor Branch team from a Caribbean Sea sponge, may be up to 80 times more potent than Taxol, a chemotherapy drug initially derived from the bark of yew trees and often used to treat breast and ovarian cancer. There's also some evidence that combining the compound with Taxol produces more powerful results than using either one alone. A synthetic

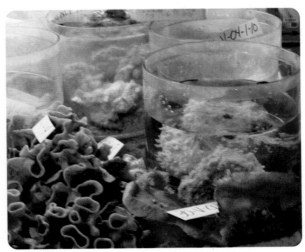

Harbor Branch marine scientists catalogue a sea sponge collected by a submersible for later study.

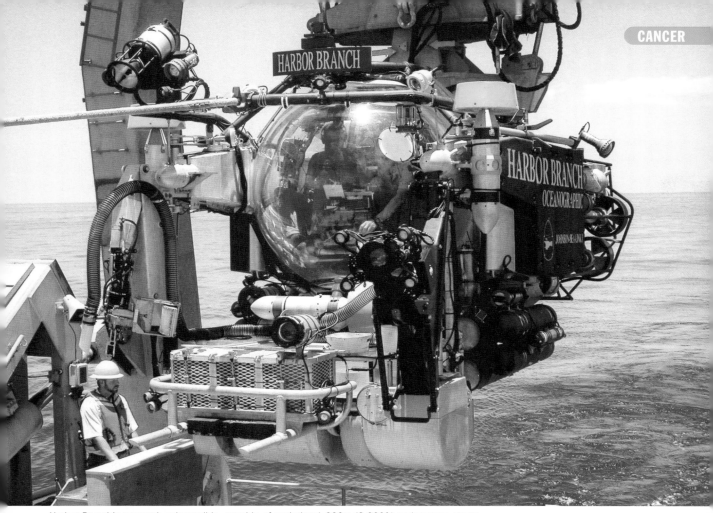

Harbor Branch's research submersible, capable of exploring 1,000m (3,000ft) underwater, starts a dive. Its mission: to find marine sources of new drugs.

version of discodermolide entered the first phase of human clinical trials for pancreatic cancer in late 2003 at the Cancer Therapy and Research Center in San Antonio, Texas. Other cancer killers from the sea currently under investigation include:

- A synthetic drug called ecteinascidin, which mimics a molecule found in sac-like sea squirts that live on Caribbean coral reefs. Early studies indicate it could be hundreds to thousands of times more powerful than any cancer drug now in use. The drug is being tested in human clinical trials in Europe.
- Dolastatin-10, isolated from a sea hare found in the Comoros Islands in the western Indian Ocean. It is undergoing clinical trials in the United States for treating a variety of cancers.
- Bryostatin 1, isolated from a tiny, plantlike marine invertebrate found off the coast of California. It is being studied in more than 40 clinical trials throughout the United States

and appears to prevent the growth of numerous tumours, including those of melanoma, non-Hodgkin's lymphoma, and kidney cancer.
- Halichondrin B, isolated from a sponge that's part of the Lissodendoryx species, found in New Zealand. It is currently undergoing testing in animals for its ability to combat numerous cancers.

All told, more than 5,000 new compounds have been derived from marine organisms in the last decade alone, says Dr Wright. Her own division has discovered more than 300 bioactive compounds (compounds that have effects on other living organisms) and has filed more than 100 patents on them. Most recently, she and her colleagues have begun exploring deep-sea sites in the Gulf of Mexico, including abandoned oil rigs and an ancient shoreline – the first time such research has been conducted on the biomedical potential of the deep-sea life in that body of water.

General cancer

Another reason to eat your spinach

You can bet that Popeye the Sailor Man never had cancer. That's because the enormous quantities of spinach he ate probably did more than just keep him strong: they also may have helped to prevent prostate and bladder cancer.

That's the finding from two studies presented at a major cancer meeting in April 2004, both of which found that getting vitamin E from food can significantly reduce your risk of either of these cancers – and spinach is a great source.

Food, not supplements If you're used to getting your vitamin E from a gel cap, that won't do the trick here. The studies, one from the USA's National Cancer Institute (NCI) and the other from the University of Texas M. D. Anderson Cancer Center in Houston, found that only vitamin E from food made a difference. The NCI study, which looked at blood samples of 100 Finnish men, found that those with the highest concentrations of a form of vitamin E called alpha tocopherol were 53 per cent less likely to get prostate cancer. Those with the highest concentrations of the other major form of vitamin E, gamma tocopherol, were 39 per cent less likely to get prostate cancer.

The Texas study found that for those with the highest alpha tocopherol concentrations, the risk of bladder cancer was reduced by 42 per cent, but no amount of gamma tocopherol had any effect.

Because vitamin E is available in relatively few foods, it is thought that most people do not get enough from their diet. It's not hard to obtain, however: 28g (1oz) of sunflower seeds contains about 14mg. Other important sources include almonds (8mg per tablespoon), spinach (6mg in one package of frozen spinach), wheat germ oil (26mg in one tablespoon), greens (1mg per cup of chopped raw greens), green and red peppers (about 1mg per large pepper), and canola oil (about 4mg per tablespoon).

Liver cancer
Diabetes raises liver cancer risk

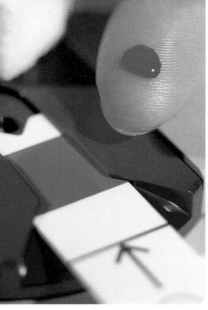

People with diabetes may now want to have liver enzyme tests annually as well as monitoring their blood sugar.

Researchers have known for years that there is a connection between diabetes and liver cancer, because people with diabetes have more cases of liver cancer and other liver disease than those without diabetes. Now, results from the largest study of its kind have put a figure to the risk: having diabetes doubles the risk of liver cancer and chronic liver disease.

The findings may have tremendous public health implications because of the growing epidemic of diabetes in the West, says lead researcher Dr Hashem El-Serag, associate professor of medicine at Baylor College of Medicine in Houston and the Houston VA Medical Center.

Behind the connection Diabetes is linked to obesity, which is an established risk factor for numerous cancers. Although they don't know for sure why liver cancer and diabetes are linked, researchers do know that people who are overweight and have diabetes are more likely to develop a condition called nonalcoholic fatty liver disease (NAFLD). It's probably related to fat accumulating in the liver because the organ can't transform enough of the fat into a form that can be eliminated.

By itself, NAFLD usually isn't dangerous. However, it can develop into what Dr El-Serag calls an uglier condition – NASH, or nonalcoholic steatohepatitis, in which inflammation of the liver damages liver cells, in some instances leading to cirrhosis and liver cancer. This may be what's happening with diabetes patients.

What it means 'If even a small percentage of those with diabetes develop NASH and liver cancer, it will translate into a very large number of patients,' says Dr El-Serag. In the meantime, he notes, it's important that people with diabetes or other insulin-related conditions, such as insulin resistance, have annual blood tests to track their liver enzyme levels, which can indicate liver disease.

Enzyme signals better test for bowel cancer

Researchers from Giessen University in Germany have devised a new screening test for bowel cancer. The test looks for an enzyme, called Tumour M2-PK, which is produced by the cancer as it grows and ends up in the faeces. The researchers found that the levels of the enzyme not only confirmed a diagnosis of bowel cancer, but indicated how advanced the disease was.

The current test for bowel cancer is the Faecal Occult Blood Test, which detects blood in the faeces. However, the FOBT does not distinguish between blood from a tumour or from a minor condition such as piles and it is estimated that only six out of every 100 people with a positive FOBT will have bowel cancer. This high level of false positives means that many people undergo invasive treatment, such as colonoscopy, when they do not need to. Also the FOBT misses some bowel cancers since not all tumours bleed.

The German researchers believe that testing for Tumour M2-PK would improve the accuracy of screening. Dr Philip Hardt, the study's lead researcher said: 'This enzyme has the potential to be an excellent safety net. It could detect more cases of the disease and possibly save unnecessary medical procedures due to fewer false positives.'

Lung cancer
An aggressive weapon
against aggressive cancer

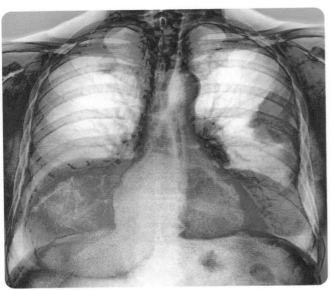

In people with certain genetic profiles, lung cancer (red and green shadings) is particularly vulnerable to the drug Iressa.

An article in the *Boston Globe* in 2002 caught the attention of the director of the Massachusetts General Hospital Cancer Center and was to result in one of the most important developments in lung cancer treatment in the past year.

Dr Daniel Haber Ph.D. read about a patient's amazing recovery from terminal lung cancer in 2002, after she was treated with the then-experimental drug gefitinib (Iressa). He was intrigued. He knew that Iressa worked in only about 10 per cent of patients and that genetics were the likely reason, but no one knew which genes made some patients so responsive to the drug. Dr Haber set out to find out, with the help of some colleagues. What the doctors found could mean that more patients who could be saved by the drug will get it sooner.

How it works Iressa, approved in 2003 for patients with non-small-cell lung cancer, works by blocking signals within the cancer cells, thus preventing a series of chemical reactions that cause the cells to grow and divide. Specifically, it works through structures known as epidermal growth factor receptors (EGFRs). Proteins called epidermal growth factors attach to these receptors, triggering reactions that enable the cells to grow and divide. Iressa blocks the receptors, halting the process.

Dr Haber and his colleagues, as well as a group of researchers at Dana Farber Cancer Center in Boston who were working separately on the problem, found that patients in whom Iressa worked had genetic mutations in the EGFRs. The mutations made the cells grow much faster and more aggressively than 'normal' cancer cells. Additionally, the mutant receptors seem to bind more tightly to Iressa, in effect creating a tighter seal against cancer growth. In other words, although the mutations make the cancer more aggressive, they also make it more susceptible to the drug.

What it means The discovery is already changing the way some people with lung cancer are treated. 'Right now, all lung cancer patients are treated the same way,' Dr Haber says, 'but now we know that if you have a certain genetic mutation, you're so likely to respond to Iressa that it should be part of your first line of treatment.'

EGFRs are found on several other types of cancer cells, including breast cancer, cancer of the bowel and prostate cancer. In theory Iressa could be used to treat these cancers, too, and current trials aim to explore the drug's potential against them.

In the UK the drug is available only to people who are taking part in clinical trials. It can be prescribed on a 'named patient basis' – when a specialist thinks it may help a particular patient.

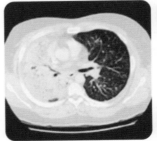 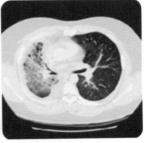

Left: CT scan shows cancer in a patient's right lung. Right: marked improvement after six weeks on Iressa.

Prostate cancer

Radiation for prostate cancer: the earlier, the better

Thousands of lives could be saved each year if doctors began treating recurrent prostate cancer with radiation immediately, a practice that rarely occurs. That's the finding in a groundbreaking paper published in the *Journal of the American Medical Association* (JAMA) in March 2004.

In the UK around 27,000 men are diagnosed with prostate cancer each year. Even when the prostate is removed, the cancer can return – often in the bones. Once it recurs, only radiation will cure it but few men are offered the treatment in time – in the USA, largely because radiation is not considered effective for aggressive recurrent tumours. Instead, doctors tend to prescribe hormone therapy, which slows the cancer's growth but doesn't kill it. In the UK, radiotherapy for recurrent prostate cancer is usually aimed at relieving pain, particularly if the cancer has spread to the bone.

Now, the largest ever evaluation of radiation as a treatment for recurrent prostate cancer has found that given early enough, radiation *can* cure the cancer, or at least significantly improve a patient's prognosis, say researchers from Baylor College of Medicine in Houston.

PSA levels not enough Part of the confusion stemmed from a misunderstanding about what it meant when levels of PSA, a protein released by prostate cells, rose after the prostate was removed. For years, doctors assumed that rising PSA rates meant the cancer had spread to other organs and was thus incurable. The new study found that this wasn't necessarily true.

The findings highlight the need for men to stay vigilant about their care for prostate cancer after surgery, says Dr Mitchell S. Anscher, a radiologist at Duke University Medical Center in Durham, North Carolina. Dr Anscher wrote an editorial about the study that appeared in the same issue of JAMA.

'They need to be aware of the findings at the time of surgery and whether they're really in a group that has a very high chance of being cured just with surgery or are in the group that is at risk of a recurrence.'

That means tracking their PSA levels after surgery, finding out their Gleason scores – an indication of the cancer's severity – and learning if there were positive margins (cancer cells) at the edges of the tissue that was removed. The main reason a man wouldn't qualify for radiation would be that the cancer had spread to his lymph nodes.

US experts hope the findings will mean that men will be sent for evaluation much earlier to see if they qualify for radiation. Dr Kevin M. Slawin, the study's lead author, is creating a formula to help doctors decide if a patient should have radiation after a cancer recurrence.

In the UK, a new trial funded by the Medical Research Council has just begun. It will compare hormone therapy and radiotherapy with hormone therapy alone for advanced prostate cancer.

RESEARCH ROUND-UP

More confusion about PSA results

One of the most controversial screening tests for cancer is the PSA blood test, used to check for prostate cancer. It indicates levels of prostate specific antigen (PSA), a protein released by prostate cells. When healthy men should be tested and how the results should be interpreted in both healthy men and those with cancer are subjects of debate. In April 2004, the waters got murkier with the publication of a study finding that even low PSA levels in men who already have prostate cancer could have serious implications.

Typically, PSA levels of 4.0 or less are thought to be relatively benign, even in men being treated for cancer. This study, from researchers at the University of Chicago, found that cancer specimens from men with levels less than 4.0 were still clinically significant, indicating that they required treatment. The findings mean that doctors should not rely on PSA readings alone to determine the status of a man's cancer nor assume that a low-PSA cancer doesn't require immediate treatment.

147

New way to predict the spread of **skin cancer**

The incidence of malignant melanoma, the deadliest form of skin cancer, continues to rise around the world. Currently, about 132,000 melanoma skin cancers occur globally each year, resulting in more than 33,000 deaths. In the UK, about 7,000 people are diagnosed with malignant melanoma each year. The cancer is more common in women than in men and the risk of being diagnosed increases with age (rates are highest in the over 75s). Although easily curable if caught early, the risk of death from the malignant melanoma dramatically increases if the cancer has the chance to spread (metastasize) to other organs. Now, researchers at Bristol University think they've found a new way to predict whether a melanoma will spread.

How it works To date, doctors have focused on the thickness of a melanoma, believing that the thicker the cancer, the more likely it is to metastasize. But only one in four thick melanomas spread, while many thin ones metastasize as well. Most melanomas, if they spread, travel to nearby

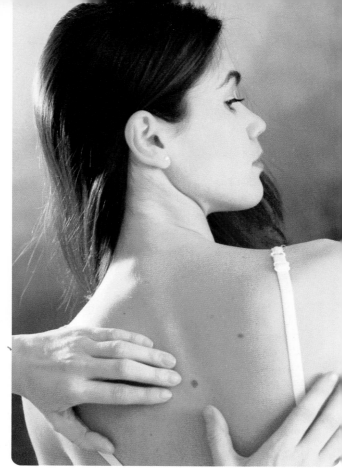

The earlier skin cancer is detected, the better the chance that it can be cured before it spreads to other organs.

lymph nodes through lymph vessels – vessels that connect lymph nodes, carrying lymph fluid in and out. Knowing that in animals the growth of lymph vessels is associated with the spread of cancer, the British researchers focused their efforts on those vessels. They recorded the density of lymph vessels surrounding melanoma samples from 21 patients, then followed the patients for at least eight years. As predicted, the denser the lymph vessels were, the more likely the patient was to develop additional cancers. In fact, the correlation between lymph vessel density and cancer metastasis was much greater than the correlation between melanoma thickness and cancer metastasis.

Availability Because this was a small study, the researchers now have to wait and see if their findings hold up in a study of hundreds of patients. If verified, the findings could provide important information to doctors about which patients should receive more extensive treatment and be more closely followed for signs of metastasis – and which are free to breathe a sigh of relief.

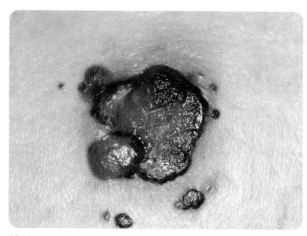

Melanomas are typically asymmetrical with an irregular border. They tend to be multicolored and ¼in wide or more.

Skin cancer
Melanoma can't hide from new vaccine

It sounds crazy – deliberately killing healthy skin cells in order to treat skin cancer. But a group of Mayo Clinic researchers in Rochester, Minnesota, believe it may be a powerful new approach to making the body's immune system destroy melanoma tumours. In fact, they tried it on mice and it eradicated the tumours.

Using therapeutic 'vaccines' to get the immune system to kill cancer cells hasn't worked very well in the past. (Although they're called vaccines, they are intended to treat people with cancer.) The vaccines are designed to teach the immune system to recognize malignant cells so the body can destroy them, but that's a tough job because cancer cells look so much like healthy cells. The Mayo Clinic scientists tried a new approach involving healthy, pigment-producing skin cells called melanocytes, the same cells that later change into melanoma.

How it works The scientists placed melanoma tumours in mice, then injected the mice with a vaccine composed of the antiviral drug ganciclovir and two types of DNA – one that codes for an immunity-boosting protein called heat shock protein and another that codes for an enzyme that attracts ganciclovir, which then kills melanocytes.

As the cells died, the heat shock proteins spilled out, sending 'help' signals to immune system cells called T cells. The T cells charged in and began destroying the melanocytes. Then, since melanoma cells look identical to melanocytes (at least to T cells), the T cells turned on the melanoma cells and began destroying them, too. The researchers published their findings in the August 2004 issue of the journal *Nature Biotechnology*.

Study co-author and Mayo oncologist Dr Gregory A. Daniels Ph.D. and his team hope their approach might work with other cancers. He notes, however, that not all tumours grow from nonessential cells. You wouldn't want to kill healthy lung tissue, for instance, in order to mount an immune response against lung cancer. Nevertheless, he thinks there may be a way to induce the immune response without actually having to kill the normal cells – something he and his team are working on.

Availability The researchers hope to begin human clinical trials on their vaccine approach sometime in 2005.

INBrief

▶ Early infections fight leukaemia

If you worry because your child seems to get sick all the time, you can take some comfort. A French study found that children who had any common infection before the age of 1 were 20 per cent less likely to get a common form of childhood leukaemia than children who never got sick. If the child's infection was related to the stomach – for instance, gastroenteritis – the risk dropped by 90 per cent. Not surprisingly, the earlier children attended nursery, the less likely they were to get leukaemia, probably because children in day care are exposed to more infections.

▶ A new reason to dust under the bed

Numerous studies find that regular exercise can keep cancer at bay. Now, a new study from Vanderbilt University and the Shanghai Cancer Institute in China has found that routine household tasks – dusting, laundry, cooking and cleaning – performed four or more hours a day cut a woman's risk of endometrial cancer by 20 per cent. Can't stand to clean house? An hour a day of walking cut the risk by up to 40 per cent.

▶ New drug for prostate cancer

Abarelix (Plenaxis) has been approved in America, the first in a new class of drugs designed to treat prostate cancer that has spread. Given by injection, it belongs to a class of drugs called luteinizing hormone-releasing hormone antagonists. They work by shutting down the production of testosterone, which feeds prostate cancer cells. Unlike similar drugs, abarelix doesn't cause an initial surge of testosterone, which can result in tumour growth and bone pain. Some people may be severely allergic to it, however, so doctors must enrol in an education programme before prescribing it.

DIGESTION
AND METABOLISM

Researchers have made a number of important discoveries on the
diabetes front

First the bad news: there are millions of people who are unaware that they have *pre*-diabetes – a condition that can turn into full-blown diabetes – because it is usually symptomless and is not routinely tested for.

On the bright side, research points to new ways to use food to lower your risk of diabetes – by eating antioxidant-rich foods, drinking coffee (especially decaf), and sprinkling cinnamon on your food. If you do develop diabetes, a breakthrough drug that's based on the saliva of Gila monsters can help control your blood sugar. Also, there's new evidence that being physically fit will help you live longer – even if you're overweight.

Another bit of news to digest: researchers have discovered links between emotional health and bowel disorders. People with inflammatory bowel disease may reduce flare-ups by avoiding or treating depression, and those with irritable bowel syndrome can find years of relief with a few sessions of hypnotherapy.

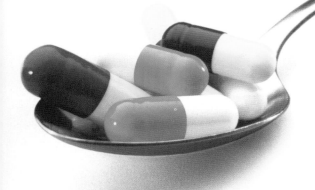

Bowel problems

Antibiotics may increase the risk of Crohn's disease

Experts know little about what causes Crohn's disease, a type of inflammatory bowel disease. It seems to run in families and there's increasing evidence of a genetic link. But it's becoming more common, suggesting that something may trigger the disease in susceptible people. Researchers have been looking for that trigger, and scientists at the Queen's Medical Centre, University of Nottingham, have discovered clues that point to antibiotics.

Using cases from a vast, computerized medical database that contains detailed records on approximately 5 per cent of the UK's population, researchers compared the histories of 587 patients who'd been diagnosed with Crohn's with those of 1,460 healthy people. They found that 71 per cent of people with Crohn's had taken antibiotics in the two to five years before their diagnoses, compared with 58 per cent of people without Crohn's. The study was published in the journal *Gut* in February 2004.

This study doesn't prove that antibiotics cause Crohn's but suggests the drugs are associated with the disease. More studies are needed to confirm a link. Antibiotics may contribute to Crohn's by killing off beneficial bacteria found in the digestive system, the authors say.

TOP trends

TODDLING TOWARDS DIABETES

Diabetes UK estimates that if current trends of increasing obesity and sedentary lifestyles continue, especially with the increase in Type 2 diabetes and an ageing population, that up to 20 per cent of people could potentially develop diabetes at some point in their lifetime. This prospective rise in diabetes is mirrored elsewhere in the Western world, especially in the USA.

Babies who were born in the United States in 2000 face a 'substantial' probability of developing diabetes at some point in their lives, according to research published in the *Journal of the American Medical Association* in October 2003. Overall, males have almost a 33 per cent chance of developing the disease, and females have more than a 38 per cent chance. Unfortunately, these estimates may be low, since they don't take into account the people who will develop diabetes but won't be diagnosed.

IN THE GUT BUG WAR YOU NEED TO FEED THE TROOPS

You may well have heard of probiotics – the beneficial bacteria found naturally in the gut that boost the immune system and stave off intestinal troubles by keeping 'bad' bacteria in check. A variety of yoghurts and dairy drinks containing colonies of the 'good' bugs have been on sale in Britain for years. The idea was that the yoghurt or drink contained enough probiotics for some to survive digestion and make it to the intestines where they supplemented your natural flora. But the gut bug war has just stepped up a level – now you can 'feed' the good bacteria that live in your gut by eating food laced with 'prebiotics'. Prebiotics are special food ingredients that nourish only the good bacteria, encouraging them to multiply at the expense of the harmful bacteria. The overall effect is a healthier digestive system.

Kellogg's, the breakfast cereal giant, has been the first to market a prebiotic kids' cereal in the UK. The product, Rice Krispies Muddles, contains a prebiotic called inulin, which is a plant carbohydrate extracted from chicory roots. Inulin is not digested in the stomach and so passes into the large intestine intact where it is food for the good bacteria living there.

In the USA yoghurt maker Stonyfield Farm says it adds inulin to its yoghurts as well as some fruits and vegetables. Horizon Organic Dairy adds a type of soluble fibre called NutraFlora, which also acts as a food for healthy bacteria, to its children's yoghurts.

Worm
your way out
of IBD

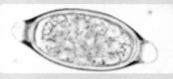

It may not be very appealing, but a dose of worm eggs may reduce the symptoms of inflammatory bowel disease (IBD), according to a recent study at the University of Iowa. The placebo-controlled trial involved 54 patients who had ulcerative colitis.

Every two weeks, for 12 weeks, researchers gave 30 patients a drink containing 2,500 eggs from the *Trichuris suis* worm, which normally infects pigs' intestines. The remaining 24 patients received a placebo.

At the end of the trial, 48 per cent of the patients receiving the ova experienced an improvement in their symptoms, compared to 15 per cent of the control group.

Gastroenterologist Joel Weinstock, who ran the trial, believes that the worms help the body by triggering a healthy immune response. His theory is that our immune systems have evolved to cope with parasites and can become overactive without them – leading to IBD. The worm eggs release larvae into the intestine, but they are eliminated from the body after a few weeks.

Bowel problems
IBS patients have a good gut reaction to hypnosis

Your tummy is getting *verrry* sleepy… Researchers have known for some time that in the short term, hypnotherapy can help relieve the symptoms of irritable bowel syndrome (IBS), which is characterized by abdominal pain, bloating and alternating constipation and diarrhoea. Now, a British study has shown that such therapy can offer long-term relief lasting five or more years.

The researchers at South Manchester University Hospital gave questionnaires to 204 IBS patients before, immediately after, and up to six years after treatment with hypnotherapy. The participants were asked about their symptoms, anxiety levels and quality of life.

Seventy-one per cent of the patients improved 'very much' or 'moderately' immediately following the therapy, which consisted of up to a dozen hour-long sessions. Of those people, 81 per cent maintained that improvement years later. The patients who responded to hypnotherapy also had lower anxiety scores on completion of treatment and reported that they needed fewer visits to the doctor and used less medication.

How it works Hypnotherapy helps patients enter a relaxed, dream-like state in which they're more open to suggestion. For treating IBS, patients are encouraged to imagine themselves calming their troubled digestive systems. This may involve placing their hands on their abdomens and envisioning a feeling of warmth, as opposed to pain. The study participants then regularly practised self-hypnosis at home with the help of a CD or tape.

Part of the benefit of hypnotherapy may come simply from the stress relief it provides. Studies suggest that hypnosis may also help a person damp down muscle activity in the gut and even the sensitivity of the gut lining – factors that aren't usually under conscious control and that contribute to IBS symptoms.

Availability Using hypnosis to treat IBS hasn't become common yet, although some gastroenterologists are beginning to recommend it. If you're interested in trying it, ask your GP for referral advice.

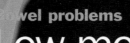

Bowel problems

Low moods linked to IBD flare-ups

People with inflammatory bowel disease (IBD) are prone to depression, but those who remain more upbeat and less anxious may have fewer relapses, according to an Austrian study.

Researchers at the University Hospital of Vienna followed 60 adults with Crohn's disease and ulcerative colitis for 18 months. At the start of the study, 28 per cent of the patients were found to be depressed. These patients had their first relapses an average of 97 days later, compared with nearly a year for those who weren't depressed. The more depressed the people were, the sooner their relapses occurred. The depressed patients also had more flare-ups during the study period. Having anxiety was also associated with more frequent flare-ups.

Since these diseases can't yet be cured, the goal in treating them is to reduce flare-ups, the researchers note. Thus, people with IBD should also be screened and treated for depression as part of treatment for their bowel disease.

RESEARCH ROUND-UP

Montezuma gets an extra measure of revenge

If you're not careful while travelling to Mexico, you may bring home a lasting but unwanted souvenir of your trip: irritable bowel syndrome (IBS).

In a study conducted at the University of Texas-Houston Medical School, 98 American students responded to a survey six months after they visited Mexico. Sixty-two had suffered from diarrhoea while travelling; about 10 per cent of these students reported that they later developed symptoms of IBS, such as diarrhoea, constipation and crampy abdominal pain only relieved by a bowel movement.

None of the students who stayed diarrhoea-free while travelling had IBS symptoms six months later. Whether the delayed symptoms were a result of some infectious organism or a lingering response to the infection is unknown, says lead researcher Dr Pablo Okhuysen of the university's General Clinical Research Center.

To reduce your risk, follow the usual advice for eating and drinking while holidaying abroad, particularly in developing countries: drink bottled water only, stick with cooked foods and fruits you can peel, and avoid buffets and drinks with ice. If you have a digestive upset while travelling, and it persists after you return home, talk to your GP, suggests Dr Okhuysen.

Too much iron has heavy consequences

Iron plays a crucial role in health, since it helps your blood carry oxygen around your body. Having too much iron, however, may raise your risk of diabetes.

Harvard researchers checked the records of more than 32,000 women from the long-running Nurses' Health Study and found that those who developed diabetes had significantly higher levels of ferritin, a protein that stores iron in the body. The higher your ferritin levels, the more stored iron you have. Women with the highest ferritin levels were more than twice as likely to develop diabetes as women with lower levels.

It's uncertain why iron may contribute to diabetes, and more research is needed, but the researchers point out that the mineral is thought to increase the activity of free radicals (molecules that damage cells). The damage may decrease the body's sensitivity to insulin, leading to high blood sugar.

The research echoes the results of a 1998 Finnish study of 1,000 middle-aged men. Researchers found raised serum insulin and blood glucose in men who had high concentrations of ferritin in their blood.

Diabetes
Fitness is more important **than weight**

It's possible to be overweight yet physically fit. If you need convincing, just watch professional rugby players in action. Those massive forwards are certainly hefty, yet they're aerobically fit enough to tear up and down the field. Now it turns out that among overweight men with diabetes, those who are physically fit live longer than those who aren't and maybe just as long as those who aren't over-weight, according to a study led by Dr Tim Church Ph.D., medical director of the Cooper Institute in Dallas.

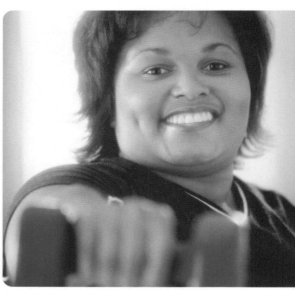

Another reason to exercise: if you have diabetes, even if you're overweight, your chances of living a long life are improved if you're in good shape.

What the study showed The study involved nearly 2,200 men who were followed for up to 26 years. Their fitness levels were rated based on their performance on treadmill tests. During the study period, normal-weight men who were the fittest were six times less likely to die than those who were least fit. Even among overweight and obese men, the fitter the men, the better their chances of a longer life. In fact, the study suggests that the obese men who were 'somewhat' to 'very' fit were no more likely to die prematurely than the fittest normal-weight men.

'I was really surprised that weight had a far lesser role than fitness,' says Dr Church. The study didn't look at causes of death or exactly how fitness protected the participants, but diabetes does increase a person's risk of heart disease and stroke, and staying in shape reduces those risks.

How much exercise is enough? Maintaining a fitness level that can improve your health doesn't require marathon-level training, says Dr Church. Just half-an-hour of moderate physical activity (such as brisk walking) five times a week can do the trick.

But before you pack some doughnuts as a mid-training snack – beware. Although you can be fat and fit, most people aren't. If you are overweight your GP will probably advise you to lose the excess pounds, especially if the weight is concentrated around your abdomen. However, these findings suggest that the most important thing is to be active. With regular exercise and a balanced diet excess weight will soon disappear.

Diabetes
Lizard spit inspires cutting-edge diabetes drug

Gila monsters, the venomous lizards with a nasty bite, have never been known for their healing powers, but now a hormone derived from their saliva is the basis for what could be the next breakthrough drug for Type 2 diabetes.

The drug, exenatide, is a synthetic version of a compound found in the mouths of Gila monsters. It does a lot of impressive things, according to Dr Steve Edelman, professor of medicine at the University of California, San Diego, who has been involved in clinical trials of the drug.

Exenatide can lower blood sugar without dropping it low enough to cause hypoglycaemia, a condition marked by shakiness and dizziness. It also leads to weight loss – which many people with diabetes need – and it may even rejuvenate cells in the pancreas that make insulin, a boon to people with diabetes who don't make enough of the hormone naturally, Dr Edelman says.

How it works Exenatide functions much like the human hormone GLP-1 (short for glucagon-like peptide), which is produced in the gut. GLP-1 stimulates the pancreas to produce insulin after a meal so that the insulin can help keep blood sugar levels from rising too high as the food is digested. People with Type 2 diabetes have trouble making or using their own insulin.

Existing drugs to reduce blood sugar can work *too* well, causing hypoglycaemia, but exenatide works more like a dimmer switch. Its effects taper off as blood sugar drops towards normal levels.

'If you were to design something to treat diabetes, that's what you might design,' says Dr John Eng, who discovered that Gila monsters carry the compound used in exenatide. The drug is delivered by one or two daily injections. In the most recent studies, the highest tested dose of exenatide reduced people's haemoglobin A1C – a long-term measure of glucose control – an average of 1 per cent, which is a sizeable drop. (A 5 per cent A1C level is normal. Patients in the study started at an average of 8 per cent.) The most common side-effect was nausea. Subjects also lost an average of 2 kilos (4.4lb) over 30 weeks, which is unusual as many medications that improve blood sugar levels cause weight gain.

Availability The developers of exenatide have completed phase III trials – the studies on large groups of people that are required before a drug can be licensed in the US; the next step is to gain approval by the US Food and Drug Administration (FDA). Exenatide is likely to be the first medication of its kind to hit the market, but other companies are working on drugs that are similar to GLP-1.

Diabetes
Antioxidant-rich foods may lower diabetes risk

Researchers in Finland have found more reasons why you should eat your vegetables and whole grains: the antioxidants they contain may steer you away from Type 2 diabetes.

The researchers analysed the eating habits of more than 4,000 men and women who were surveyed in the late 1960s and early 1970s. Based on this data, they were able to calculate the amounts of several different antioxidants the people consumed, including vitamins E and C and various carotenoids (substances found in red, yellow and orange plants and vegetables).

During a 23-year follow-up period, 383 of the men and women developed diabetes. The study authors calculated that people who consumed the most vitamin E were roughly 30 per cent less likely to develop the disease than those who consumed the least. And those who ate the most b-cryptoxanthin, a type of carotenoid that's converted to vitamin A in the body, were roughly 40 per cent less likely to develop diabetes. The results were published in the February 2004 issue of *Diabetes Care*.

The people in the study got most of their vitamin E from whole grain foods, vegetable oils, and margarines, says Jukka Montonen M.Sc., the lead study author and a researcher at the National Public Health Institute in Helsinki. Vitamin E is also found in leafy green vegetables and nuts. Most of the healthy

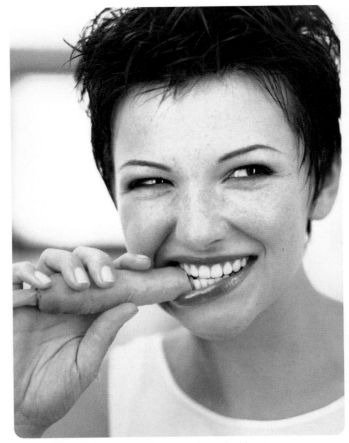

Count on carrots, as well as other colourful vegetables, to help protect you from diabetes (not to mention heart disease and cancer).

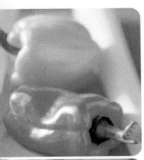

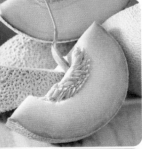

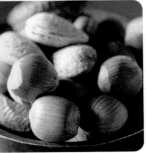

Finns' carotenoids came from red and yellow vegetables, Montonen says. Good food sources of vitamin A and carotenoids include carrots, red bell peppers and cantaloupe.

Explaining the effect Antioxidants may protect against diabetes by neutralizing free radicals (unstable oxygen molecules that damage cells), says Montonen. One way free radicals may contribute to diabetes is by damaging beta cells in the pancreas, which produce the insulin that helps blood sugar enter cells. Beta cells are particularly susceptible to free radical damage, and if they stop producing insulin as they should, blood sugar rises. Another way free radicals could contribute to diabetes is by causing cells in the body to take in less blood sugar.

The anti-diabetes effects of the antioxidant-rich foods may also have been due to other protective components of the foods, such as fibre, Montonen says, as well as the possibility that people whose diets contain plenty of beneficial foods have healthier lifestyles overall.

Diabetes

New **diabetes fighters,** already in your kitchen

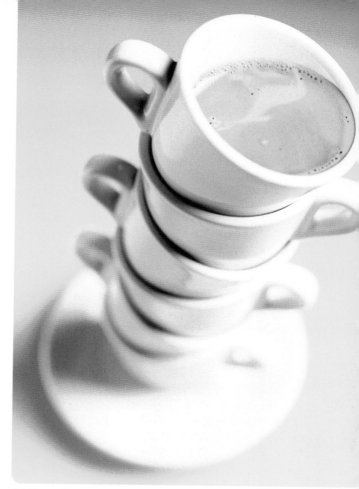

Drinking coffee – a lot of it – seems to lower the risk of diabetes. Two other staples, wine and cinnamon, can lower blood sugar.

Want to fight diabetes? Reach for a cup of java, a glass of Cabernet, or even a slice of apple pie. Groundbreaking new research suggests that coffee, wine and cinnamon may all be strong weapons against the disease.

Protection in a mug Several recent studies show that people who drink coffee – the most popular beverage in the world – have a lower risk of Type 2 diabetes. They also offer several reasons why the drink may pack a disease-fighting punch.

One study, published in the January 2004 issue of the journal *Annals of Internal Medicine*, looked at data on roughly 42,000 men and 84,000 women who participated in large-scale studies that tracked their diets and the diseases they developed. When the researchers took into account the volunteers' age, weight and other risk factors for diabetes, they found that men who drank at least six cups of coffee daily had less than half the diabetes risk of men who drank none. Women who drank at least six cups daily had roughly a 30 per cent lower risk than women who drank none.

Another study, published in March 2004 in the *Journal of the American Medical Association*, looked at nearly 15,000 men and women in Finland, which leads the world in per capita coffee consumption, over the course of about 12 years. It also found that the more coffee people drank, the lower their risk of developing diabetes.

Why coffee reduces diabetes risk is not known, although experts agree that caffeine isn't the force at work. The authors of the first study speculate that the potassium, niacin, magnesium and antioxidants in coffee may improve glucose metabolism (the way the body uses blood sugar) and lower insulin resistance (which contributes to high blood sugar).

The authors of the second study were backing on a chemical called chlorogenic acid, which may disrupt an enzyme that regulates the release of glucose from the liver. It may also keep blood sugar in check by limiting the ability of cells in the intestines to move sugar into the bloodstream.

These studies don't *prove* that coffee prevents diabetes, and the authors don't recommend that you start drinking it for diabetes prevention. Diabetes UK seconds that view, recommending that the results should be treated with caution. It suggests further research should be carried out to find out what is causing the surprising results. Drinking large amounts of coffee will have other side effects and the long-term effects of high coffee consumption remain unknown.

If you already have a coffee habit, though, the new research may make you feel better about it. You might want to switch to decaf, however, since there's evidence that caffeine impairs the ability of insulin to do its job of clearing the bloodstream of glucose.

Tasty spice, especially nice Cinnamon does more than lend flavour to apple pie and other baked treats: it may also help lower your blood sugar when

157

you make it part of your daily diet. Pakistani volunteers swallowed capsules containing either cinnamon or wheat flour every day for 40 days. After that time, those who took cinnamon had blood sugar reductions of between 18 and 29 per cent. The study authors think that the spice may make the body more sensitive to insulin, the hormone that allows blood sugar to be taken in to cells.

Since cinnamon is nearly calorie-free, the authors suggest that people who have diabetes, or those who wish to prevent it should regularly sprinkle the spice on their food. As little as ½ teaspoon a day could do the trick.

Diabetes UK would like to see more research in this area before recommending that people spoon on large amounts of the spice.

Vintage medicine People with diabetes were once told to avoid alcohol, but according to a French study, components of red wine can actually help lower high blood sugar – at least in laboratory animals. For six weeks, researchers fed healthy and diabetic rats either pure alcohol extracted from wine, polyphenols (a type of antioxidant) extracted from wine, both, or neither. The diabetic rats that consumed both the polyphenols and the alcohol had about the same blood sugar levels after a meal as healthy rats. The animals that received only alcohol had better blood sugar levels than those that received only polyphenols or neither substance. Both alcohol and polyphenols may work by increasing cells' sensitivity to insulin.

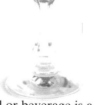

Diabetes UK acknowledges that wine, especially red wine, may offer health benefits. However, it warns that there is insufficient evidence to suggest that it is worth taking up drinking if you are teetotal. And, of course, no food or beverage is a substitute for taking your diabetes medication or getting more exercise and eating right.

More of us need to worry about **pre-diabetes**

It has been estimated that more then 300 million people worldwide are oblivious to the fact that they have conditions that could lead to heart disease and diabetes. The conditions, known as impaired glucose tolerance (IGT) and impaired fasting glucose (IFG), are often referred to as pre-diabetes. IGT and IFG indicate that glucose (sugar) is not being processed efficiently by the body. Research has shown that people with pre-diabetes have a 50 per cent chance of developing Type 2 diabetes within 10 years, while the risk of developing cardiovascular disease is doubled.

Pre-diabetes is marked by blood glucose levels that are higher than normal, but not high enough to warrant a diagnosis of diabetes. People are often unaware that they have this condition because there are no obvious symptoms.

According to the International Diabetes Federation, IGT and IFG are more likely to be found in people with:
- A family history of diabetes;
- Obesity;
- High blood pressure;
- High cholesterol.

Certain communities also have a greater incidence of the condition, including Asian Indians, Chinese, and indigenous Australians.

Grave implications High blood sugar may be a symptom of a larger problem, often referred to as insulin resistance syndrome. It's generally found in people who are sedentary and overweight, with fat accumulation particularly around the waist. Insulin resistance occurs when the body's cells don't respond as they should to the hormone insulin, which helps the sugar from foods enter the cells. When the sugar can't enter cells, it builds up in the bloodstream. Insulin resistance is linked to an increased risk of unhealthy cholesterol levels, build-up of plaque in the arteries, and a resulting higher risk of heart disease and stroke. According to the

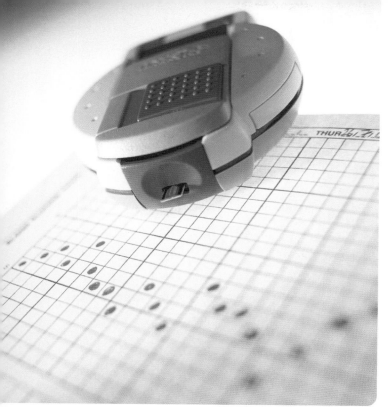

Should you be considering a blood sugar test? People with pre-diabetes – marked by higher-than-average blood sugar levels – are at increased risk of developing full-blown diabetes.

IN*Brief*

▶ Coeliac disease and mental illness may travel together

A Danish study has found that having coeliac disease – or a family history of it – may be a risk factor for schizophrenia. In coeliac disease, eating grains containing a protein known as gluten causes damage to the small intestine.

Researchers compared nearly 8,000 people with schizophrenia who were admitted to a psychiatric unit with 200,000 people who did not have schizophrenia. When they looked at the incidence of coeliac disease in both populations, they found that people with the digestive disorder were more than 200 per cent more likely to have schizophrenia than those who didn't have coeliac disease.

▶ Video capsule pinpoints hidden bleeding

If you have gastrointestinal bleeding, swallowing a camera in a pill could help you and your doctor find out what's causing it. An Italian study found that tiny capsules containing cameras and lights identified the source of bleeding in 92 per cent of people who had visible digestive bleeding. This technology – called capsule endoscopy (CE) – allows doctors to see portions of the small intestine that can't be viewed by putting a scope down the oesophagus or up through the rectum.

The authors say that CE is best for people whose bleeding is ongoing, whether it's visible to the eye – as with bloody bowel movements – or hidden in the stool and discovered through stool tests.

American Heart Association, adults with diabetes are up to four times more likely to have heart disease or strokes than those without diabetes.

Another condition linked to insulin resistance is polycystic ovary syndrome (PCOS), a cause of infertility in women. Up to 70 per cent of women with PCOS, which is marked by lack of ovulation, may have insulin resistance.

How do I know if I have pre-diabetes? Pre-diabetes is not routinely tested for in the UK, but you might consider asking your GP for a test if you are over 45 and have any of the risk factors already mentioned. The two basic blood tests that diagnose diabetes can also indicate pre-diabetes. Both measure the glucose levels in the blood. A fasting plasma glucose test is where you will be asked not to eat anything before a blood sample is taken. A two-hour plasma glucose test also requires fasting, after which you consume a measured amount of glucose and blood samples taken, with a final bood test two hours later. IFG is diagnosed when a fasting test gives a result of between 6.1 and 7.0 mmol/l. IGT is indicated after the two-hour test if the result is between 7.8 and 11.1 mmol/l.

What should I do now? If you have IGT or IFG it does not necessarily mean you will definitely develop diabetes. You can cut your risk by losing weight (if you are overweight), taking more exercise and eating healthily.

EYES

AND EARS

As millions of 40-somethings reach for their first reading glasses a new, minimally invasive, procedure may **restore vision**

Called conductive keratoplasty, it is the first medical procedure officially approved to correct presbyopia, which begins to affect most people as they approach the age of 50.

Older eyes affected by age-related macular degeneration may benefit from a host of new therapies, including common and experimental medications, radical surgery that involves moving the retina, and a miniature telescope that is actually implanted in the eye. And, it transpires, if you are taking drugs to reduce high blood pressure, you'll be protecting yourself against dry-eye syndrome.

One day in the future, doctors might be able to restore failing hearing by growing tiny new sensory hair cells. Meanwhile, heavy drinking has been implicated in hearing damage as has hormone replacement therapy. Even being of shorter than average stature may put people at risk of hearing loss.

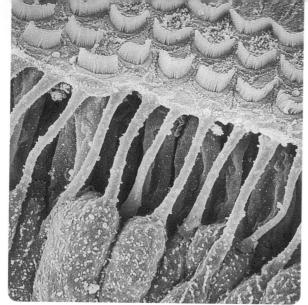

When microscopic hairs in the inner ear are bent by sound waves, they release chemicals that generate nerve impulses. These impulses travel to the brain, where they are interpreted as sound.

Hearing impairment

Growing hair to repair **hearing**

Some human hairs are not even visible, yet their loss causes far more distress than a balding patch on a middle-aged head. They are tiny hair cells in the inner ear, and they are responsible for your hearing. When sound waves move the fluid in the inner ear, the hairs vibrate, causing nerve cells below the hairs to generate electrical impulses which are sent to the brain and interpreted there as sounds.

When too many of the 15,000 or so sensory hair cells in each ear are damaged – most frequently as a consequence of ageing, heredity or the use of particular antibiotics – hearing is permanently lost. Reptiles and birds are able to regenerate sensory hair cells but humans cannot. Now, though, modern medicine may have come up with a solution.

A future cure for hearing loss? European scientists working on a research project called the Bionic Ear have taken the first steps down a path that could lead to replacement sensory hair cells for the human ear. They isolated inner-ear hair cells from adult mice and, by exposing them to proteins that promote cell growth, induced the cells to multiply – something they would never do under normal circumstances. The scientists were also able

to manipulate them into becoming different types of cells necessary for the transmission of sound, including auditory nerve cells and glial cells, which nourish the nerve cells.

This means that the cells which the scientists isolated in the mice were stem cells – the 'master' cells that have the capacity to turn into other types of cells and multiply indefinitely. (Unlike embryonic stem cells, which have been the subject of heated political debate for several years, these stem cells exist in adults, so there is no moral dilemma associated with their use.)

The researchers expect to find similar stem cells in the ears of humans and hope to nudge them in the laboratory into becoming sensory hair cells – and perhaps producing a cure for hearing loss.

What's next? Finding out whether such new hair cells could replace damaged ones in the human ear – and working out how to get them to do it – will involve many years of research, but this discovery may pave the way to therapy that could restore hearing using a patient's own hair cells.

TOP trends

JEWELS IN YOUR EYES

Remember the advent of eyebrow piercing and tongue studs? Just when it seemed that humans were running out of body parts to adorn with jewellery, surgeons in the Netherlands have begun implanting 'jewels' into the eyes.

People who have the desire to adorn their eyeballs can choose from shapes such as hearts and half-moons. The tiny ornaments, called JewelEye, have been designed specially for implantation in the conjunctiva, the mucous membrane that lines the front of the eyeball. The brief surgical procedure is performed by a ophthalmic surgeon using a local anaesthetic and an operating microscope. According to the Netherlands Institute for Innovative Ocular Surgery, which developed it, the implant does not interfere with the normal functioning of the eyes, and no adverse effects have been reported from its use.

But British eye experts are concerned that this type of surgery could irritate the eye. 'The stud could move around and migrate because the tissue in the conjunctiva is quite loose,' says John Dart, a surgeon at Moorfields Eye Hospital in London. 'Any movement is likely to cause inflammation. If it moves, there will be scar tissue and you could get some bleeding.'

Heavy drinking hurts hearing

By now you have probably heard that moderate drinking is good for your heart. Heavy drinking, on the other hand, has been shown to cause all sorts of problems, including increased risk of heart disease and liver damage. If you need yet another reason to keep your drinking in check, consider this: German scientists have found evidence that heavy drinking causes hearing loss.

Two groups of men were recruited for the study: one made up of heavy drinkers and one of moderate social drinkers. All the participants answered questions about their consumption of alcohol and were given blood and hearing tests. Then, in each participant, the scientists recorded and evaluated electrical currents in the brain that are responses to sound. They found that in the heavy drinkers it took longer for the brain stem to process sound.

Short on hearing

People who are shorter than average may be more prone to hearing loss than taller people, according to researchers at Gothenburg University in Sweden. They tested the hearing of 479 men aged 20 to 64 who were exposed to noise in their jobs. Among them, short men were three times more likely to have worse hearing for their age than taller workers. The researchers also tested 500 randomly selected men who were born in 1974. In that group, men with hearing loss were twice as likely to be short as men with normal hearing.

The researchers suspect that adult hearing loss can be traced back to what happened in the womb: a low level of a particular growth hormone during the development of the foetus may lead to a reduced number of cells at birth, resulting in short stature and early onset of hearing loss.

Hearing impairment
Hormone therapy may harm hearing

In recent years, hormone replacement therapy (HRT) – in addition to bringing many benefits – has been reported to increase women's risk of developing heart disease, stroke, breast cancer and dementia. Now it appears that the therapy may be associated with hearing loss.

In a small study at the University of Rochester and the Rochester Institute of Technology in New York, three separate hearing tests were given to women who had had HRT and women who had not. Women in the HRT group performed worse on all three tests, but the most dramatic difference was discovered in a test of how well the brain processes sounds detected by the ear. Women in the HRT group did 30 per cent worse than women in the non-HRT group. A deficit in the brain's ability to filter and prioritize sounds is most noticeable in situations where there is a great deal of background noise.

The researchers had expected that, since the ear contains receptors for the hormone oestrogen, HRT might help women's hearing, not make it worse. The team has begun researching a number of questions raised by their finding, including why the therapy may be linked to hearing loss, how much and what type of therapy may be to blame, and whether hearing improves when HRT is stopped.

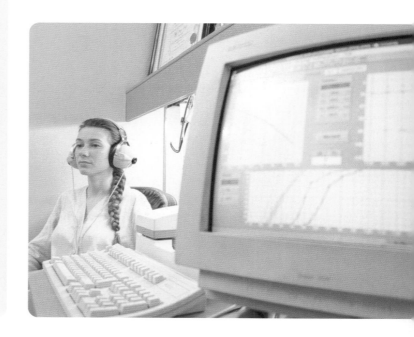

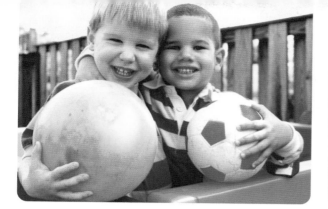

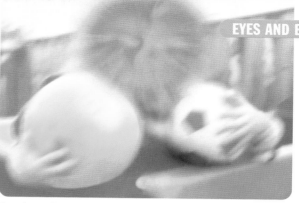

Two views of the same scene: as it would appear to a person with normal vision (left) and to a person with macular degeneration.

Macular degeneration

A two-stage assault on advanced eye disease

Many people approaching retirement dream of a future of gazing at their grandchildren and enjoying all those books and films that they never had time for while they were still working. But, for the unlucky ones, age-related macular degeneration, may rob them of the vision they need to enable that future to unfold.

Macular degeneration spares peripheral vision but steals the sharp central vision necessary for recognizing faces, reading and other activities. At its worst, central vision is replaced by a black blotch. Nobody knows what causes it, and there is no cure. One treatment for advanced macular degeneration, called photodynamic therapy, uses medication and a laser to slow down or stop the disease, but it rarely improves vision. Many who receive it continue to lose sight despite multiple treatments – and once their central vision has gone, it has gone for good.

A radical, two-part surgical procedure, developed and refined at Duke University in North Carolina, is now helping some people with advanced macular degeneration. It is not capable of restoring 20/20 vision, but patients who had little hope of seeing again have regained enough central vision to continue their normal activities.

Dr Cynthia Toth, a professor at Duke, says that the vision of people who have had the procedure improves on average by one line on an eye chart and their reading speed improves by about 25 words per minute. That may not seem like much, but it is significant for many people faced with a visionless future. 'Most patients get back to reading using reading glasses – they're able to sit down and read a book again,' says Dr Toth, who has performed hundreds of the procedures. 'Patients are telling us it has an impact on their quality of life at home.'

How it works Macular degeneration affects the macula, the central part of the retina, where light-sensitive cells are concentrated. In advanced macular degeneration, scarring and leaky blood vessels form underneath the retina and begin to damage the macula. The two-phase procedure – which is technically known as macular translocation surgery with 360-degree peripheral retinectomy – moves the retina away from the diseased area of the eye wall to a spot with healthy tissue before more damage can occur.

As a first stage, fluid is injected underneath the retina, which is cut away from the eye wall. The optic nerve is left intact and acts as a pivot when the retina is rotated away to a healthy area and leaky blood vessels are removed. After this, the patient's vision is tilted because of the rotation. Two months later, when the eye has healed, a second procedure corrects the tilt by detaching and repositioning four of the six muscles that hold the eye in place.

Limits and risks The surgery is available only to patients with advanced macular degeneration who are already blind in one eye and have lost vision in the other within the previous six months. The procedure is performed on the less damaged eye.

Complications do occur. At the Duke University eye centre there is a 10 per cent risk of retinal detachment, which can cause permanent vision loss. Some patients have double vision or some residual tilting after the surgery, which can be treated with special glasses or additional surgery.

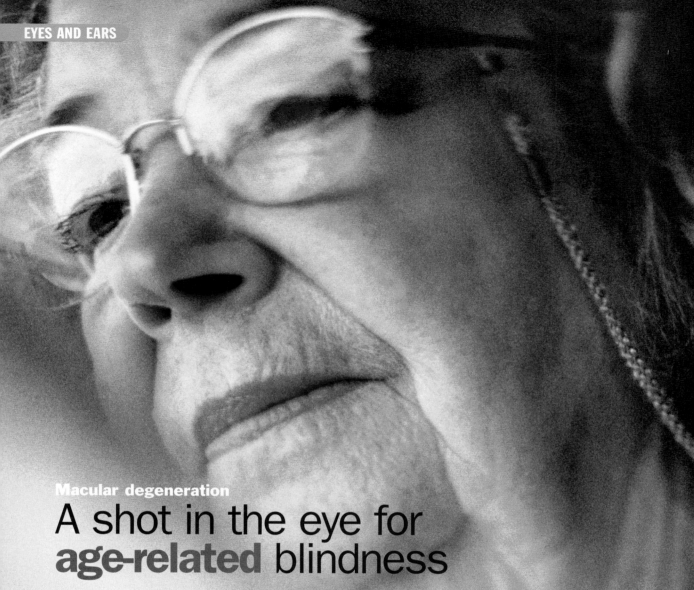

Macular degeneration

A shot in the eye for age-related blindness

People in the USA suffering from severe age-related macular degeneration may soon be able to get help from two new medications, pegaptanib (Macugen) and ranibizumab (Lucentis), as long as they are brave enough to take a shot in the eye – literally.

The drugs treat the 'wet' form of age-related macular degeneration, which affects more than half a million people in the UK alone and can destroy vision in a few months. Both drugs are undergoing clinical trials in America, which means that hundreds of people with this form of the disease have endured multiple injections into their eyeballs.

In the latest clinical trial of Macugen, the drug was found to be 27 per cent more effective than a placebo (dummy injection) at limiting vision loss in patients with wet macular degeneration. Patients treated with Lucentis for about three months had small gains in vision, while those who received standard care (observation or a laser treatment called photodynamic therapy) lost the ability to see an average of five letters on an eye chart.

How they work In wet macular degeneration, abnormal vessels grow behind the retina and leak blood and fluids, ultimately destroying the centre of the retina (the macula), where light-sensitive cells are concentrated. Crucial to the development of Macugen and Lucentis was the recent discovery of vascular endothelial growth factor (VEGF), a protein that helps to stimulate the formation of new blood vessels. Both drugs block VEGF, preventing it from activating vessel-forming cells.

Availability Macugen and Lucentis are still in clinical trials in the USA, but no plans have been reported to test them in the UK.

Macular degeneration
A telescope for 'black holes' in vision

Forget the Hubble. There is a new telescope that can see right around black holes – and it is so tiny that it can fit inside a human eye.

The telescope is the Implantable Miniature Telescope (IMT), and the black holes it sees around are caused by age-related macular degeneration, a condition in which the macula – the central portion of the retina – deteriorates. In its advanced stage, the disease causes a permanently blurred or blind spot in the centre of the visual field. Peripheral vision is not affected, but anything requiring 'straight-ahead' vision, such as reading, becomes nearly impossible.

About 300 people in Europe and the USA have had the telescope implanted in their eyes during clinical trials. The average improvement in vision has been two or three lines on an eye chart (three lines represent double the vision capacity – say, from 20/100 to 20/50), allowing patients to resume some of their normal activities.

'This is an amazing technology. Even I have to admit that this is particularly cool,' says Dr Baruch Kuppermann, an investigator in the clinical trials who has been involved in eye research for 15 years.

How it works

The IMT is implanted in the eye's lens during a one-hour outpatient procedure. The device magnifies images to two to three times their normal size and projects them over a wide field of the retina, beyond the damaged parts. The implant is made in the eye with

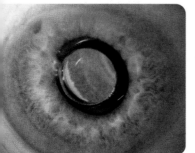

A tiny telescope six weeks after implantation in an eye.

poorer vision, while the other eye is left untreated to handle peripheral vision (although this is reduced in comparison with having side vision in both eyes).

Dr Kuppermann, who is based at the University of California at Irvine, says that his patients feel no difference in the eye with the IMT. 'But you see a little glint in their eye,' he adds. 'The implant extends just beyond the pupil.' Natural eye movements can be used to see with the telescope, but patients need training to make the most of it. Once the device has been implanted, the eyes do not work together any more because the brain is unable to merge the larger image from the telescope with the normal-sized image from the other eye.

Patients typically work with a low-vision therapist for about six weeks after the procedure, learning to suppress the smaller image and focus their attention on the larger one – which is similar to what people do when they look through an ordinary telescope.

Availability The telescope is being evaluated for safety and effectiveness in a two-year clinical trial at 28 ophthalmic centres across the USA. The manufacturer, VisionCare Ophthalmic Technologies, expected to seek Food and Drug Administration (FDA) approval of the device after the study's first year, near the end of 2004. If approved, the IMT would be available in late 2005 at the earliest.

RESEARCH ROUND-UP

Inflammation in the body may be linked to eye condition

Inflammation measured by a 'marker' protein called CRP signals an increased risk of heart disease and stroke. New research shows that high CRP levels are also linked with age-related macular degeneration. Inflammation has no cure, but stopping smoking, taking regular exercise, losing weight and eating more oily fish seem to help. A British study has revealed that foods rich in the natural food pigment lutein, found in dark green vegetables, pumpkin and red pepper, may slow the development of macular degeneration.

Eye damage affects sleep

Sleeping is no easy matter for people with optic nerve damage. Researchers at Washington University in St Louis, Missouri, studied sleeping and waking cycles in 25 visually impaired young people between the ages of 12 and 20 and in 12 young people with normal sight. Those with optic nerve disease were 20 times more likely to have daytime sleepiness than those with normal sight, and nine times more likely to have daytime sleepiness than those with vision impairment not involving the optic nerve. People with optic nerve damage had trouble falling asleep, and woke up at all sorts of times.

Recent research has found that the retina contains nonvisual, light-sensitive cells that determine light levels and communicate with the part of the brain that is involved in sleeping and waking cycles. These cells are concentrated at the head of the optic nerve. People with optic nerve disease may have difficulty using daylight to synchronize their internal rhythms with what is occurring in the outside world, say researchers.

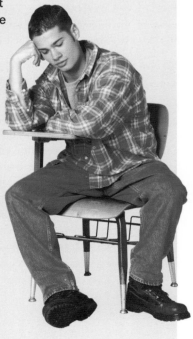

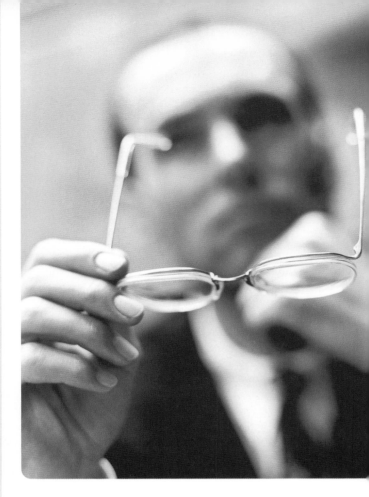

Vision impairment
Over 40?
Can you read this without glasses?

'What a drag it is getting old,' sang the Rolling Stones, and many people approaching their half-century are likely to nod their heads in agreement. Millions of them need reading glasses – or will need them within the next ten years. The reason? A condition called presbyopia, which is caused by the stiffening of the eye's lens and which makes it difficult to see clearly up close. Most people first notice the problem in their forties, and by the age of 50 nearly everyone has it.

Now, for the first time, there may be an opportunity to avoid those reading glasses – thanks to a procedure called conductive keratoplasty, which has been granted official approval for the treatment of presbyopia and farsightedness. It is now available, at a price, at more than 200 clinics worldwide, including several in the UK.

'The procedure is minimally invasive and very safe,' says Dr Penny Asbell of Mount Sinai Medical Center in New York. 'It's not a laser, and no tissue is removed.'

How it works In conductive keratoplasty, a probe thinner than a human hair is used to apply radio waves to the cornea, the outer layer of the eye. Like an electrical current, the radio waves seek to complete a circuit and return to their source. When they meet resistance – in this case, the cornea – they produce heat, which is used to shrink the corneal tissue in a circular pattern. The cornea becomes more dome-shaped and near vision is brought back into focus.

The procedure is typically performed in just one eye in order to restore close vision without compromising distance vision. Some people who need bifocals to correct both their distance and near vision can have conductive keratoplasty done in both eyes, with a small correction for the 'distance vision' eye and more correction for the 'near vision' eye.

In clinical trials, 87 per cent of people who had conductive keratoplasty had 20/20 vision after the procedure and were able to read the sort of print that appears in the telephone book. A minority were not totally successful, says Dr Asbell, who was a researcher in the trials and performs the surgery

herself. But, she says, 'We're talking about getting good vision for most activities. We're not going for extremes. Most days, we're not reading the smallest letter on the chart – that's not normal, everyday vision.' In fact, most people would be happy to be able to read the morning newspaper without having to hold it at arm's length.

Does it last? Conductive keratoplasty is not likely to resolve your vision problems for ever. Although the procedure is permanent, the eyes continue to age. Some people need further treatment every few years – 'maybe as often as they would upgrade their glasses,' says Dr Asbell.

Adjusting the focus: a probe thinner than a hair corrects vision by shrinking corneal tissue with radio waves.

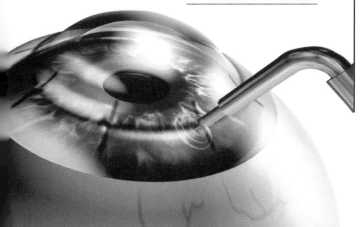

INBrief

▶ Blood pressure drugs for dry eyes

Blood pressure drugs called angiotensin-converting enzyme (ACE) inhibitors seem to reduce the risk of dry-eye syndrome, a condition common in elderly people. When researchers followed nearly 2,500 people who did not have the syndrome over a period of five years, only 9 per cent of those taking ACE inhibitors to lower their blood pressure developed dry eyes, compared with 14 per cent who were not taking them. The protective effect of the drugs may derive from their anti-inflammatory properties. It is not known whether taking an ACE inhibitor can provide relief after dry-eye syndrome has developed.

▶ Early treatment best for eye disease in premature babies

A leading cause of vision loss in premature babies is a disorder called retinopathy of prematurity, the growth of abnormal blood vessels at the back of the eye. A study of 317 infants at high risk of retinopathy showed that early and aggressive treatment, involving the use of a laser or freezing the retina to reduce the number of blood vessels, is the most effective. Infants who, based on current recommendations, would have been treated later were shown to retain better vision with early intervention.

HEART
AND CIRCULATORY SYSTEM

Researchers continue to investigate newer and better ways of getting heart disease under **control**

Gene therapy is set to improve angina symptoms by growing brand new blood vessels to feed the heart. Statin drugs and implanted defibrillators are saving the lives of more people with heart failure. Researchers have also discovered how they can help to prevent cognitive problems in people who undergo bypass surgery.

Surgery, less popular now than angioplasty (the newer, less invasive approach to dealing with clogged arteries), may actually be the better option, at least when performed by the best surgeons, because it delivers longer-lasting results. This conclusion surprised even researchers who conducted a study of the procedure.

On the low-tech side, there are new reasons why alcohol and the Mediterranean diet are both good for the heart: they control inflammation of the arteries, now thought to be intimately connected with heart disease. Recent studies found that people who drink moderately, and those following the traditional Mediterranean diet, have lower levels of CRP, a protein that indicates levels of inflammation.

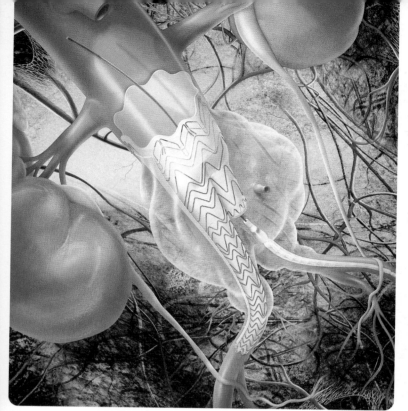

A tiny support structure called a stent is inserted via a catheter into a bulging abdominal aortic aneurysm. The stent's two branches extend into the arteries that lead toward each leg.

Aneurysms

Stent is better than traditional aneurysm surgery

An abdominal aortic aneurysm (AAA) is a dangerous bulge in the part of the body's largest blood vessel located in the belly. Although aneurysms often aren't detected until it's too late, there are actually two ways of repairing these deadly bubbles: traditional 'open' surgery and a less invasive approach that involves a catheter threaded through a small incision. For years, the experts have passionately debated which approach is better, but now the argument may be over. A study shows that compared with the open surgical technique that many doctors had come to rely on, the newer, less invasive technique gets high marks for improving chances of survival and promoting quicker recovery.

The traditional procedure, which involves making a long incision in the abdomen and stitching up the aneurysm, was the only option until the early 1990s when UK surgeons began

TOP trends

HEART SURGERY GETS A NEW 'THEME SONG'

Many surgeons like to play music while they operate, and now some heart patients at renowned hospitals – including Columbia University Medical Center in New York City, the Cleveland Clinic in Ohio and Cedars-Sinai Medical Center in Los Angeles – are getting their own audiotapes to listen to, via headphones, while they're under the knife. These aren't just any old tapes, though; they are designed to help patients through their surgeries and possibly speed recovery.

The tapes deliver positive messages geared to specific surgical procedures. The voice on the recording might reassure patients about tubes or medical devices or have them imagine that their arteries are becoming wider and more flexible. The patients listen to the tapes before, during and after their operations. (Research suggests that people are able to process information while under anaesthesia.)

To find out how well the tapes work, doctors at Columbia have launched a study involving coronary bypass patients. The patients will be given either standard care, standard care plus relaxing music, or standard care plus music and targeted messages. They will be assessed after their operations to see whether the messages helped to alleviate postsurgical depression – a common problem with bypass surgery – and the need for pain medication, among other outcomes.

WEST NILE ALERT

Over the past four years the West Nile virus has spread across North America and parts of Europe, including two cases in Ireland, and there are fears that the virus could reach the UK. The virus is normally contracted via a bite from an infected mosquito but it can also be transmitted via blood transfusions. In 2003 there were six confirmed cases and three more possible cases of Americans who became infected in this way. In Britain, the National Blood Service has introduced a screening test for the virus for blood donors who have recently travelled to the USA or Canada. The Department of Health still believes that the chances of the virus arriving in the UK are low.

TOP trends

SAY 'ADIOS' TO ANGIOGRAMS?

Scientists are developing more and more sophisticated ways to peer into your body to find out whether you have heart disease – meaning better information for your doctor and minimum discomfort for you. The latest generation of high-tech imaging machines includes '16-slice' computed tomography (CT) scanners that capture details of the body in tiny, ½mm slices. These scanners are being used to look inside blood vessel walls with little risk or discomfort for patients. Several hospitals and cardiac centres in the UK are already using the stunning images produced by these super-fast (and super-expensive) CT machines to diagnose heart ailments. They could make the angiogram (which requires threading a catheter into the coronary arteries in order to inject a dye) a thing of the past.

using a device called a stent graft. The device is a collapsible reinforcement for the aorta that's shaped like a tiny pair of trousers; it's designed to be positioned inside the aneurysm and extend slightly down into the artery that leads to each leg. The graft is inserted via a long, thin catheter inserted through

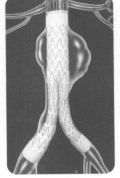

an incision in the groin. For doctors who took to the new minimally invasive technique, the idea of open surgery started to look outmoded and extreme, but surgeons who swore by the older method considered the new technique too iffy to become the new standard.

The first study to compare the two, published in January 2004, analysed information from thousands of AAA repairs performed in hundreds of hospitals in New York State over a two-year period. The bottom line: use of the stent graft boosts a person's chances of

AAA stent repair improves recovery times and survival rate.

surviving the procedure. Fewer than 1 per cent of stent recipients died, compared with 4.2 per cent of those treated with surgery. The study also showed that people who had the stent-graft repair were able to return home in less than four days and needed to recover for only about two weeks. People who underwent open surgery stayed in the hospital an average of ten days and needed up to two months of recovery time to get back to their normal activities.

Angina
Homegrown blood vessels relieve angina

For people with angina, any exertion – walking, talking, and even simply standing – can bring on debilitating chest pain caused by reduced blood flow to the heart. Think of what happens when traffic flow on a motorway narrows because one lane is closed: fewer cars can get through.

Likewise, when coronary arteries narrow due to the build-up of plaque (made up largely of cholesterol), less blood can get to the heart. Now, there may be a way to help the body add more 'lanes' by injecting a gene that encourages extra blood vessel branches to sprout out from the coronary arteries.

How it works The gene, called Ad5FGF-4, is delivered by way of a harmless virus (a modified, deactivated version of the common cold virus), which is injected directly into the heart with a syringe. The gene can stimulate growth of both heart muscle cells and cells lining the arteries. The therapy had previously been studied in animals, and in 2003 researchers, led by Dr Cindy Grines of William Beaumont Hospital in Royal Oak, Michigan, took the big step of testing it – successfully – in people.

All the patients taking part in the study, published in October 2003 in the *Journal of the American College of Cardiology* had angina that was not responding to medicines; none could have surgery. Thirty-five patients received gene therapy and 17 received placebo injections. Eight weeks after the single gene injection, the areas of the heart that showed low blood circulation were reduced by an average of 4.2 per cent in the people who had the gene therapy. Those who received the placebo treatment experienced no such improvement. The researchers hoped that blood circulation would continue to improve within the hearts of the gene therapy patients.

Availability Two larger clinical trials, involving 450 patients each, are starting up in order to gather more information on long-term, symptom-

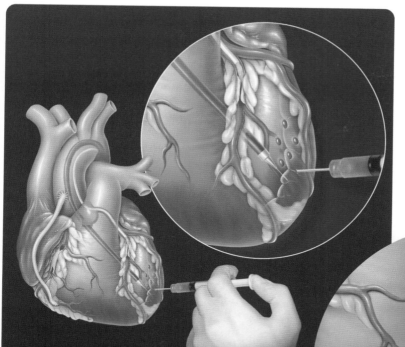

Genes that encourage the growth of new blood vessels are injected directly into the left ventricle of the heart (left). The new blood vessels provide improved circulation to the heart muscle (below), relieving angina.

relieving effects of the gene therapy. If all goes well, the treatment could be approved in America within the next five years. In the UK, a trial is also under way at Papworth Hospital in Cambridge to see if the therapy is able to help patients with refractory angina who are not responding to medication and cannot have bypass surgery. The results of this study should be available in about two years time.

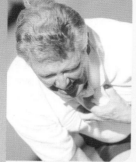

RESEARCH ROUND-UP

A new pill for chest pain

Chest pain that isn't life-threatening can still affect a person's quality of life. Millions of people experience chronic chest pain caused by reduced blood flow to the heart, a condition called angina. This difficult-to-treat problem, usually a result of heart disease, can reduce a person's ability to exercise, work and enjoy regular daily activities. For more than a quarter of angina sufferers, the most commonly prescribed medications, such as nitrates and beta blockers, just don't help.

Now there's an experimental drug, called ranolazine, that could benefit people who don't respond to other medicines. It's thought to work by helping the heart get more mileage out of less oxygen by increasing its ability to use glucose to produce energy. In studies, ranolazine let people exercise longer without experiencing angina and reduced the overall number of angina attacks.

The company that makes ranolazine, CV Therapeutics, has completed two Phase III trials (one with ranolazine as a sole treatment and the other with the drug used in combination with standard angina drugs). Approval has been sought from the European Agency for the Evaluation of Medicinal Products and if successful ranolazine may soon be more generally available.

Atrial fibrillation

Putting dangerous arrhythmia on ice

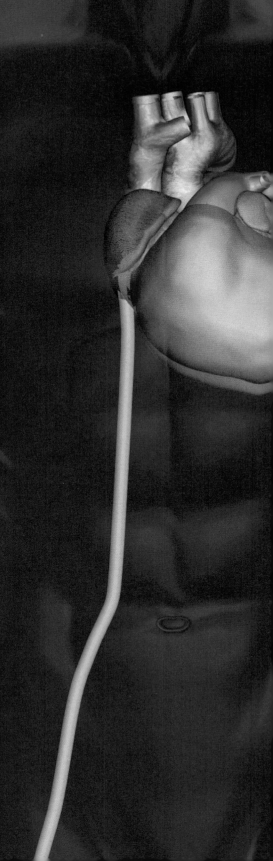

A new 'cool' treatment for uncontrolled atrial fibrillation (the most common form of heart rhythm abnormality) may be safer than the standard surgical approach. Atrial fibrillation (AF) can cause heart palpitations, shortness of breath, dizziness, and, perhaps most worrisome, an increased risk of stroke due to blood clots. (Blood clots can form when an uneven heart rhythm allows blood to stagnate between beats instead of being evenly pumped and mixed.) Some types of AF can be controlled with drugs, but when AF is 'permanent', when it is not responding to drugs or electrical treatment to reset the heart's rhythm, the next step is surgery.

The standard surgical fix uses radiowaves to generate heat that selectively scars the heart, creating 'inactive' spots that interrupt the electrical signals that cause the arrhythmia. But this approach (called radiofrequency ablation) can actually lead to the blood clots that the procedure aims to prevent, because intense heat has a coagulating effect on blood cells. In addition, the inactive sites must be relatively large in order to effectively stop atrial fibrillation, and the risk of clotting grows along with the size of the treated areas.

Luckily, applying heat is not the only way to interrupt the erratic electrical signals from an arrhythmic heart. Early studies of a new treatment device called CryoCor show that freezing tiny areas of heart tissue appears to be as effective as using heat. And the cold method does not seem to lead to clot formation.

Like radiofrequency ablation, the cold treatment uses a minimally invasive technique to thread a catheter through an artery and into the heart. Once in position, the tip of the catheter delivers a medical refrigerant gas that can reach temperatures as low as −116°C (−176°F), low enough to freeze small bits of heart tissue.

Availability CryoCor is already available in Europe, and more than 300 patients have been treated with the new technique so far.

Sudden death warning

An Illinois woman named Shalon Gardner was only 17 years old when she suddenly developed a very rapid heartbeat. Dr Preben Bjerregaard, a cardiologist at St. Louis University Hospital, recalls that when he looked at her electrocardiogram (ECG), a test that measures the electrical signals during each heartbeat, 'I saw this incredible, short QT interval, which I had never seen before.' The QT interval is the length of time separating electrical impulses in the heart. People with long QT intervals are known to be at higher risk for sudden death, but based on Ms Gardner's symptoms of heart palpitations and her short QT measurements, Dr Bjerregaard feared she might face the same tragic fate.

Dr Bjerregaard was surprised to discover that Ms Gardner's mother and brother also had short QT intervals, indicating a family propensity for serious heart trouble. To head off sudden death, each Gardner family member had a defibrillator surgically implanted. If erratic heart rhythms occur, the devices will kick in and save the day.

The short QT interval has also been identified in some families in Europe and is most likely related to a rare genetic defect. Dr Bjerregaard advises anyone with a family history of sudden death, especially among younger family members, to have their QT intervals measured with an ECG.

A catheter with a special tip that can freeze tissue is threaded through the groin and along an artery into the heart, where it is carefully positioned against a vein in the left atrium.

A 'mapping catheter' with a ring-shaped tip is used to confirm electrical activity in the vein before tissue is frozen to interrupt the electrical signals that can lead to atrial fibrillation.

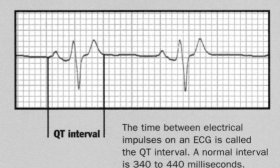

QT interval

The time between electrical impulses on an ECG is called the QT interval. A normal interval is 340 to 440 milliseconds.

Cardiovascular disease
Greek diet reduces **inflammation**

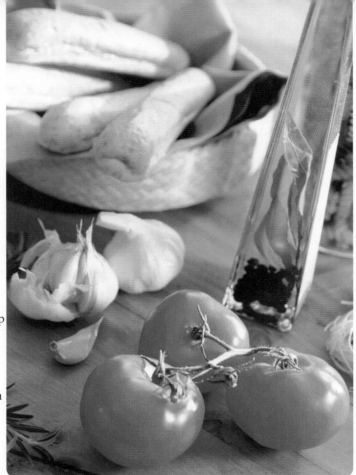

Scientists may have just uncovered the mystery of the Mediterranean diet. Since the 1970s, doctors and nutritionists alike have praised the traditional Greek diet as being particularly heart healthy, but exactly how a cuisine rich in olive oil, fruits, fish and vegetables (and short on red meat) might help the heart was not totally clear. Some experts believe the diet's effect on blood pressure is responsible; others point to cholesterol reduction. They may all be right – but according to new research, the Mediterranean diet does something else, too: it fights inflammation, a major contributor to heart disease.

A study involving more than 2,000 healthy Greeks used a specially developed food questionnaire to track the participants' food preferences. The participants were then divided into groups based on how closely they followed a traditional Greek-style diet. When given blood tests, the top Greek-style eaters showed 20 per cent less C-reactive protein (CRP) in their blood than people who ate a diet that was less rich in vegetables, olive oil and other foods associated with the classic Greek diet. CRP is a chemical that indicates chronic, low-level inflammation, including inflammation within artery walls. Elevated levels of CRP are now known to signal an increased risk of heart disease, because the inflammation ultimately leads to dangerously fragile blockages in the blood vessels, which could lead to a heart attack. Those who ate the traditional Greek cuisine also had fewer other signs of inflammation.

Another recent Greek study offered more proof of the heart-protecting power of the Mediterranean diet. Researchers at the University of Athens Medical School followed more than 22,000 volunteers for 44 months. Those who most closely followed the traditional Greek diet had a much lower risk of death from heart disease.

RESEARCH ROUND-UP

Tummy tuck tissue to heal hearts?
Body tissue extracted during tummy tuck procedures may one day be put to good use in healing damaged hearts. Tissue generally referred to as 'body fat' also contains large numbers of non-fatty (stromal) cells that can be separated from tissue removed through procedures such as liposuction. According to test-tube research being performed by scientists in France and the United States, these stromal cells can be coaxed to develop into other types of tissue, including blood vessel and heart tissue.

Researchers believe that these cells could then be injected (using a catheter) into areas needing repair and improved blood flow, such as a damaged region of the heart or a blocked artery. One major benefit of this approach is that unlike a transplanted heart, for instance, the stromal cells won't be rejected by the immune system because the body recognizes them as its own.

Cardiovascular disease
Controversial **calcium scans** have their day

Many heart attacks occur without any warning. How can you know if you're at risk? One way is to have a scan that detects calcium deposits within the coronary arteries. The scans, known as electron-beam computed tomography (EBCT), are available only at a few private clinics in Britain and have been considered by some doctors to be an expensive waste of time. Now, however, new research shows that for some people – those seemingly at moderate risk of heart disease – they may indeed be worth the money.

In EBCT, a beam of electrons (invisible particles of energy) is aimed at targeted parts of your heart as you lie flat on a table that glides into position within the scanning machine. Powerful magnets detect the electrons as they pass through your body. The images that result can show minute details, including calcium deposits on the lining of the arteries. Some doctors think that those layers of calcium – which have nothing to do with your dietary calcium intake – form around plaques in order to keep them from bursting and causing a heart attack. But regardless of why they form, the bottom line is clear: the more calcium deposits you have in your arteries, the more plaques you have.

Who can benefit? EBCT scans are worthless for people who already know they are at high risk for heart attacks. What would be the point of further proof? Their doctors already know that they need aggressive treatment. The scans are probably also a waste of time and money for people who already know their risk is very low (for instance, those who are under 45, have never smoked, and have low cholesterol levels, low blood pressure and no family history of heart problems). It's the 'in-betweeners' who, according to findings from three US medical schools, could benefit from the additional information an EBCT scan provides.

How do you know if you're in-between? A person's risk of cardiovascular disease is usually measured by a grading system called the Framingham scale, which takes into account risk factors including cholesterol levels, smoking, blood pressure, family history and diabetes. People with high Framingham scores are considered at high risk; those with low scores are considered at low risk.

About 40 per cent of adults have a Framingham score somewhere in the middle – neither dangerously high nor safely low. Their risk may not be considered high enough to warrant treatment with drugs – unless the EBCT shows trouble.

The new study, published in the *Journal of the American Medical Association* in January 2004, followed more than 1,400 people who were at risk for heart disease. All of them were scored on the Framingham scale and received EBCT scans. They were then contacted yearly for eight years. In the end, among people with mid-range Framingham scores, those with the highest arterial calcium levels also had the greatest risk of heart attack or death from heart disease.

What it means If you think you're at moderate risk for a heart attack, consider asking your GP about where you might be able to have an EBCT scan. Be aware, however, that currently the test is unavailable on the NHS and you will have to pay for it. Also know that if your scan shows no calcium deposits, it doesn't mean you can feel free to eat all the hamburgers and chips that you want; in the study, seven of 195 'moderate-risk' people with calcium scores of zero had heart attacks.

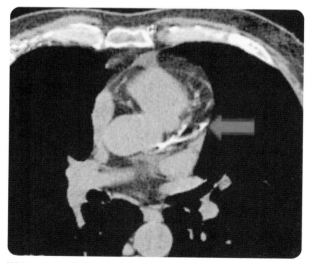

White areas of this scan indicate calcium deposits – meaning there is plaque in the arteries, increasing heart attack risk.

Deadly heart attack
gene discovered

If you could take a simple blood test that would let you know if you were at greatly increased risk of a heart attack and stroke, would you do it? Scientists have found a gene mutation that nearly doubles the risk of both. The discovery was made by a team led by deCODE Genetics, a developer of drugs and diagnostic tests, during a study of 296 families in Iceland.

The mutation is a change in the genetic code of a gene called ALOX5AP, which is involved in inflammation – now considered a leading cause of heart disease. The mutated gene is believed to increase the production of a chemical identified in the blood of people who have a history of heart attack. The researchers speculate that the chemical, leukotriene B4, is an indicator of inflammation in artery walls, which contributes to plaque formation.

A test to detect the chemical isn't currently available, since developing such tests often takes two to three years. Meanwhile, the deCODE group has also begun clinical trials of a drug designed to inhibit the gene's activity and dampen its damaging effects.

Other genes that increase the risk of cardiovascular disease have also been identified. If you learn through genetic testing that you have an increased risk of heart attack, it's all the more important to be vigilant about maintaining a heart-healthy lifestyle by exercising, eating a balanced diet and keeping stress levels down.

Cardiovascular disease
New reasons to **imbibe** a bit

Doctors know that moderate drinking – a daily glass of wine, beer, or spirits – lowers the risk of a heart attack. No one's exactly sure why, but alcohol does seem to raise levels of HDL (the 'good' cholesterol that sweeps up LDL, or 'bad' cholesterol), while helping to 'thin' the blood to prevent dangerous blood clots. But according to new research, alcohol may also counter a process now thought to be intimately linked with heart disease: inflammation.

Inflammation is the body's response to injury, whether from a cut, invasion by bacteria, or some other assault – such as the attack on artery walls by LDL cholesterol. Researchers have recently linked heart attacks to arterial inflammation, a process that encourages plaque to accumulate inside artery walls and causes clumps of plaque to burst. In the body, inflammation can be measured indirectly by determining levels of chemicals called C-reactive protein (CRP) and interleukin-6 (IL-6).

Researchers in Italy measured these chemicals in 2,574 men and women aged 70 to 79. The volunteers also filled out questionnaires detailing their drinking habits. Sure enough, levels of CRP and IL-6 were lowest in people who drank one to seven alcoholic beverages each week.

Don't take the news as permission to drink with abandon, however. The researchers found that people who had eight drinks or more a week were more likely to have higher levels of CRP and IL-6, possibly because regular consumption of more than about one unit a day may lead to early-stage liver disease – indicated by increased levels of the two inflammation markers measured.

Mentally, men fare better after bypass

Men and women can both benefit from bypass surgery, but for women, the benefits may be smaller. A study at Duke University Medical Center in North Carolina looked at a group of men and women who were about to undergo the surgery. Before surgery and a year later, each patient took a series of tests that measured life-quality factors, including depression, anxiety and perception of health. At the one-year mark, the women had more depression and anxiety and felt that their ability to carry out their daily activities had decreased since the surgery.

Why the difference? One reason may be that the surgery just doesn't help women as much as it helps men. Women have smaller arteries, and the blood vessels used in bypass surgery tend not to last as long. After surgery, women typically show less improvement in angina symptoms and spend more days in bed.

Cardiovascular disease

Bypass surgery? Tell your doctor to **cool it**

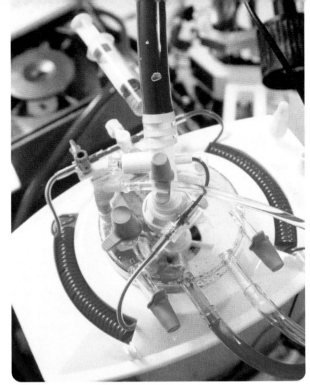
A heart-lung machine adds oxygen to a patient's blood, removes carbon dioxide, and returns the blood to the body.

If you're about to undergo coronary artery bypass, consider this: people who have the surgery may have memory and concentration problems afterwards. In fact, up to one-third of bypass patients report some mental impairment following surgery. Now, researchers at Duke University in Durham, North Carolina, think they have worked out what the problem is – as well as a solution.

Bypass surgery typically involves using a heart-lung machine to temporarily take over for the heart by mechanically pumping blood throughout the body. This allows the surgeon the advantage of working on a motionless heart. (Technology now allows some bypass surgeries to be performed on beating hearts, but most still rely on heart-lung machines.) When blood is circulated through the machine, it is cooled to a relatively low temperature – approximately 30°C (86°F) – to help protect the brain and other organs from damage during surgery. When the surgery is over, the blood must be rewarmed to normal body temperature; the heart-lung machine does this by gradually increasing the temperature of the blood as it passes through the pumping equipment.

Heating the circulating blood too quickly can cause the core of the brain to become overheated. This overheating, called hyperthermia, is known to cause cognitive problems. According to the Duke researchers, who analysed more than 6,000 cases of bypass surgery, nearly all patients who underwent bypass before 1993 became hyperthermic. The analysis exposed the problem of overheated blood, and Duke doctors now take the necessary steps to rewarm patients' blood more slowly.

The researchers hope to spread the message of the danger of rapid blood rewarming to other medical centres. They recommend that doctors spend an extra 10 to 15 minutes warming blood slowly to avoid overheating delicate brain tissue.

British surgeons are also aware of the problem and studies have been carried out to determine the best way of monitoring blood temperature in the brain. Researchers at Queen Elizabeth Hospital in Birmingham found that conventional peripheral measurements of blood temperature may underestimate the real temperature in the brain.

RESEARCH ROUND-UP

Good mates protect your heart

Engaging in 'male' activities – think watching football and tinkering with the car – can be good for the heart, at least when men do them together. According to a Swedish study, men who have a support group of friends are much less likely to develop heart disease than those who tend to go it alone. The researchers followed 741 50-year-old men for 15 years. The men who regularly spent time with good friends were almost half as likely to be diagnosed with heart disease as those with the least social interaction. Researchers also discovered a greatly reduced heart disease risk in the men who were most emotionally attached to their friends. So boys, now you have the perfect excuse for a lads' night out – you'll be doing your heart a favour.

Cardiovascular disease

Bypass may (still) be better for you

Sometimes a new, 'easy' way to get something done just isn't as reliable as a time-honoured technique. Although angioplasty is the more modern, less invasive treatment for coronary artery disease, a surprising study showed that bypass surgery saves more lives.

Bypass uses open-heart surgery to literally bypass the damaged artery by stitching in a healthy section of blood vessel. Angioplasty, on the other hand, is much less invasive and requires a fraction of the recovery time. In angioplasty, instead of cutting open the patient's chest, the doctor reaches the blocked artery by inserting a catheter via a narrow slit (usually in the groin, sometimes in the armpit), then uses tiny tools to clear out the blocked arteries and prop them open with miniature wire tubes called stents.

In recent years the number of angioplasties performed in Britain has increased while bypass surgery has remained static. Current Department of Health target rates for the two interventions are roughly 50:50.

Why bypass may be better Heart doctors who regularly perform angioplasty, including Dr Sorin J. Brener, a cardiologist at the Cleveland Clinic in Ohio, were extremely sceptical of the idea that open-heart surgery might be preferable for the highest-risk patients. However, the study led by Dr Brener that compared the two procedures showed that traditional bypass surgery delivered longer-lasting results than angioplasty, which opens up relatively small sections of artery. The results were published in the May 2004 issue of the journal *Circulation*.

'My own findings surprised me,' says Dr Brener. He found that for nearly 900 patients 'at the worst end of the illness spectrum' (people with heart disease plus diabetes or high blood pressure), the potential surgical complications and tougher recovery were worth it. Five

In coronary bypass surgery, healthy blood vessels are taken from the leg and grafted onto the heart. This bypasses clogged arteries, improving blood flow to the heart.

years after surgery, patients who had their diseased or blocked arteries completely bypassed had close to half the risk of dying from heart disease compared to similar patients who had undergone angioplasty.

Choose the right hospital Where a patient has the surgery matters. Dr Brener says that the results of his study were greatly influenced by the Cleveland Clinic's above-average rate of surgical success – the clinic boasts bypass-related mortality rates that are about a third of the US national average. Bypass performed at another hospital with less experienced staff may not be the better option compared with angioplasty at the same location, he says. If choosing between bypass surgery and angioplasty, Dr Brener suggests requesting as much information as possible about the hospital's rates of complication and death. In the UK, hospital performance statistics are already widely available, and can be accessed on the internet at: www.nhs.uk/Root/Performanceratings/Default.asp

Heart failure
Statins for heart failure

You probably think of statins as cholesterol-lowering drugs, but a study published in February 2004 showed that these drugs may also dramatically reduce the risk of death from heart failure when added to standard treatment.

Millions of people around the world have heart failure, in which the heart loses the ability to pump enough blood through the body. There are between 600,000 and 900,000 people with heart failure in the UK, who are at risk of hospitalization and death from the condition. 'New heart failure medications are urgently needed,' says Dr Gregg Fonarow, professor of medicine in the division of cardiology at the University of California, Los Angeles, and coauthor of the study. 'Our research shows that statins offer the potential to provide additional benefits to patients who are already on standard medical treatment for heart failure,' he adds.

Statins, which include atorvastatin (Lipitor) and pravastatin (Lipostat), are often prescribed to treat both high cholesterol and coronary artery disease, but medical experts have been unsure whether the drugs would help or hurt heart failure patients.

First of all, people with heart failure frequently have low cholesterol, so using a cholesterol-lowering drug didn't seem to make much sense. In addition, some researchers worried that statins might have negative effects when used for heart failure, because the drugs lower levels of coenzyme Q_{10}, a heart-protective substance produced by the body.

Other experts, though, had a suspicion that statins could save the lives of some patients. Dr Fonarow and his colleagues followed 551 people with heart failure. In addition to taking standard medication, nearly half of the group was also taking statins to treat other heart-related problems. Over the course of one year, those taking statins had a reduced need for heart transplants and a substantial 55 per cent reduction in the risk of dying from heart failure.

How it works Statins may help heart failure patients in a number of ways, says Dr Fonarow. They may reduce inflammation in the heart and blood vessels, rejuvenate damaged heart tissue by improving blood flow to the area, or somehow improve the way the nervous system controls heart function. All of these effects could help reduce the incidence of heart attack and death. Adding statins to existing treatment is safe for people with heart failure, the researchers concluded.

Availability In the UK you can now buy simvastatin (Zocor) without prescription, in consultation with your pharmacist.

Implanted defibrillators: more people could benefit

For people who have had heart attacks due to heart failure, surgically implanted defibrillators – those 'guardian angels' that monitor heart rhythm and automatically administer an electric jolt if it should go awry – are godsends. But according to a recent study, even more people could benefit from them, including those with moderately severe heart failure who have never had heart attacks.

The study, sponsored by the US National Heart, Lung and Blood Institute, looked at more than 2,500 patients at nearly 150 hospitals in the United States, Canada, and New Zealand. The participants had all been diagnosed with heart failure; 52 per cent had had heart attacks, and 48 per cent had heart failure stemming from viral heart infections. The study showed that defibrillators reduced sudden death by 23 per cent. After five years, only 28.9 per cent of people who had implanted defibrillators had died, compared with more than 36 per cent of those who didn't have the devices.

The US study also compared the benefits of defibrillators with that of a drug that can prevent irregular heartbeat. People who got only the anti-arrhythmia drug had a 28 per cent chance of dying from the problem, substantially more than the 17 per cent chance for those who had defibrillators.

There's a catch, of course. Although you can't put a price on saving a life, defibrillators cost around £10,000 (not including the cost of surgery). In the UK implanted defibrillators are used only in patients who have a history of serious dysrhythmias who are at very high risk of sudden cardiac death.

Say goodnight to high blood pressure

If you have high blood pressure, you may want to check your body clock. A small study at the Netherlands Institute for Brain Research showed that men with high blood pressure lowered their nighttime readings with regular use of melatonin, a hormone often used in supplement form for insomnia and jet lag. 'Melatonin could be a very good candidate for future therapeutics,' said Dr Nelson Chong, Coulson lecturer in molecular cardiology at the University of Leicester. 'It is one that has been pretty much overlooked previously, as most people have associated it only with sleep disorders.' Researchers stress, however, that anyone with high blood pressure should continue with their medication until larger studies clarify who might benefit from melatonin.

Hands up for better blood pressure

Want lower blood pressure? Just raise your hand. A study featured in a January 2004 issue of the journal *Annals of Internal Medicine* tested the blood pressure of 100 men and women when they had their arms raised to chest level and then dangling at their sides while they were standing, seated and lying down.

The researchers found that regardless of their overall body position, the test subjects' blood pressure was lower when their arms were raised than when their arms were resting at their sides.

The researchers did not make any suggestions as to how patients should hold their arms during a blood pressure reading. Current best practice when taking blood pressure is to ensure that the arm is supported and held horizontal at the level of the heart. If the arm is below heart level systolic and diastolic pressure will be overestimated and if it is held above heart level the readings will be underestimated.

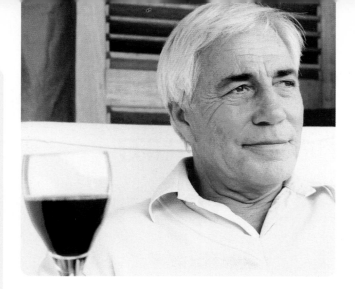

High blood pressure
The pressure is off: moderate drinking is okay

If you have high blood pressure, your doctor has probably warned you that drinking alcohol could put you at risk for even higher blood pressure or other health problems. According to new research, though, the heart-protective benefits of moderate drinking may outweigh any negative effects on blood pressure.

Researchers from the University of Massachusetts Medical School analysed data from the Physicians' Health Study, a huge initiative involving more than 80,000 male doctors who contribute to medical research by submitting annual health questionnaires. Specifically, they looked at some 14,000 men who had past or current high blood pressure but no history of heart attack or stroke at the outset of the study. The men who drank alcohol regularly – lightly or moderately – had a lower risk of death from heart disease than those who didn't.

'Alcohol does not lower blood pressure per se,' says Howard Sesso, M.P.H., Sc.D., assistant professor of medicine at Brigham and Women's Hospital in Boston and coauthor of the study. 'However, we found that among men with hypertension, drinking no more than one drink a day reduced their risk of dying from cardio-vascular disease.' Dr Sesso says it is most likely the ethanol (the type of alcohol in all alcoholic beverages) that does the trick. Scientists believe that ethanol may protect the heart by raising good cholesterol and preventing dangerous blood clots.

High cholesterol
Super-low cholesterol a super idea

Think your cholesterol is low enough? Think again, because 'low enough' may be getting lower. A recent experiment showed that cutting cholesterol to well below the current recommended level could significantly reduce the risk of death from cardiovascular disease.

The eye-opening study was led by researchers at Harvard and Brigham and Women's Hospital in Boston. They found that for people with unstable angina or those recovering from heart attacks, a drug that aggressively lowers 'bad' LDL cholesterol – far below the level currently recommended – kept arteries clearer and prevented more heart disease-related deaths than the standard cholesterol-lowering drug. The findings may mean that all of us could benefit from cholesterol levels that are even lower than those previously considered safe.

The power of high-dose statins The study was the first to pit the older statin drug pravastatin (Lipostat) against the newer and more potent atorvastatin (Lipitor). Pravastatin was designed to reduce LDL cholesterol to 100mg/dL (milligrams per decilitre of blood), the accepted target for people at high risk. With high-dose atorvastatin, the aim was to get LDL levels down to 70mg/dL.

More than 4,000 people who had heart attacks or chest pain at 350 hospitals in eight different countries took part. People who got atorvastatin typically saw their LDL cholesterol drop right down to 62mg/dL – and it paid off. After two years, only 22.4 per cent of those people had further heart-related problems, while more than 26.3 per cent of people who took pravastatin had either died, had heart attacks or strokes, required bypass surgery, or been hospitalized for severe angina.

Not surprisingly, the super-powered statin drug is more expensive and carries a slightly higher risk of side effects. The benefits of the stronger drug regimen, however, may outweigh any of those concerns, according to Dr Christopher Cannon, Harvard cardiologist and lead researcher for the study. 'Starting today, patients going home after a heart attack should be given a high-dose statin regimen,' he says.

Benefits for everyone? Dr Cannon and his colleagues later completed an analysis of people taking atorvastatin six months after their heart attacks – when their conditions had stabilized. The results showed that atorvastatin delivered the same powerful cholesterol-lowering, heart-protecting benefit, suggesting that the drug could be useful as a preventive measure in people with no history of heart trouble. But there are dangers associated with low cholesterol levels; some studies have associated very low cholesterol levels with severe depression, anxiety and a risk of suicide. Therefore doctors are unlikely to recommend that everyone take statins as a preventive measure for heart disease.

Nevertheless people who are at high risk of coronary heart disease (even though they have had no previous events) may benefit from the approach. If you fall into that category you should discuss the situation with your GP.

Lowering cholesterol, improving survival

Lowering heart attack patients' cholesterol below current standards improves their survival, says a new study. It suggests that the newer, more potent statin drug, atorvastatin, works better with high-risk patients than the older statin drug pravastatin.

Percentage of patients taking 40mg of **pravastatin** daily who died or experienced a cardiac event, such as a new heart attack.

Percentage of patients taking 80mg of **atorvastatin** daily who died or experienced a cardiac event, such as a new heart attack.

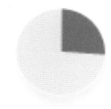

26 per cent

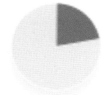

22 per cent

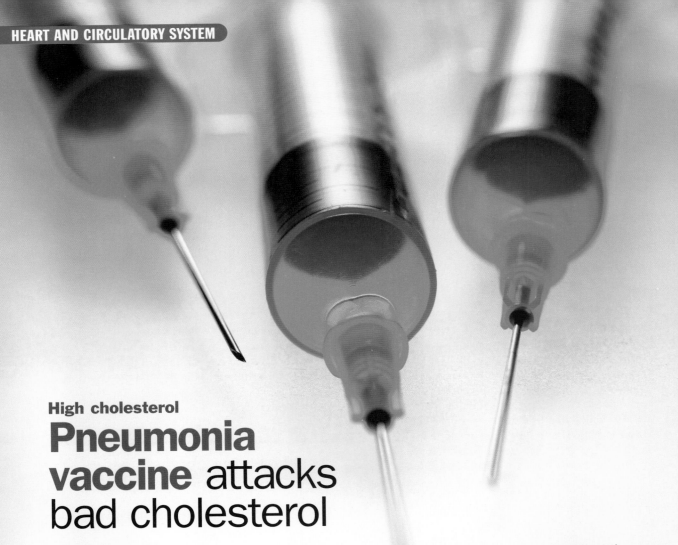

High cholesterol
Pneumonia vaccine attacks bad cholesterol

High cholesterol may someday be treated – or even prevented – with a familiar, low-tech vaccine that will protect your arteries from sticky plaque.

Immunologists and cholesterol experts working together at the University of California, San Diego, have found that in mice, a simple pneumonia vaccine can help protect against heart disease by increasing the body's immune response to 'bad' LDL cholesterol. Mice that were vaccinated against pneumonia showed a 21 per cent reduction in plaque build-up compared with unvaccinated mice.

How it works The vaccine works by activating a naturally present antibody – the antibody for the pneumonia bacterium. Antibodies 'flag' dangerous substances by attaching to them so the body can attack and destroy them. The pneumonia vaccine also works against LDL cholesterol because, as it turns out, the surfaces of both the pneumonia bacterium and LDL have an identical chemical marker. When the immune system is 'primed' by the pneumonia vaccine to recognize the pneumonia bugs, it also spots the bad cholesterol and binds with it. The connection disables the cholesterol and makes it less likely to stick to artery walls.

This isn't the first study to link vaccines with better heart health. A study of 286,000 elderly people hospitalized for heart disease or stroke found that they were able to leave the hospital sooner if they'd had flu shots.

What it means Should you run out and roll up your sleeve for a pneumonia vaccine to defend yourself against heart disease? Study co-author Dr Gregg Silverman says it's possible that current pneumonia vaccines deliver such a benefit, but no one is certain. 'The vaccines we studied were not specifically designed to boost this response. Based on what we now know, a more focused vaccine could be made for treating or even preventing cardiovascular disease in patients.' Research in primates is now under way.

Sickle cell disease
Treat high lung pressure – stay alive

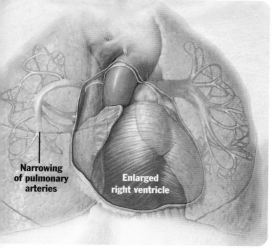

Narrowing of pulmonary arteries

Enlarged right ventricle

Pulmonary hypertension: lung arteries narrow, and the overworked heart enlarges.

Anyone with sickle cell disease should be regularly screened for high blood pressure in the arteries that deliver oxygen to the lungs. Not only is this problem very common in people with sickle cell disease – a genetic blood disorder that distorts the shape of red blood cells – but it can also be deadly.

High blood pressure in the lungs, called pulmonary hypertension, affects 20 to 40 per cent of people with sickle cell disease. Researchers believe that it's caused by sickle cell related changes that break down red blood cells and leave excess haemoglobin (the blood component that carries oxygen) floating in the bloodstream. The extra haemoglobin binds to nitric oxide, a chemical that is important for keeping blood vessels open. Without enough usable nitric oxide, blood flow in the lungs can become restricted, leading to sudden death.

A study by researchers from the USA's National Institutes of Health (NIH) recently confirmed the lifesaving value of treating pulmonary hypertension. They followed 190 men and women with sickle cell for 18 months. At the end of that period, 12 of the 62 people with pulmonary hypertension had died (20 per cent of that group), compared with only two of the 128 sickle cell patients without the lung condition (less than 2 per cent).

The increased risk of death was very high even in people with only mild or moderate pulmonary hypertension, leading one researcher to call the lung condition the 'number one predictor of sudden death syndrome' for people with sickle cell disease.

What it means to you If you or someone you know has sickle cell disease, be sure to ask about testing and treatment for pulmonary hypertension. The NIH researchers used noninvasive Doppler echocardiology, a form of ultrasound, to spot the condition. They recommend aggressive treatment, including medications that increase nitric oxide in the blood, inhaled nitric oxide gas, and blood transfusions. Drugs called calcium channel blockers (which relax blood vessels and allow more blood to get through) may also help.

FUTURE BREAKTHROUGHS

A six-in-one heart pill
Imagine popping a single pill every day that contains six powerful protective medicines to stave off heart attack and stroke. Cutting the incidence of cardiovascular disease by as much as 80 per cent is the grand idea behind the proposed Polypill, which would contain a cholesterol-lowering statin drug, three blood pressure medicines, the heart-friendly vitamin folic acid, and a small dose of clot-melting aspirin. The pill would be recommended for people aged 55 and up regardless of heart disease risk factors, since everyone stands to benefit. Clinical trials have not yet begun, however, so it could be several years before the super pill becomes available.

Red wine in a pill
If you prefer the natural approach to heart health but want or need to forgo red wine, you may soon be able to get the same benefits in a pill. Researchers at the Pavese Biochemical Institute in Pavia, Italy, have begun freeze-drying wine and condensing it into alcohol-free pills that, they say, could provide all of the known benefits of a glass of wine, including protection against heart disease. The ingredients include wine's antioxidants, which neutralize cell-damaging free radicals, contributors to heart disease. Not only would swallowing a pill be faster than drinking a glass of wine, you'd still be able to pass muster as a designated driver.

MUSCLES
BONES AND JOINTS

An ageing population: that means more cases of **osteoporosis**

So it's good news that taking a common vitamin – either singly or in a multivitamin – can help keep your bones strong and fracture-free. According to other research, supplements that contain red clover or components derived from tofu can also help, thanks to their oestrogen-like plant chemicals.

For aching joints, science is bringing out the big guns. By pairing two rheumatoid arthritis drugs never before used together, researchers have come closer to stopping the crippling disease. Thinking bigger, other researchers have taken a giant step toward using stem cells to repair joints damaged by arthritis. And one team has a startling theory about what causes most cases of osteoarthritis – one that could lead to treatments and preventive measures, previously unimagined.

In the war on pain, two old favourites for joint pain relief, glucosamine and ibuprofen, turn out to be like Astaire and Rogers, working better together than either one alone. And speaking of old favourites, there's now another reason to love Botox, the popular toxin: new research shows it works wonders for eliminating certain types of back pain.

Arthritis
Stem cells shown to reverse arthritis

Goats have joined the growing list of animals involved in stem cell research. Unlike the cats, sheep, and mice that have been cloned using stem cells, however, these goats aren't being replicated. Instead, scientists are using stem cells to cure the animals' arthritis.

The stem cells involved are not the controversial embryonic stem cells culled from the earliest stages of life. Rather, they are adult stem cells that survive throughout life in bone marrow, muscle tissue and the bloodstream.

How it works Like embryonic stem cells, adult stem cells seem to have the ability to become just about any type of tissue in the body, and they are capable of replicating almost indefinitely. Thus, they serve as remarkable little 'repair engines'. Researchers had already shown that adult stem cells can be used to repair some human organ tissues, such as the heart. Up until now, though, it was uncertain whether they could successfully mend the notoriously hard-to-repair cartilage and bone found in joints. The goats have helped to answer that question.

Researchers from Osiris Therapeutics in Baltimore, USA, extracted stem cells from the goats' bone marrow and allowed them to multiply in a petri dish. Then they injected some 10 million of the

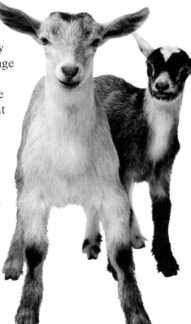

Arthritis hope. Stem cells repaired worn tissue in goats' knees.

TOP trends

ARTHRITIS? YOU'RE NOT ALONE

According to the Arthritis Research Campaign (ARC) the number of people with arthritis could be far greater than previously thought. The ARC had estimated that around 8 million people suffer from arthritis and joint pain in the UK, but a recent MORI poll revealed that 13 million people believe they are affected by the condition. The discrepancy is thought to be due to the way the data was collected. The previous figure had been based on the number of people visiting their GP about the condition. The MORI survey asked people directly about their current health and so produced a higher number.

It would appear that many people are often simply treating themselves with painkillers rather than consulting their GP – a real concern as there is now so much that can be done to help the condition and new treatments are being developed all the time. So the best advice is to take yourself to a doctor's surgery as soon as you suspect anything is wrong.

KNEE REPLACEMENT SURGERY KICKS OFF

In the UK, knee-replacement operations have more than doubled in the last decade, according to Bristol University's Department of Social Medicine. The figures, published in the July 2004 issue of the *Annals of Rheumatic Diseases*, were revealed after researchers examined hospital statistics in England between 1991 and 2000. First-time knee replacements more than doubled while the number of people having repeat surgery rose by 300 per cent.

But the data also highlighted a worrying inequality of access to the operation. It found that people who are the most well off are more likely to have the surgery irrespective of need. This seems to suggest that those who can afford to do so are having private operations rather than enduring the NHS waiting lists.

Rates of primary surgery were higher among women and among those aged between 65 and 79. With an ageing population and improving techniques, the authors say, it is likely that the very elderly will soon be considered suitable for surgery.

The future of arthritis relief?

A close-up of a goat's knee tissue shows early-stage arthritis damage (top) and repair after stem cell treatment (bottom)

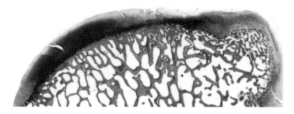

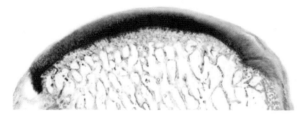

cells into the goats' arthritic knees. The result? Joint tissue that had been worn away by arthritis began to grow back. The progression of cartilage damage was significantly slowed, and bone erosion was reduced.

The study also showed that stem cell therapy may be useful for preventing knee arthritis as well as treating it, since timely joint repair discourages cartilage damage from progressing to full-blown arthritis. The results were published in the December 2003 issue of the medical journal *Arthritis and Rheumatism*.

Availability Since goats aren't people, a lot of work must be done before stem cell transplantation becomes a proven and safe treatment for human arthritis. Several human studies are already under way. Scientists from the Avon Orthopaedic Centre in Bristol are hoping to treat osteoarthritis patients with the therapy. Patients requiring a hip or knee replacement will have stem cells harvested from their bone marrow. The cells will be cultured in laboratories and replaced in the joint where it is hoped they will grow into the natural joint tissue, effecting a repair. Meanwhile researchers at Leeds University are aiming to develop the in situ 'tissue engineering' so that they can repair the cartilage in knee joints, eventually allowing younger patients to avoid a total knee replacement until later in life.

Arthritis

Two-drug mix may knock out rheumatoid arthritis

In rheumatoid arthritis, the joints are attacked by the body's immune system and systematically destroyed. For the 600,000 people who have to endure the cripplingly painful symptoms of rheumatoid arthritis in the UK, there is no single drug that can halt the disease, although medicines known as DMARDs (disease-modifying anti-rheumatic drugs) and TNF (tumour necrosis factor) inhibitors can ease symptoms and slow the damage. Now it appears that an unusual approach – using both types of drugs at the same time – is much more effective than using either type alone. The drug regimen works so well, in fact, that it seems to stop the disease in its tracks.

That's what Swedish researchers found when they studied 686 rheumatoid arthritis patients from across Europe and Australia. The patients were divided into three groups. One group received both the DMARD methotrexate (Maxtrex) and the TNF inhibitor etanercept (Enbrel); the others received either one drug or the other.

After one year, joint damage was slowed significantly more in the volunteers who were treated with both drugs. More than 33 per cent of those patients virtually stopped having arthritis symptoms while on the drugs, compared with 13 per cent on methotrexate alone and 16 per cent on etanercept alone. The study results were published in the British medical journal *The Lancet* in February 2004.

How it works The two drugs tackle the condition in different ways. Methotrexate works by suppressing the overactive immune system that triggers the rheumatoid arthritis. Etanercept has a different mechanism – it works by interfering with the activity of TNF, a protein that's a major culprit in the swelling and joint damage caused by this type of arthritis. Having

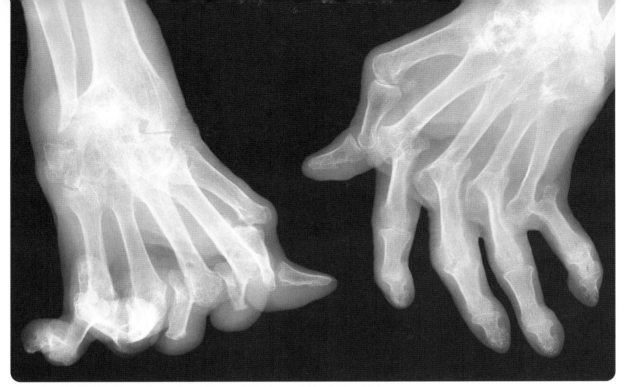

The red on this X-ray indicates fingers bent abnormally by rheumatoid arthritis. Joints damaged by the disease can become inflamed and painful, limiting movement.

different methods of action doesn't necessarily guarantee that medications can work together effectively and doctors would not normally prescribe medication in this way. But the Swedish study has shown that the two drugs in this particular combination have a 'synergistic' effect (the two together work better than either on its own).

'If we initiate treatment with etanercept in combination with methotrexate, we can stop the inflammatory process,' says study author Dr Lars Klareskog Ph.D., from the Karolinska Institute in Stockholm. 'The body recovers and can begin to heal.'

Availability You can ask your GP now about combination therapy, but the study authors expect progress toward routine use of the treatment to be gradual. Further studies are needed to determine long-term safety and identify which patients are most likely to benefit from the therapy.

Studies are planned to test the drug combination's effectiveness in people who have been recently diagnosed as having rheumatoid arthritis. (The Swedish study looked at patients who had had the disease for an average of 6½ years.) The hope is that treating the disease with the two drugs very early in its progression will be effective enough to actually heal joint damage.

RESEARCH ROUND-UP

Arthritis medications' heart-saving bonus

The drugs you're taking for rheumatoid arthritis may be reducing your risk of heart disease, including heart failure. One of those drugs, the immune system suppressant methotrexate (Maxtrex), is already known to do so. Now, new research, published in the March 2004 issue of the *American Journal of Medicine*, shows that drugs called TNF inhibitors, such as infliximab (Remicade) and etanercept (Enbrel), also help guard against heart disease. This is a welcome finding, since the drugs were previously suspected of worsening certain heart conditions.

The protective effect of the drugs will also be a source of comfort, since this and previous studies have shown that having rheumatoid arthritis raises the risk of heart failure and other kinds of heart disease, including fatal heart attacks. The reason behind this has long puzzled the scientific community and researchers from the University of Leicester are currently trying to find an answer. They will be looking to see if a genetic factor is involved.

Arthritis

A new powerful hitter in the **anti-arthritis** line up

A rheumatoid arthritis drug that works wonders for one person may be useless to another. That's why doctors depend on having a variety of options to choose from. The next option that may one day be added to the doctors' 'box of tricks' is a powerful drug that suppresses the immune system. It's so powerful, in fact, that it's currently used to prevent organ rejection in transplant recipients. Since rheumatoid arthritis is caused by an overactive immune system, immunosuppressants make up a key treatment category.

The drug, tacrolimus (Prograf), is already being prescribed for arthritis 'off-label' – that is, outside the use for which it was approved – in a number of countries. Most doctors in the UK, however, would need the drug to be approved specifically for rheumatoid arthritis before prescribing it for that purpose. But a recent study, reported in the British medical journal *Rheumatology* in March 2004, brought that approval a step closer.

What the study showed A team of researchers from Arizona recruited almost 900 rheumatoid arthritis patients to the study. All of the participants had been treated unsuccessfully with disease-modifying anti-rheumatic drugs (DMARDs), the most common class of rheumatoid

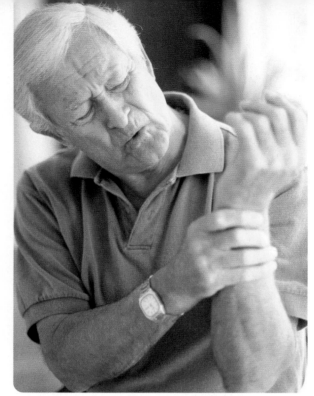

Not satisfied with your current rheumatoid arthritis medicine? A powerful new alternative is on the way.

arthritis medications. All of them were given Prograf daily. After 14 months, the researchers found that the drug benefited a significant portion of these users: about 26 per cent showed at least a 70 per cent improvement in swollen and painful joints. However, many of the volunteers reported side effects, such as headache and diarrhoea. Other serious side effects have been connected to the drug including pneumonia and even diabetes.

Availability The drug was expected to be approved for rheumatoid arthritis treatment in Japan by the end of 2004. In Europe and the United States, where more studies were still under way in 2004, approval will take a year or two longer.

Want arthritis relief?
Treat your depression

If you feel better, so will your joints, suggests a study of more than 1,800 depressed elderly people in five American states, which found that aggressive treatment of depression has a welcome side effect: less arthritis pain. A lot of people stand to benefit from this discovery as four out of five adults over the age of 70 have arthritis and about one in six has depression.

Researchers have known for a while that some antidepressant drugs can reduce pain under certain circumstances but their success as pain relievers has been inconsistent. This latest study showed that people who took antidepressants and underwent psychotherapy experienced less arthritis pain (not to mention fewer depressive symptoms) after 12 months than people who simply took medication. No one fully understands why.

Arthritis
Double-barrelled relief for **joint pain**

Millions of people take glucosamine to prevent damage to bones and cartilage. The supplement (a synthetic version of a substance found in the body) has also been shown to help repair joint damage. Now, researchers from Temple University in Philadelphia have discovered that glucosamine has a third trick up its sleeve: providing relief from joint pain. The only catch is that you need to combine it with ibuprofen.

Glucosamine appears to have no pain-blocking effect of its own (although, of course, reducing joint damage lessens pain, which is why people taking the supplement often feel better). When the researchers tested glucosamine along with ibuprofen on mice, it noticeably boosted the power of the pain reliever. This 'drug synergy' didn't happen when glucosamine was teamed with other painkillers, such as aspirin.

The next step is to find out whether the combo has the same effect in humans. Studies are already under way. The result may be a single pill containing the optimal doses of both ibuprofen and glucosamine to deliver immediate pain relief along with ongoing joint benefits. Meanwhile, it may be best to consult your GP about using the two together, particularly if you are taking other medications. Glucosamine is now available on prescription.

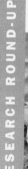

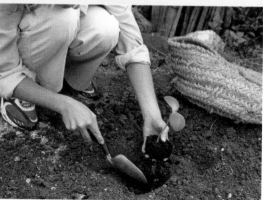

RESEARCH ROUND-UP

Squatting – a risk factor for arthritis of the knee?

Amateur gardeners in the Western world and typical residents of China's capital city have at least one thing in common: they squat a lot. As a result, they're statistically more likely to have arthritis of the knee later in life. According to a study of more than 1,800 Chinese men and women over age 60, the more you squat in early adulthood, the higher your risk of eventually developing knee arthritis (a specific type of arthritis called tibiofemoral osteoarthritis).

Rheumatologists had often wondered why knee arthritis rates are higher in China than in the West, even though obesity (a major arthritis risk factor) is less of a problem there. The answer seems to be that squatting is a traditional resting and working position in China. In the study, many residents of Beijing reported having squatted for more than three hours a day in their 20s. Those people were twice as likely to develop knee arthritis in their 60s as people who reported squatting less often.

The study, published in April 2004, confirms previous British research showing that people whose work involves squatting have a greater risk of developing arthritis.

Is it rheumatoid arthritis?
An earlier test can tell you

Is the joint pain that's been bothering you caused by osteoarthritis or the more serious disease rheumatoid arthritis? It often takes years before your doctor can determine which it is. And since rheumatoid arthritis (a malfunction of the immune system) is treated differently to the age-related osteoarthritis, a delayed diagnosis also means a delayed prescription for the drugs that can help. The situation is highly undesirable, since the sooner rheumatoid arthritis is treated, the less damage the joints sustain.

That's about to change. Dutch researchers have announced that with a new diagnostic test, which measures blood levels of an antibody called anti-CCP, it's now possible to predict accurately whether early-stage arthritis will develop into rheumatoid arthritis.

In results of a 936-patient study, 93 per cent of people who tested positive for anti-CCP at the early stage of joint pain went on to develop rheumatoid arthritis within three years, compared with only 25 per cent of those who tested negative for the antibody.

An anti-CCP test is already available in the UK. Known as the DIASTAT anti-CCP assay, it is being produced by Axis-Shield UK, based in Dundee. Ask your GP for more details.

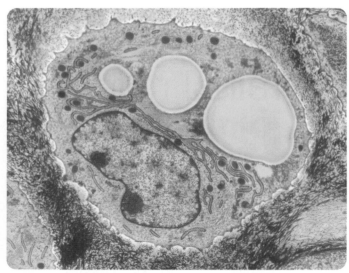

A new theory holds that ageing cartilage cells lose their ability to replicate, possibly causing arthritis. Antioxidants could extend the life of these cells.

Arthritis
What really causes arthritis?

If you have osteoarthritis, the most common form of arthritis, you've probably been told that simple wear and tear is to blame – that the cartilage that keeps the bones in the joints from rubbing against one another has been worn away by a lifetime of mechanical stress. In other words, your joints hurt because you've used them so much. That's the usual explanation, but it could be all wrong.

Research presented to the American Academy of Orthopaedic Surgeons in March 2004 points to an entirely different explanation for osteoarthritis that may assign the wear-and-tear theory to the dustbin of medical history. According to a team led by Dr Joseph Buckwalter, professor of orthopaedics at the University of Iowa in Iowa City, the cartilage damage of osteoarthritis has little to do with wear and tear and lots to do with ageing cartilage cells and that ubiquitous health 'baddie' known as oxidation.

That view, if proven correct, could open up a whole new universe of preventive strategies, treatment options, and perhaps even a cure. 'Within a few years, we hope to have some important new ways of decreasing the risk of osteoarthritis,' Dr Buckwalter says. One preventive step might be as simple as taking supplemental antioxidants such as vitamin C. This view is supported by researchers from the University of Manchester. In their study, published in the July 2004 issue of the *Annals of Rheumatic Diseases,* found that people whose diets were lacking in fresh fruit and vitamin C were more likely to develop inflammatory polyarthritis.

The real problem After analysing cartilage tissue in patients ranging in age from 1 to 87 years, Dr Buckwalter and his colleagues concluded that a major reason cartilage breaks down is that cartilage cells, known as chondrocytes, lose their ability to generate new tissue with age. The solution? Discover a way to postpone the chondrocytes' retirement. The professor and others are now working on it. 'We're already getting some interesting results in our efforts to prolong the functional life of chondrocytes,' he says.

Dr Buckwalter's analysis also pointed to another arthritis culprit: free radicals. Experts have long known that these unstable oxygen molecules, released as by-products of natural chemical reactions in the body, harm cells. The damage they cause to chondrocytes, Dr Buckwalter says, hastens the ageing of those cells and increases the risk of osteoarthritis. Joint injuries, because they bring oxygen to the cartilage as blood rushes in to heal the damage, also speed the death of chondrocytes.

A potential solution If free radicals contribute to the problem, antioxidants, which neutralize them, could be part of the solution. Antioxidants, such as vitamin C, vitamin E, and beta-carotene, are abundant in many fruits and vegetables and other foods, as well as in green tea and dietary supplements. 'Antioxidants, especially vitamin C, are useful for protecting your entire musculoskeletal system,' says Dr Nick DiNubile, clinical assistant professor of orthopaedic surgery at the Hospital of the University of Pennsylvania, Philadelphia.

A joint effort: eating fruits and vegetables that are rich in vitamin C, vitamin E, and beta-carotene may help to fend off osteoarthritis.

RESEARCH ROUND-UP

Osteoporosis drugs may do double duty

Could osteoporosis drugs such as alendronate (Fosamax) and risedronate (Actonel) also help protect against arthritis and help ease joint pain? According to one study, the answer is a resounding 'Yes'.

Researchers at the University of Tennessee studied more than 800 women, most of whom reported knee pain from osteoarthritis, the most common type of arthritis. All were 69 or older and most took some kind of medication for osteoporosis – either raloxifene (Evista), the hormone oestrogen or a bisphosphonate drug such as Fosamax or Actonel.

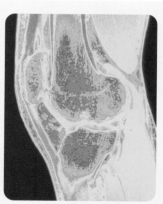

MRI scans showed that women who took osteoporosis drugs called bisphosphonates experienced less severe arthritis.

MRI scans showed that women who had taken bisphosphonates in the months or years preceding the study had, on average, less severe knee arthritis than those who'd either been taking another type of osteoporosis drug or weren't taking any medication for osteoporosis.

The bisphosphonate users also tended to have less knee pain and suffered less from arthritis-related problems, such as bone marrow swelling, bone spurs and the wearing away of the bone itself. The apparent slowing of arthritis progression may come from the drugs' ability to reduce damage from inflammation.

Back and neck pain

Simple injections
ease back pain

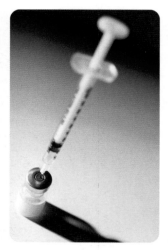

Injections to soothe your aching back may have just become cheaper and easier. Australian researchers say that the most effective ingredient in common ligament injections to treat back pain may very well be the needle itself. That surprising possibility arose in January 2004, when published study results revealed that patients who were given 'prolotherapy' injections every other week for three months reported no more improvement than those who were injected with a simple saline solution.

Prolotherapy involves injecting a substance such as phenol, glycerin, or glucose, usually blended with a local anaesthetic, directly into the ligaments in the area of pain. The prolotherapy agents are thought to speed recovery by strengthening the ligaments. But researchers from the University of Queensland found that in a group of volunteers with chronic back pain, those who received inert saline injections got the same amount of pain relief at the same rate as those who received prolotherapy.

If prolotherapy is no more helpful than saltwater, why does either treatment provide any benefit at all? 'The effect may lie in the needle rather than the specific injection solution,' say the study authors. In other words, it's possible that the needle produces a counter-irritant effect. In this phenomenon, the body's response to a new, less severe pain effectively blocks the nervous system's response to pre-existing pain.

A Swedish study has shown that sterile water injections can relieve lower back pain during the first stage of labour. Whether they work because of the counter-irritant effect or some other action, these injections disrupt what orthopaedists call the pain/spasm cycle. (First, a muscle spasm causes pain, then the body's reaction to that pain causes a spasm.) Blocking that cycle temporarily helps your body focus on healing the underlying cause of the pain. The Australian study suggests that it may be worth asking your doctor about using such an approach for your back pain.

Back and neck pain

Artificial disc
is no pain in the neck

Just a few months after having an experimental disc surgically inserted between two of her neck vertebrae, a female study volunteer accidentally drove her van into a tree. She survived, thanks to the vehicle's airbag. The artificial disc weathered the impact so well that the A&E staff called the study leaders to ask, 'What is that thing?'

The thing in question was a synthetic version of the shock-absorbing discs that keep the vertebrae in the neck from rubbing against each other and from pinching nearby nerves. These artificial discs are already being used in the UK and could save tens of thousands of people from having to choose between excruciating pain caused by damaged vertebral discs and a surgical procedure that drastically limits freedom of movement.

The indication of the artificial disc's durability provided by the woman's accident is what medical researchers call anecdotal evidence – an interesting story to be sure, but not exactly scientific proof that the disc works. In March 2004, however, researchers at Loyola University in Chicago unveiled the results of a laboratory study in which the disc withstood impact forces far beyond anything a person's spine will probably ever experience in the real world. That *does* count as scientific evidence.

How it works When our ancestors began to walk upright, they bucked the trend among mammals. Thanks to gravity, modern sedentary ways, and ever-increasing life spans, that move pretty much guaranteed that by the 21st century, virtually all adults over 40 would suffer from degeneration of the spongy disc tissue that serves as a buffer between vertebrae in the spine.

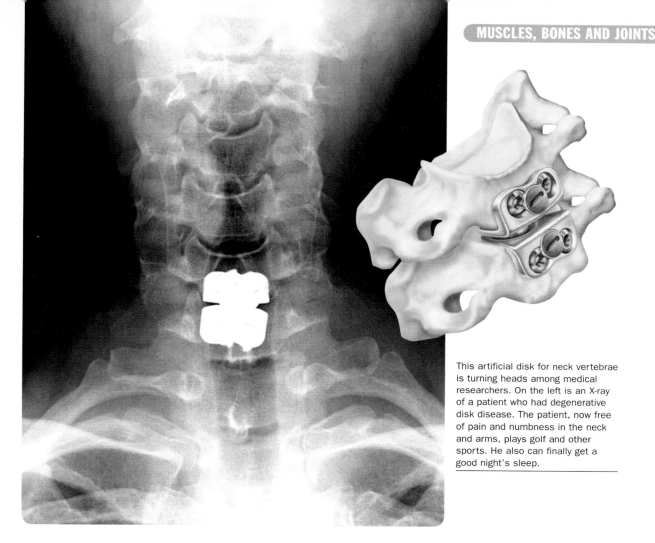

This artificial disk for neck vertebrae is turning heads among medical researchers. On the left is an X-ray of a patient who had degenerative disk disease. The patient, now free of pain and numbness in the neck and arms, plays golf and other sports. He also can finally get a good night's sleep.

When the problem occurs in any of the seven upper vertebrae that run from the base of the skull to the top of the back, it's called cervical disc disease. And it can hurt a lot.

Until recently there was only one surgical solution, known as fusion. This gives up on saving the damaged disc, instead removing it and fusing the two neighbouring vertebrae together with the help of bone grafted from the hip. Since the surgery leaves the patient with limited ability to make up-and-down or side-to-side neck movements, it is usually reserved for people whose pain has become unbearable or who are in danger of suffering serious nerve damage.

The artificial disc changes all that. Although made of metal, it serves the same protective function as a real disc. Thus, unlike fusion surgery patients, artificial disc recipients are literally as good as new, enjoying full freedom of movement. The cervical disc's design differs from that of an artificial disc meant for the lower back (lumbar disc), which has been used for several years. The new disc includes tiny screws to help firm up its placement in the neck area, where there's much more spinal movement to accommodate and less natural pressure to help hold it in place.

Availability The researchers are so pleased with the preliminary results of the ongoing study that they predict US government approval as soon as a year after the final results are evaluated in 2006. Dr Russ Nockels, one of the study leaders, thinks the availability of an artificial disc will bring about a new approach to dealing with the pain of cervical disc disease. 'The balance between the positive and negative aspects of surgery will change,' he says. 'More people will say, "Why wait?"'

In Britain similar research has been carried out into the use of cervical discs. At the London Spine Clinic, an artificial cervical disc has completed clinical trials and is already in general use.

Back and neck pain

The latest wrinkle in back pain relief: **Botox**

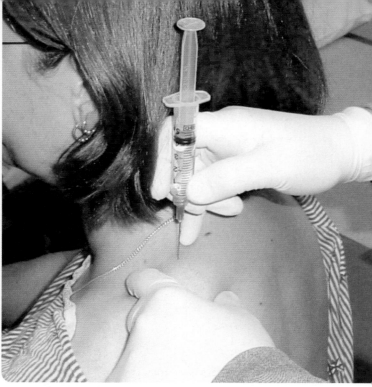

Botox injections into neck and upper back muscles give some patients relief from persistent pain for six months to a year.

Botox injections have been successfully used to treat everything from facial wrinkles and migraine headaches to bladder problems and even body odour. So why not back and neck pain as well?

Eight weeks after 25 volunteers in Georgia received injections of botulinum toxin directly into the muscles causing their persistent neck and upper-back pain, the average reported pain level dropped by nearly 40 per cent.

Botox makes perfect sense as a back pain treatment. It was, after all, originally developed to relax muscle spasms, which are often responsible for back pain. And study author Dr Amy Lang, a rehabilitation medicine specialist from Lawrenceville, Georgia, thinks the effect of Botox on upper-back muscles can go beyond pain relief. Her research appeared in the January 2004 issue of the *Journal of Pain Management*. In many cases, she says, Botox helps correct postural imbalances that may be causing the spasms.

How it works Botox's original fame as a wrinkle smoother has left the impression that it 'freezes' or 'paralyses' muscles. Instead, injecting it into painfully tense upper-back or neck muscles actually relaxes the muscles as it inhibits the release of chemicals that trigger the contraction of muscles. Further pain relief may come from Botox's interference with proteins that carry pain messages to the brain.

As Botox relaxes upper-back and neck muscles, it lengthens them from their contracted state, making it easier for them to be strengthened with physical therapy and exercise. By selecting the appropriate muscles for Botox injections and strength training, doctors can help the body realign itself, putting an end to posture-induced pain.

The number of shots needed for pain relief varies from person to person. According to Dr Lang, some people get relief for six months to a year with just one injection session. Others need regular follow-ups. The patient's attitude about the treatment counts. 'The ones who do the best are the ones who make a commitment to their own recovery,' she says. 'It's not just a matter of getting a few shots. You need to follow your physical therapy programme and make whatever ergonomic or other lifestyle adjustments needed.'

Availability A single treatment of Botox costs around £200 and this has meant that it is not routinely available on the NHS. However, it has been successful in alleviating some of the severe back pain associated with certain conditions, such as multiple sclerosis or cerebral palsy. Private clinics do offer the treatment, of course, and have been using it for lower-back pain, encouraged by other recent studies that show it relieves spasm-induced pain for as long as three to four months. The new study, although small, suggests that similar treatments make sense for the upper back and neck.

Dr Kevin Markham, a pain specialist at BUPA's Clare Park Hospital in Farnham, Surrey, says that although the treatment is not a cure, patients see more than a 50 per cent reduction in pain. If you suffer from back pain, talk to your GP about being referred to the nearest centre that is offering this treatment – but you will probably have to pay for it.

Carpal tunnel syndrome

A pain-free way to sound out **carpal tunnel**

Ultrasound, the same technology that provides expectant parents with wavy moving pictures of their developing foetuses, may soon be the diagnostic tool of choice for spotting the condition known as carpal tunnel syndrome. This condition is associated with tingling or numbness in the hand and pain in the wrist and forearm.

Egyptian researchers assembled 78 people who had carpal tunnel syndrome and 78 people who did not. They then used electromyography and ultrasound to diagnose all of them. Electromyography, which involves the insertion of wire electrodes into muscle tissue and mild electric shocks to the fingers and wrist, is an established diagnostic procedure for carpal tunnel syndrome.

The Egyptian study showed that ultrasound, which uses soundwaves to create images of the nerve that runs through the carpal tunnel in the wrist, was as good as electromyography at revealing nerve damage. But ultrasound was the clear winner in pinpointing the exact cause of the damage.

Typing and other repetitive hand movements are common causes of carpal tunnel syndrome. On the left, a patient undergoes an ultrasound scan to test for compression of the median nerve, which runs through the carpal tunnel in the wrist.

For example, ultrasound could 'see' whether the pain was the result of an inflamed tendon sheath pressing on the nerve, damage within the nerve itself, or some other cause. The study also showed that ultrasound is more effective in evaluating how well carpal tunnel patients respond to treatment.

In the UK doctors use a nerve conduction test to diagnose carpal tunnel syndrome. The test is painless, unlike electromyography, but not very reliable. With the new ultrasound technique, doctors now have a third diagnostic option that is not only painless and easy to carry out but also more reliable and more extensive in the information it provides.

Osteoporosis

Time to bone up on vitamin B_{12}

Here's yet another reason to make sure you take a multivitamin every day: the B vitamins it contains could very well help you avoid debilitating fractures. One of the 11 members of the B-vitamin family – vitamin B_{12} – has recently been shown to play a bigger role than previously thought in keeping bones strong as you grow older, fending off osteoporosis and the serious fractures that often go with it.

New research from the University of California, San Francisco, looked at how much vitamin B_{12} was circulating in the bloodstreams of 83 volunteers age 64 and up. Measurements taken over a six-year period yielded a clear finding: those who had the highest blood levels of B_{12} showed the least loss of bone density in their hips over that period, while those with the lowest levels of B_{12} showed the most bone loss.

How it works No one knows for sure why lack of B_{12} would speed bone loss. Like folate, another B vitamin,

B_{12} helps reduce levels of the protein homocysteine which has recently been linked to osteoporosis risk (as well as heart attack risk). But additional factors, as yet unknown, could be at work.

What it means to you The finding is especially important because B_{12} deficiency, rare in younger adults, is much more common in women over 60, the people who are most at risk for osteoporosis and hip fractures. If you think you may not be getting enough B_{12}, ask your GP if it's a good idea to have a blood or urine test to determine how much of the vitamin is circulating in your system. If the levels are low, you need to find out why.

Vitamin B_{12} deficiency is sometimes due to pernicious anaemia, a serious condition that requires medical treatment. It's also possible that you're simply not getting enough shellfish, milk, cheese, eggs, organ meats and other sources of vitamin B_{12} from your diet. More likely, your digestive system just isn't absorbing the vitamin B_{12} from those foods the way it used to, which means you'll need a B_{12} supplement.

The recommended daily intake of vitamin B_{12} for people aged 50 and over is 2.4mcg. Most multivitamins offer more than that, prompting the study authors to note, 'Our data indicate that long-term use of multivitamins may be an effective means of reducing B_{12} deficiency in older women.'

A rising star among bone boosters

On the periodic table of elements, you'll find strontium occupying the same vertical row as calcium and magnesium. Just like its close cousins, strontium plays a role in bone formation. Now, after decades of trying, medical researchers have discovered a way to use strontium's bone-building capacity in an osteoporosis treatment.

In January 2004, French researchers published results of a study showing that a patented strontium compound – strontium ranelate – not only increases bone density in women who have osteoporosis

but also reduces their risk of vertebral fractures. The researchers followed 1,442 women with osteoporosis who took strontium ranelate for three years. Their risk of new vertebral fractures was cut almost in half, and the bone mineral density in their lower spines increased by 14.4 per cent.

Strontium ranelate has proven so effective in recent studies that it's expected to become available in Europe sometime in 2005 in the form of a daily pill called Protelos. In the UK, strontium ranelate is currently being appraised by NICE (the National Institute for Clinical Excellence) who are scheduled to issue their decision in January 2006.

Osteoporosis
Early warning for osteoporosis

Scans and X-rays can reveal whether your bones are brittle, but by then the damage is pretty much done. The fact is, it's far easier to prevent osteoporosis than to try to cure it – but few people take the threat seriously enough to do anything to protect their bones while they still can. That could change in the coming years, now that researchers have discovered a gene variation that triples the osteoporosis risk of anyone who has it.

All of us carry the gene, dubbed BMP2 by biotech scientists at the Icelandic company deCODE Genetics, but it exists in several different variations. Three of those variants signal high osteoporosis risk. If you discover you have a high-risk variation, you'll have all the motivation you need to start taking preventive measures. Those include high calcium intake (up to 2,500mg a day), adequate vitamin D (10mcg to 15mcg a day), regular exercise, and bone-protecting prescription medication such as alendronate (Fosamax), risendronate (Actonel), or raloxifene (Evista).

Two factors were key in connecting the BMP2 gene with high osteoporosis risk: the recent completion of the human genome map and the easily traceable genealogy of Iceland's population. By scanning the genomes of 207 Icelandic families, the deCODE team was able to isolate genes common to the osteoporosis patients (living and long dead) who were analysed. The finding does not mean that BMP2 is 'the' osteoporosis gene, since researchers suspect that several other genes have variants that also contribute to osteoporosis risk. Nor does it doom its owners to brittle bones and certain fractures. It does, however, issue a loud wake-up call to people with any of the three high-risk variations of the gene, the most significant genetic risk factor for osteoporosis yet discovered.

Availability A genetic test for BMP2 won't be ready until 2006 at the earliest. First, scientists must confirm the gene's role as a risk marker in broader

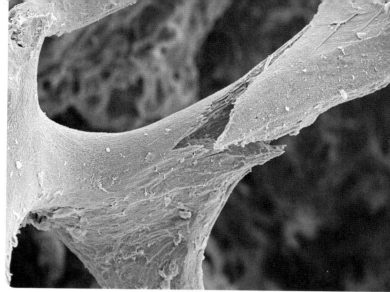

This is a magnified image of fractured bone tissue from a patient with osteoporosis. Genetic tests may soon reveal who is at high risk.

RESEARCH ROUND-UP

Safer oestrogen for your bones?

The popularity of oestrogen replacement therapies plummeted among postmenopausal women when it was shown to increase the incidence of breast cancer and heart disease. But many women over 50 have wondered if there may be a way to take advantage of oestrogen's bone-saving properties without the risks. Soon, the answer may be yes.

In August 2003, a University of Connecticut study revealed that ultra-low doses of a type of synthetic oestrogen called micronized 17 beta-estradiol clearly increased bone mineral density in older women without the negative effects associated with oestrogen. For example, none of the 167 women involved in the study developed breast cancer over the three-year study period. The rate of other unwanted side effects, such as breast tenderness and abnormal mammograms, was similar in women who took estradiol and those who took placebos (dummy pills).

As promising as this form of oestrogen seems, though, it won't be considered an osteoporosis treatment option until larger studies assess its safety over a longer period of time as well as its effectiveness in preventing fractures rather than just bone loss.

and more varied populations than Iceland's. Meanwhile, a much more limited test of fracture risk, based on a previously verified genetic marker called collagen 1A1, will be introduced in 2005.

For bone strength tofu in a capsule

Tofu, the jelly-like form of soy that's held an exalted place in Asian diets for centuries, has a new role: osteoporosis prevention. The best part is that you don't need to change your diet to benefit from tofu's bone-saving powers. A study by Israeli researchers has shown that a tofu-derived supplement boosts bone mineral density in postmenopausal women, reducing their risk of osteoporosis and the fractures that often go with it.

Researchers gave 98 volunteers either a 344mg or a 644mg daily dose of the supplement, dubbed DT56a for now, over the course of a year. While the low-dose group showed no improvement, those who received the higher dose had a significant 3.6 per cent increase in bone density in their lower spines.

Tofu's health value is attributed to its rich concentration of phytoestrogens, plant chemicals that provide many of the same benefits as the human hormone oestrogen – including bone density improvement – but without the risks that oestrogen supplementation carries.

DT56a works so well because it preserves all of the key phytoestrogens in their natural form. As a dietary supplement, DT56a is already available in capsule form in Britain, sold as Tofupill and available in health food shops.

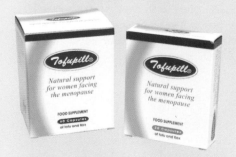

Osteoporosis
Diuretics – the new treatment for bones?

Diuretics are making a big comeback. Recently, a panel of experts designated these age-old urination-promoting medications as the first-choice treatment for high blood pressure. Now, a new study has shown that taking diuretics is also an excellent way to protect against hip fractures.

Dutch researchers studied the medical records of nearly 8,000 men and women over the age of 55. The scientists concluded that those who had been taking diuretics for at least a year had, on average, half the risk of hip fractures than those who hadn't been taking the drugs.

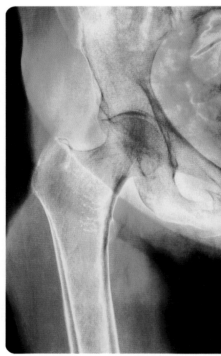

Diuretics, typically prescribed for high blood pressure, may have a welcome side effect: fewer hip fractures.

The finding makes sense because diuretics are known to slow age-related bone loss by cutting down on the amount of calcium excreted in urine. However, this study, published in the September 2003 issue of *Annals of Internal Medicine,* was the first to connect diuretic use with protection against hip fractures, which are often the consequence of the bone-wasting disease osteoporosis.

The study also found that the fracture-prevention benefits of diuretics disappear soon after you stop taking the drugs. Although the study authors consider long-term diuretic use to be safe under a doctor's supervision, they say further study is needed before diuretics can be recommended as an osteoporosis treatment for people who don't have high blood pressure.

Osteoporosis

Bone strength is boosted by clover

Worried about thinning bones? Take a tip from hungry cows. They like to graze on red clover, and it turns out that this common pasture herb packs a bone-boosting wallop. Available in supplement form, red clover is teeming with isoflavones, plant compounds that deliver the bone-protecting benefits of oestrogen without the risks associated with hormone replacement therapy. In a recent British study of 200 women aged 49 to 65, those who took red clover supplements daily lost much less bone density in the lower backbone after a year than those who didn't take them.

How it works Low oestrogen levels after menopause take much of the blame for the increased risk of osteoporosis after age 50. Since hormone replacement therapy increases the risk of heart disease and breast cancer, researchers have been looking at so-called plant oestrogens such as isoflavones as alternatives. Scientists have yet to prove the safety of these compounds, but researchers are encouraged by the relatively low rates of breast cancer and heart disease among Asian women, who eat large amounts of isoflavone-rich soy.

The British researchers didn't use soya beans as their isoflavone source, as most previous studies had. Rather, they used a supplement derived from red clover, which could explain why this was the first well-designed study of significant size to clearly show the bone-saving benefits of isoflavones. Red clover is not only richer in isoflavones than soy, it also contains different kinds of isoflavones.

Availability The researchers, who published their study results in the February 2004 issue of the *American Journal of Clinical Nutrition,* are looking for a few more answers before they'll recommend red clover to help prevent or treat osteoporosis. They want to see proof that the isoflavones will reduce fractures in addition to helping to maintain bone density. They also want to confirm that red clover's isoflavones work as well on hipbones as they do on the backbone. Since bone mass is greater in the hip, a longer study period is needed to come to any conclusions.

Red clover is available over the counter at chemists and health food stores in various forms, including teas, tinctures, capsules and tablets. The red clover product used in the study was Promensil, which is typically used to relieve menopausal discomforts.

RESEARCH ROUND-UP

Love cola? Your bones don't!

Sipping cola may be refreshing but it could also be weakening your bones. It doesn't matter if your favourite cola is Pepsi or Coke, diet or caffeine-free; a survey of the drinking habits of more than 2,500 volunteers showed that those who consumed more than three 12oz servings a day of any kind of cola had up to 5.1 per cent lower bone mineral density in their hips than those who didn't drink that much. It does matter whether you're a man or a woman, though; only women showed low bone mineral density as a result of drinking cola.

Fizzy drinks have long been suspected of weakening bones and some studies have blamed it on their caffeine content. But this study, reported in September 2003, is the first to single out colas. The research, from Tufts University in Boston, also challenges earlier assumptions by pinning the blame on cola drinking itself rather than on a concurrent decrease in calcium-rich foods, such as vegetables and dairy foods. The problem, the study leaders suspect, is that colas are loaded with phosphoric acid, which can interfere with bone formation.

IN*Brief*

▶ A blood test predicts fracture risk

Bone density tests can help reveal how vulnerable your bones are, but the calcium content they measure is not the only indicator of fracture risk. Another kind of test may soon be available to help your doctor decide early on if you need medication to combat osteoporosis. The new test measures blood levels of a protein known as RANKL; low levels of the protein indicate that there's less than a 1 per cent chance of a fracture in the next five years.

REPRODUCTION

AND SEXUALITY

Many of this year's advances have a common theme: improving the quality of **life for women**

In the arena of infertility treatment, frozen eggs have resulted in several successful pregnancies, and it is clear that egg freezing could allow women to delay childbearing or to conceive after undergoing cancer treatment. Even more remarkably, doctors have used frozen pieces of ovarian tissue to produce viable eggs, which may mean more options for women who face an early menopause because of cancer treatment.

For women with exceptionally heavy periods, there is a new technique that uses microwave energy to remove the uterine lining permanently, significantly reducing bleeding or even stopping it entirely. There is also a new birth-control pill that reduces episodes of withdrawal bleeding from 13 to 4 a year. Meanwhile, the search for a female Viagra continues, but has so far failed to yield satisfactory results.

Also, an over-the-counter fertility supplement has been proven to work and a common allergy drug helps relieve hot flushes.

Contraception
New pill means fewer 'periods'

Women in the USA taking a new contraceptive pill will have many fewer withdrawal bleeds than is the case with the conventional birth control pill. In September 2003, the Food and Drug Administration approved Seasonale, an oral contraceptive designed to cut the number of bleeds a woman experiences each year from about 13 to about 4. (These episodes are often referred to as 'periods' but, as the FPA, the British birth-control association points out, 'You don't have proper periods when you are on the pill. What you have is called a "withdrawal bleed". The bleeding – which doesn't always happen – is caused by you not taking hormones in the pill-free week.')

How it works Seasonale is exactly the same as any other birth control pill containing the hormones oestrogen and progesterone. Essentially, it tricks the body into thinking it is pregnant so that the ovaries don't release any eggs, making a real pregnancy impossible. The uterine lining builds up more or less as it would in preparation for pregnancy (although not as much) and then it is shed when the woman stops taking the hormones for a week. The only difference between Seasonale and traditional oral contraceptives is how the pills are taken. With traditional birth control pills, the woman takes the hormone pills for 21 days, then takes no pills or inactive pills for a week, during which

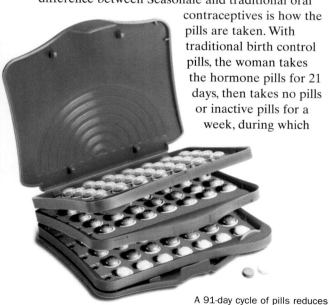

A 91-day cycle of pills reduces withdrawal bleeds to four a year.

TOP trends

BIG RISE IN TEENAGE PILL USE

Almost one in four girls aged 16 and 17 in Britain now takes the contraceptive pill – with the proportion rising from 17 to 24 per cent in the four years from 1999 to 2003, according to a survey by the Office for National Statistics. Among girls aged 16 and 17, condom use by partners also rose, from 18 to 23 per cent in four years – an important development given the rise in sexually transmitted infections.

'The survey results are very encouraging in terms of the nation's sexual health,' says Anne Weyman, the chief executive of the FPA (formerly the Family Planning Association). 'The increase in Pill use across all age groups shows that women's confidence in this highly safe and effective method continues to grow, and that they are taking less notice of the many unfounded scare stories about it.'

Although Britain has the highest rate of teenage pregnancies in Europe, the rate in girls under 18 has declined by 9.4 per cent since 1998. The increase in contraceptive use among teenagers is probably a result of improved sex education and access to services for young people, says the FPA. The number of women aged 16 to 49 who had taken the 'morning-after pill' once during the previous year was 5 per cent – a small decrease on the previous year.

FAKE VIAGRA SALES THREATENED

More and more people are buying prescription drugs online – including some 600,000 Britons annually, according to a 2003 National Audit Office report – and the popularity of some of these drugs, especially the anti-impotence medication Viagra, has spawned a multitude of illegal internet pharmacies, many selling fake pills. In August 2004, in response to this growing trade, the drug giant Pfizer, the makers of Viagra, began a legal campaign against online pharmacies pushing counterfeit versions of the drug.

The campaign aims to seize sites selling fake pills and to stop spammers sending messages offering Viagra for sale. Many of the spam messages refer to so-called generic versions of the pill. Pfizer says that there is no such thing as legal generic Viagra because such a version of the drug has not been approved by the US Food and Drug Administration. People are also warned about the health dangers of taking illegal pills or pills obtained without a doctor's prescription. Viagra should only be taken on medical advice since it could exacerbate existing health problems.

she has a withdrawal bleed. With Seasonale, women take the active pills for 12 weeks (84 days) in a row, followed by one week of inactive pills. While taking Seasonale as recommended, women will have only four bleeds a year, but initially they may have some breakthrough bleeding until their bodies adjust.

Mixed reactions The concept of a drug that enables women to have fewer 'periods' has stirred up controversy in the USA, with some women's groups expressing concern about the long-term health implications of Seasonale. They also criticize statements by the drug's manufacturer, Barr Pharmaceuticals, that menstruation has a negative effect on women's lives.

On the other hand, Michael P. Goodman, an obstetrician and gynaecologist in Davis, California, who has been practising for more than 34 years, says Seasonale is not a big shift. For years, he and other

doctors have been prescribing regular, 28-day oral contraceptives to be taken 'back to back' – that is, without the week of no pills or inactive pills – for women who have very heavy periods or who want to skip their periods for some reason. 'It's amazing the drug companies have waited so long to bring something like this to market,' says Dr Goodman, author of *The Midlife Bible: A Woman's Survival Guide*. 'I've been telling patients to take birth control pills this way for years.'

His belief in the safety of taking hormones for several months without a break is endorsed in the UK by the FPA, who think that such a routine could also reduce oral contraception failure rates. As it is, for those women who take a week's break between packs, it is much easier to forget to take the first one when starting a new pack. It is simpler just to get into the habit of taking a pill every day.

Don't blame the pill for extra pounds

Ever since the contraceptive pill was first prescribed more than 40 years ago, it has been blamed by some women for weight gain. In fact, about 20 per cent of women either cease taking the Pill or avoid it altogether because of concerns about gaining weight. One study found that women who gave up oral contraceptives were more likely to say they had gained weight while on the Pill, even when they hadn't.

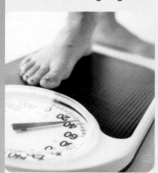

It now seems that worries have been unfounded all along. A research team in the Netherlands and North Carolina reviewed 42 studies of women on birth control pills or patches. They reported in the February 2004 issue of *Obstetrics and Gynecology* that the Pill does not appear to cause much, if any, weight gain. This backs up the findings of a Polish study involving 800 women in 2002, which found no correlation between oral contraceptives and weight gain.

Male birth control gets boost

The search for a male contraceptive has received a shot in the arm – or, rather, an implant in the arm. A December 2003 study showed that implanting tubes containing a synthetic hormone that resembles testosterone into a man's arm may be an effective form of birth control. The implants fool the brain into thinking the body is making enough testosterone, causing it to shut down production of natural testosterone, which is required for sperm production.

Called MENT, the implant is better than taking natural testosterone because it does not enlarge the prostate. The synthetic hormone is also better than natural testosterone at reducing sperm count, but it doesn't affect sexual desire or performance. In the study, the implant was left in place for 9 to 12 months, during which it continued to be effective.

However, a common problem in the search for a male contraceptive remains a lack of volunteers prepared to take part in trials. 'There's a very strong idea that women should suffer more in the service of preventing pregnancy than men,' says Mary Boyle, a clinical psychologist at the University of East London. 'That's a serious barrier to any male contraceptive.'

Fertility

Conception follows ovary transplant

In September 2004, the world's media was buzzing at the news from Brussels that a 32-year-old woman had given birth naturally – without using in vitro fertilization (IVF) – after her frozen ovarian tissue had been transplanted back into her body. This breakthrough offers hope to thousands of cancer patients whose treatment may make them infertile.

The woman was diagnosed in 1997 with Hodgkin's lymphoma. Before she received chemotherapy, some of her ovarian tissue was removed and frozen. One ovary was left untouched. When she was declared free of cancer in April 2003, the ovarian tissue was reimplanted, just below her existing ovary. Several months later she was discovered to be ovulating normally, and she became pregnant early in 2004.

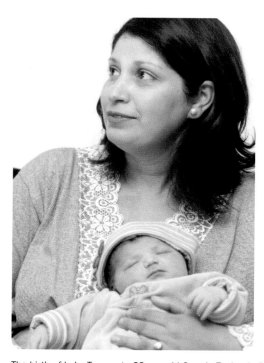

The birth of baby Tamara to 32-year-old Ouarda Touirat in Brussels has brought new hope to women with cancer. The day she was born, *The Lancet* published research from the team of scientists at the Catholic University of Louvain, who made her birth possible.

The remarkable procedure – the first successful pregnancy in a woman who has had an ovary transplant – was described in *The Lancet* by the team who pioneered the treatment, headed by Professor Jacques Donnez of the Catholic University of Louvain, Brussels. He told reporters: 'Our findings open new perspectives for young cancer patients facing premature ovarian failure.' But, as was quickly pointed out, the procedure may raise ethical issues as the technique could be used to beat the menopause

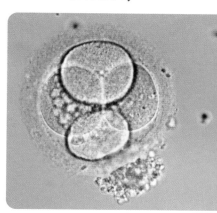

Eggs produced by transplanted ovarian tissue can be harvested and fertilized in a petri dish, creating an embryo, above.

Ovarian tissue grown elsewhere in the body
In New York Dr Kutluk Oktay of Cornell University is doing similar work. He has also successfully transplanted ovarian tissue into a former cancer patient and, in this case, the tissue was thawed and implanted under the skin of the woman's abdomen, where, after a few months, it started producing hormones and manufacturing eggs. Some were removed and mixed with sperm in a petri dish to create an embryo which was implanted in her womb.

Growing ovarian tissue in other parts of the body is not a totally new idea. A few years ago, the same researchers at Cornell University succeeded in doing it after implanting ovarian tissue into a woman's arm. But using the eggs produced by the tissue to make a viable embryo was a significant leap forward, says Dr Oktay. Although the embryo did not result in a pregnancy when it was implanted in the woman's uterus, Dr Oktay insists that he is not concerned by the outcome, as there is no more than a 10 to 20 per cent chance of pregnancy with any IVF procedure.

Optimistic outlook The procedure is preferred to egg freezing (see page 204), which requires more than a month to stimulate and extract the eggs, because ovarian tissue can be collected with a day's notice. Dr Oktay is confident it will become a regular path to pregnancy as tissue preservation techniques are perfected and pregnancies result.

Fertility

Babies born from **eggs that were frozen**

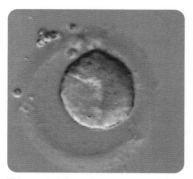

This egg has been placed in a solution that removes water from it, protecting it from damage during freezing and thawing. It has shrunk to 50 per cent of its original size.

Great advances in egg-preservation techniques mean that an increasing number of babies around the world are being born from eggs that were once frozen. In the UK, the first 'frozen-egg' baby was born in October 2002 to Lee and Helen Perry, who had been unable to conceive naturally. The birth took place two years after the lifting of a ban on this type of conception. Egg freezing holds promise for couples undergoing in vitro fertilization (IVF) as well as those who want to delay having a family. IVF treatment often results in several extra embryos (eggs united with sperm) that remain frozen for years and sometimes decades. Deciding what to do with the embryos poses ethical and moral dilemmas.

If women could have their eggs frozen, however, they could repeat the IVF procedure whenever they decided they were ready to have children – or they could dispose of the unfertilized eggs without having to deal with the issues surrounding disposal of the embryos. Egg freezing would also benefit women who must undergo chemotherapy or radiotherapy, which affect ovulation. These women could have their eggs frozen beforehand for use at a later date. Egg freezing, says Gillian Lockwood of Midland Fertility Services in the UK, may come to be seen as 'the ultimate kind of family planning'.

Although several groups around the world have been working on the problems of egg freezing, one of the most successful is Assisted Fertility Services in Indianapolis, where eight women have delivered healthy babies conceived using frozen eggs, and a ninth was expected to deliver in the autumn of 2004.

How it works The challenge with freezing eggs, says Jeffrey Boldt, the director of the Indianapolis programme, is that, unlike easily frozen sperm, an egg is a very big cell filled with water. When frozen, the water forms ice crystals big enough to 'blow the egg apart', he says. 'The trick is to get the water out of the cell before it freezes.'

To do that, scientists have devised a special solution that pushes the water out of the egg and fills the space it once occupied. They also keep the eggs in the solution longer than other researchers in this area have done previously to ensure that they have removed as much water as possible from them.

The babies born so far came from eggs that had been frozen for, on average, six to nine months. The eggs were thawed and fertilized in a procedure called ICSI, or intracytoplasmic sperm injection, in which a single sperm is injected into each egg. Researchers used ICSI because they think that freezing the egg damages its outer layer, making it more difficult for sperm to penetrate. So far, the fertilization rate for frozen eggs using ICSI is running just 5 per cent behind that for fresh eggs using the same procedure.

Availability Egg freezing is available only as an experimental procedure at a handful of IVF clinics around the world. Most clinics still require that participants pay for the fertility drugs needed to produce numerous eggs and for the egg retrieval.

RESEARCH ROUND-UP

Saliva test for ovulation

The days of urinating onto a stick and lying in bed with a thermometer in your mouth to see if you are ovulating may be over. You can now use a simple saliva test to identify the four or five days during your cycle when you are most likely to get pregnant. (Saliva is a recognized measure of the hormonal activity that takes place during ovulation.) First thing in the morning, you must place a drop of saliva on the tiny microscope that comes with the test, then peer through the lens. If a fern-like pattern appears, you are ovulating. The test is available on the internet under such names as Calista and Fertile Focus.

Fertility

Over-the-counter **fertility supplement** gets results

When the study results were unveiled, they surprised even the researchers conducting the trial. No one had expected that a cheap over-the-counter supplement would really make a difference when it came to helping women to get pregnant. But in a small pilot study of the effect of the nutritional supplement FertilityBlend on 30 women aged from 24 to 46 that is exactly what happened.

The women, who had been trying unsuccessfully to conceive for between six months and three years, were randomly assigned to receive either daily doses of the supplement or placebos (dummy pills) for three months. At the end of that time, four of the 15 women who had received the supplements were pregnant, compared with none who had received placebos. Another woman became pregnant after taking the supplement for an additional two months. Although 5 out of 15 may not sound like a very large proportion, it is statistically significant, says Dr Lynn Westphal of Stanford School of Medicine, who was one of the researchers on the study. 'I was surprised [by the results],' Dr Westphal admits. 'I think I was sceptical that a supplement could have that much of an impact.'

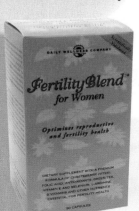

How it works The results may stem from the supplement's effects on a woman's ovulatory cycle, says Dr Westphal. FertilityBlend contains the amino acid L-carnitine, green tea extract and a

A herb in FertilityBlend affects ovulation and may increase a woman's chances of pregnancy.

handful of vitamins and minerals, but its most important ingredient is probably the herb chasteberry, which affects the levels of two hormones, progesterone and prolactin. Low progesterone or high prolactin levels can inhibit ovulation; chasteberry enhances the production of progesterone and suppresses that of prolactin.

Dr Westphal suspects that, while chasteberry affects ovulation, the other ingredients improve a woman's nutritional status, thereby increasing her chances of conception. She and the other authors of the study were so impressed with the results that they began a larger clinical trial with 100 women in early 2004.

FertilityBlend is not a cure-all. 'It's a nice thing women can take when they're trying to get pregnant,' says Dr Westphal, but if women over 35 haven't conceived within six months (with or without the supplement), they should see their doctors for testing. Also, women with blocked Fallopian tubes or other physical abnormalities probably would not benefit from the supplement.

Availability FertilityBlend is available worldwide from the company's web site: www.fertilityblend.com. The company also makes a supplement for men, which Dr Westphal and her colleagues are currently testing. Results from that trial were expected in late 2004.

Fertility

Stem cells provide male fertility hope

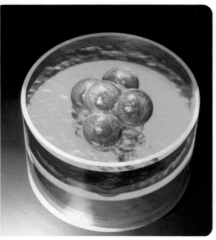

Stem cells, shown here in laboratory solution, are able to turn into virtually any kind of cell in the body.

In an experiment that could have significant implications for male infertility, Japanese researchers have transplanted frozen sperm stem cells into infertile male mice, which then went on to father live baby mice. (Stem cells are the 'genesis' cells from which all other cells grow.)

Although scientists have known since 1996 that infertile mice given sperm stem-cell transplants could make their own sperm containing their own DNA, no subsequent impregnation of females by the male mice had been recorded – until now.

By implanting the cells into very young mice, before they reached 'adolescence', researchers at Kyoto University enabled four out of eight infertile mice to father normal babies after normal sex. Those figures dropped to one in nine when adult mice were used. One in 12 adult mice given cancer drugs to destroy their sperm cells also fathered live babies after transplants. In that case, however, the sperm was injected directly into the egg in a mouse version of in vitro fertilization.

What does it mean? If the results can be duplicated in humans, the implications are particularly important for children. Since young boys do not produce sperm, they would not have any sperm to freeze before undergoing cancer treatment that might destroy their fertility. Using the new procedure, their stem cells could be frozen, then transplanted after completion of any cancer treatment. Worldwide, an estimated 1 in 650 children develop cancer during childhood and, by 2010, 1 in 250 young adults (aged 20 to 29) will be long-term survivors of childhood cancer. Between 16 and 85 per cent of them become infertile.

Sperm on demand? In another Japanese-led investigation, researchers created sperm cells from embryonic mouse stem cells. Their efforts marked the first time sperm cells have been created in a laboratory. The work may be applied to developing specialized sperm – for instance, sperm without certain genetic defects – or to adding certain traits to the sperm. Given that scientists have already turned embryonic stem cells into eggs, it opens the possibility of creating life – mouse life, at least – with no parental involvement whatsoever.

Oestrogen therapy study may have been flawed

Since 2002, some 340,000 women in Britain have given up hormone replacement therapy (HRT), following publication of American research by the Women's Health Initiative (WHI) which concluded that HRT increased the risk of heart disease and stroke.

The study involved 16,000 women, but a new report, by scientists at Yale University, suggests that it was too small to draw any statistically significant conclusions. Most of the women who participated were in their 60s and 70s, whereas previous research had suggested that HRT provided protection from heart disease for women in their early 50s.

The Yale investigators advocate more research into the exact effect of HRT on heart disease – and say that it would be wrong to dismiss the idea that it could prevent heart attacks and stroke.

Dr John Stevenson of the British Menopause Society says that the controversy had sown confusion and fear: 'We had two reasons to give HRT – for the relief of menopausal symptoms and for the prevention of osteoporosis. We knew that there was a small risk of breast cancer and a very, very small risk of blood clots, but the benefits far outweighed the risks. And nothing has changed.'

In February 2004, Professor Susan Johnson of the University of Iowa, who took part in the WHI research, said that the study's message had been widely misunderstood – and that HRT remained an effective treatment for women with severe menopausal symptoms.

Menopause
Anti-allergy drug can ease hot flushes

Relief from the discomfort of hot flushes may come from an unexpected source: anti-allergy medication. When doctors at the Baylor College of Medicine in Houston, Texas, began hearing that patients had fewer hot flushes when they took the prescription anti-allergy drug cetirizine (Zyrtec), they decided to investigate. They asked 100 post-menopausal women to take either Zyrtec or a placebo (dummy pill) for four weeks. The women also completed a daily hot flush questionnaire for one week before they started the study, establishing a 'score' based on the severity and frequency of their flushes. The score fell by 40 per cent in the women who took Zyrtec.

No one is certain why an antihistamine might have this effect. The cause of hot flushes – the most common symptom of the menopause – is unknown. Ironically, the leaflet in the Zyrtec packet warns that the drug may cause hot flushes.

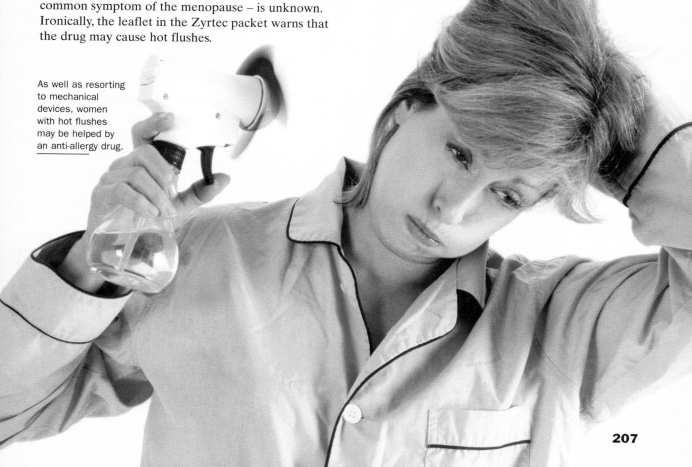

As well as resorting to mechanical devices, women with hot flushes may be helped by an anti-allergy drug.

RESEARCH ROUND-UP

How much longer will you be fertile?

Most women go through the menopause at about the age of 50, but it can happen as early as 42 and as late as 58. Scientists at St Andrews University and the Mount Sinai Medical Center in New York have now found a way to predict when it will occur using ultrasound to measure the size of a woman's ovaries.

During most of her reproductive life, a woman has many thousands of eggs in her ovaries, but the number starts to fall rapidly about ten years before the menopause. It is now possible to tell how many eggs remain – and how much longer fertility is likely to continue – by measuring a woman's ovarian size and comparing the results with an estimated average size.

The information would be useful for women who have cancer treatment when young, which could affect their fertility. It could also help women who are planning to delay having a family for professional or personal reasons.

Menstruation

Microwaves put an end to pain

For much of her life, 40-year-old Andrea Graley has suffered from excessive menstrual bleeding, sometimes using more than ten sanitary pads a day during the first days of her periods, missing work and becoming so anaemic from blood loss that she required prescription iron pills. In common with an estimated one in five women, Graley, a single mother of two from Parma Heights, Ohio, had a condition called menorrhagia.

Traditional treatments such as birth control pills did not work and, as Graley had fibroids (benign uterine cysts) and an enlarged uterus, she could not undergo surgical treatments such as balloon endometrial ablation, which destroys the lining of the uterus. Her only option, her doctor told her, was to have a hysterectomy.

Then Graley heard about a clinical trial for a new procedure for menorrhagia called microwave endometrial ablation (MEA). It uses microwave energy to permanently remove the uterine lining, the tissue that produces menstrual bleeding. Three years after the procedure, Graley has no periods at all. 'I still go through the monthly cycle but without the bleeding and cramping, and I no longer have to plan my life around one week,' she says.

How it works The brief procedure is performed in a doctor's surgery under a local anaesthetic that numbs the patient from the waist down, explains Dr Susan Wheatley of Atlanta, Georgia, who took part in the MEA clinical trials. Dr Wheatley explains how she first dilates the woman's cervix to about 8mm (the cervix dilates to 10cm during childbirth), then inserts the microwave probe and turns on the machine. She sweeps the probe back and forth inside the uterus, receiving information by means of a monitor that tells her when the tissue has been destroyed.

Studies have found that MEA causes amenorrhea (total cessation of bleeding) in over 60 per cent of women and significantly reduces monthly bleeding in 96 per cent of cases. Other forms of ablation, including the balloon procedure, in which a hot-water-filled balloon destroys the uterine lining, and cryosurgery, in which the lining is frozen off, have amenorrhea rates ranging from 13 to 54 per cent.

Microwave ablation can be performed on all women, regardless of the size or position of their uteruses (some women's uteruses are very large or 'tipped,' precluding the use of other ablation techniques). There is also some evidence that it may be successful in treating endometrial cancer.

Availability MEA has been used since 1996 in the successful treatment of women in the UK, Canada and Australia. The Food and Drug Adminstration cleared it for use in the USA in September 2003, and the company that markets it, Microsulis, is training doctors around the country in its use.

In a brief and painless procedure, microwave endometrial ablation (MEA) reduces or eliminates excessive menstrual bleeding.

Computer-controlled microwave energy heats the tip of the MEA applicator to destroy the lining of the uterus.

Pregnancy
First guidelines for **morning sickness** issued

Women have been vomiting and feeling nauseous in pregnancy since the first egg met the first sperm. Until recently, though, they received little expert advice on what to do about the problem, which affects an estimated 75 to 80 per cent of pregnant women. Now, one of the world's top gynaecological organizations has released its first-ever guidelines for treating pregnancy-related nausea, also known as morning sickness. They reflect similar advice issued to pregnant women by official bodies in the UK.

Morning sickness has always been given scant attention by researchers because women don't die from it, says Dr Murphy Goodwin of the University of Southern California Women's Hospital in Los Angeles. Goodwin chaired the committee that drafted the American College of Obstetrics and Gynecology (ACOG) guidelines. 'There has been a growing appreciation in the college that this was a problem worthy of specific attention,' he says.

This new attitude has developed because the costs – both physical and economic – are tremendous. A few women become so ill that they decide to have a termination of pregnancy, and about 2 per cent of women with morning sickness become so dehydrated that they have to be hospitalized.

As with many health conditions, the sooner that morning sickness is treated the better the outcome. But, Dr Goodwin says, 'Unless it's life threatening, most women won't take anything, and 99 per cent of doctors just tell women they'll get over it.'

Of those who do seek treatment, 90 per cent are offered therapies that aren't likely to be effective, according to one study.

The therapies advocated by the ACOG include:
- **A multivitamin taken around the time of conception** No one knows why, but studies on the benefits of multivitamins on foetal defects found that women who took the vitamins while trying to conceive also had less morning sickness.
- **Ginger** Used for centuries to quell nausea, ginger root remains one of the most successful remedies. Ginger can be taken in the form of tablets, tea, capsules, ginger ale (containing real ginger) or fresh root ginger.
- **Antihistamines** When taken as directed, these medications are safe for pregnant women and can help to alleviate morning sickness.
- **Vitamin B_6 or B_6 plus doxylamine** Vitamin B_6 is probably involved in more bodily processes than any other vitamin, doing more than 100 jobs many times a day. Studies have found that taking 75mg of vitamin B_6 daily can significantly reduce morning sickness, although no one knows why.

A prescription medication called Bendectin combines vitamin B_6 with the antihistamine doxylamine. It was used for years to treat morning sickness, but concerns about its potential role in birth defects led to its removal from the US market in the early 1980s, although it is still available in Canada under the brand name Diclectin. Studies since then have shown the drug is safe for use during pregnancy, and the manufacturer has asked the Food and Drug Administration (FDA) for permission to make it available again in the USA.

Women troubled by morning sickness should check with their doctor before taking vitamin B_6.

RESEARCH ROUND-UP

Go on, indulge – chocolate is good for your baby

A new study shows that eating chocolate during pregnancy can result in a happier baby. Finnish researchers asked pregnant women to rate their stress levels and chocolate consumption during pregnancy, then compared the data with infant behaviour six months after birth. Babies of women who ate chocolate every day during their pregnancies were more active and smiled and laughed more than babies of women who did not eat much chocolate. Also, infants of stressed women who ate chocolate during their pregnancies showed less fear when faced with new situations than babies whose mothers were stressed but did not indulge. The chemicals in chocolate that put women in a good mood seem to do the same for their babies.

Pregnancy

Women to be offered more prenatal test choice

In the past, only UK women aged 35 or older tended to be offered amniocentesis or chorionic villus sampling (CVS), invasive prenatal tests that can indicate Down's syndrome and other chromosomal birth defects. Now, in a bid to reduce the number of unnecessary amniocentesis examinations, it is NHS policy to offer all women non-invasive screening, whatever their age. If the results indicate some abnormality, they can then opt for the more precise invasive tests.

In the USA, based on clinical guidelines, insurance companies still tend to limit coverage for tests such as amniocentesis to women over 35. But this may change following a new study published in *The Lancet* which supports the case for ditching the age threshold. The risk of having a child with Down's or another chromosomal disorder rises significantly with age – a main reason why only older women were routinely offered the invasive tests, which carry a risk of miscarriage. According to the study's authors, 'This threshold was chosen because at that age, the procedure-related miscarriage risk was approximately equal to the chance that a child would be born with Down's syndrome, and the cost of offering amniocentesis would be

offset by the savings associated with preventing a birth of an infant affected by Down's syndrome.'

However, one author, Dr Miriam Kuppermann, explains that the researchers who helped to develop those guidelines assumed that women rated as equal the potential outcomes of invasive testing: having a miscarriage and giving birth to a child with Down's syndrome. 'We have shown in our previous work that this assumption is not true.'

The study, conducted at the University of California, San Francisco, was based on data from 534 pregnant women. It took account of the women's preferred outcomes (many said they would rather risk a miscarriage than give birth to a child with a chromosomal disorder). The researchers compared the cost of the tests with the benefit gained in 'quality-adjusted life years'. They concluded that the tests could be cost-effective at any age depending on a woman's 'preferences for reassurance about the chromosomal status of her foetus and, to a lesser extent, for miscarriage.'

Dr Kuppermann says her findings suggest that the woman should decide whether or not to have a more invasive test. 'You need to get information on all the tests and think about your own situation – whether that risk of miscarriage is worth getting the kind of definitive results only an invasive test can give you.'

A different approach
In the UK, by contrast, it is hoped that offering non-invasive screening, such as ultrasound and blood tests, to all pregnant women will reduce unnecessary invasive tests but alert those who may need them. The government aims to raise the detection rate for Down's from 60 to 75 per cent by 2007.

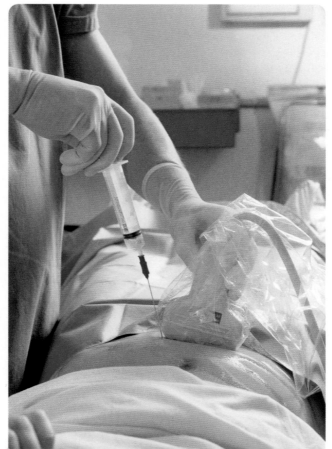

In amniocentesis, a needle guided by ultrasound is used to take a small sample of fluid from the sac surrounding the foetus.

Pregnancy

Neck thickness test can predict Down's

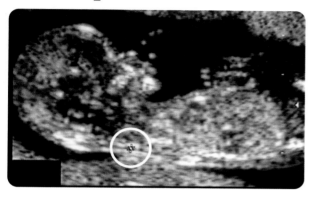

The circle on this ultrasound image indicates the baby's normal foetal nuchal translucency, or neck thickness.

The agony of waiting until almost halfway through a pregnancy to find out if your baby may have Down's syndrome could soon become a thing of the past. In the UK, it is hoped that by 2007 all pregnant mothers will be screened for the condition with a blood test as well as an ultrasound scan at 11 to 14 weeks (only some get the blood test at present) and a second blood test, and sometimes a second scan, at 14 to 20 weeks. In the USA too, this will soon be policy. A large government-funded study has found that the combination of blood testing and ultrasound in the first three months was just as effective at detecting Down's syndrome as the current second-trimester screenings.

What it is The blood test measures chemicals in the mother's blood called pregnancy-associated plasma protein-A and free-beta human chorionic gonadotropin. The ultrasound examination, performed between 10 and 14 weeks of pregnancy, measures foetal nuchal translucency, or the thickness of an area at the back of the foetus's neck, another way of detecting Down's.

Although the first and second-trimester screenings produced similarly accurate results, says Dr Mary D'Alton, one of the leading US study researchers, the advantage of the first-trimester test is that it enables parents to receive the information they need earlier.

If the result is negative, they can stop worrying about genetic defects because the risk is low. If the result is positive, they may choose to have further diagnostic tests, such as chorionic villus sampling or amniocentesis, to rule out a 'false positive'.

The study, involving more than 38,000 pregnant women at 15 US medical centres, also found that combining the first-trimester test with the traditional second-trimester screening gave significantly more accurate results than using either one alone, reducing the number of women who needed further tests to clarify the results.

Availability All pregnant women in the UK should have access to a blood test and scan at 11 to 14 weeks by April 2007.

FUTURE BREAKTHROUGHS

Press 'O' for...

No more faking it, ladies. It may not be long before you are able to have a device implanted near your spine that triggers an orgasm. About the size of a pack of cigarettes but thinner, the Orgasmatron can be permanently implanted under the skin of the lower back and is operated by remote control.

Stuart Meloy, an anaesthetist who heads a pain-management clinic in North Carolina, stumbled upon the idea while using a spinal cord stimulator to treat a woman's back pain. The device stimulates nerves that control sexual response in women, including orgasm. In a small clinical trial in the summer of 2004, nine of the ten women reported enhanced sexual feelings while using the Orgasmatron.

Dr Meloy has spoken to two interested companies about the manufacture of his invention, and has plans to begin licensing it to other doctors by the end of 2004.

Meanwhile, Liz Paul from Ilkley in West Yorkshire has devised her own, much simpler 'orgasmatron', a plastic clitoral stimulator with eight nodules which fits over the finger. Liz Paul hopes her invention, called Vielle, will help women with sexual problems: 'Women are not told how to have an orgasm and it needs explaining to them.' Clinical tests show, she says, that her device can halve the time it takes for a woman to climax, as well as intensifying her orgasm. The Vielle is sold in packs of three for under £10.

Pregnancy

Labour in water can mean less intervention

Forget about epidurals and back massages. Results of a Southampton University study, published in the February 2004 edition of the *British Medical Journal*, found that first-time mothers who spent the first part of their labour in birthing pools were less likely to need drugs for pain relief or to speed up labour than women who didn't labour in water. The study, led by Dr Elizabeth Cluett at the university's school of Nursing and Midwifery, followed 96 first-time mothers whose labours were progressing slowly. Half were given the opportunity to labour in the warm water and half received standard care. (Although some women deliver in birthing pools, many spend the early stages of labour there and get out when they are ready to push.)

Fewer than half (47 per cent) of the women who spent part of their labour in water needed an epidural, compared with almost two thirds (66 per cent) in the other group. The women in the water group were also less likely to require drugs to aid contractions (71 per cent compared to 96 per cent), and reported significantly less pain and higher satisfaction with freedom of movement. 'First-time mothers tend to get very stressed, a factor which causes hormonal changes and slow progress in labour,' says Dr Cluett. 'Our study shows that by putting these women in water, we can relax them and ease the pain. We hope that our results will provide women with an option whereby they can give birth without the need for obstetric intervention.'

Additionally, the buoyancy provided by water means that women can change positions easily, also making it easier for them to cope with labour pain.

Overall, there was an average of 6 hours between the time the women left the pool (whenever they wanted to do so) and the time when they gave birth.

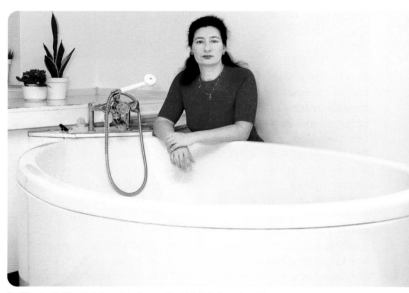

Dr Elizabeth Cluett (above) believes that birthing pools offer a more positive experience of labour – both physically and psychologically.

Caesarean delivery linked to stillbirth

A Cambridge University study has found that women with one previous caesarean delivery are twice as likely to deliver a stillborn baby in later pregnancies as those who have previously had vaginal deliveries.

Linking information on pregnant women in Scotland with a database that tracks stillbirths and perinatal deaths, researchers found that after the 39th week of pregnancy the rate of unexplained stillbirth was 1.1 per 1,000 women for those with previous caesarean deliveries and 0.5 per 1,000 for those with previous vaginal deliveries. Commenting on the findings in the medical journal *The Lancet*, Judith Lumley of the Centre for Mothers' and Children's Health in Victoria, Australia, said it was already known that previous caesarean delivery was linked with an increase in subsequent problems such as placenta praevia, where the mother's placenta becomes detached too early, and ectopic pregnancy, where a foetus implants outside the womb. 'But an association of previous caesarean section with an increase in foetal death at or after 34 weeks' gestation was not known,' she wrote. In the UK, caesarean rates have increased from an estimated 10 per cent of all births in 1987 to 22 per cent in 2002.

Premature birth
Artificial fluid to help tiny babies

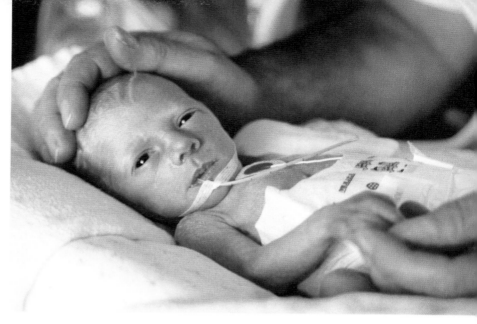

As any pregnant woman who has felt her unborn baby hiccup knows, foetuses continually gulp the salty amniotic fluid in which they float. In fact, they take in about 200 to 300ml per kilo of their weight every day until they are born. Until fairly recently, doctors did not know why. Now they believe that the fluid has an important role in the development of a foetus's immature digestive system. The finding helps to explain why babies born prematurely (and therefore deprived of the fluid) often develop life-threatening gastrointestinal problems. It also presents a potential solution in the form of artificial amniotic fluid.

An accidental discovery Two experts on the health of newborn babies at the University of South Florida in St Petersburg, USA were analysing a freezer full of amniotic fluid specimens, hoping to find hormonal clues to particular illnesses, such as infections. Instead, they found extremely high concentrations of proteins called growth factors, which enhance the production of red and white blood cells in bone marrow.

As Dr Robert Christensen explains, 'We figured that finding these growth factors in such high concentrations couldn't be an accident. There must be some purpose'. Sure enough, when Christensen and his colleague, Dr Darlene Calhoun, examined human foetal tissue, they found special sites on certain intestinal cells designed for the growth factors to 'lock' on to. These cells make up the villi, tiny fingerlike projections that line the interior of the intestine and absorb nutrients.

In premature babies, who frequently receive no nutrition by mouth for one week or more after their birth, the villi tend to atrophy. Thus, when the babies start receiving formula or breast milk, they often develop a condition called feeding intolerance, which involves vomiting, diarrhoea, bloating, bloody stools and, worst of all, a life-threatening infection called necrotizing enterocolitis (NEC).

Dr Christensen and Dr Calhoun maintained that, if they could continue introducing the growth factors into the babies' digestive tracts, they might be able to avert feeding intolerance. So they created artificial amniotic fluid – a colourless, odourless, flavourless solution of various minerals plus the growth factors. The growth factors are already available as the biomedically engineered drugs filgrastim (Neupogen) and epoetin alfa (Eprex). 'Our hypothesis is that by providing [the babies] with simulated amniotic fluid, we prevent the intestinal atrophy that otherwise would occur,' says Dr Christensen.

What the study showed Researchers tested the solution in premature babies by giving them varying amounts starting on the first day of life. Eventually, the doctors increased the dose of growth factors to mimic the amount the infants would have received in the womb. In the group's most recent study, published in the March 2004 issue of the *Journal of Perinatology*, doctors in Mexico used the solution on ten premature infants who had already been treated for NEC. All the babies tolerated the solution well, and none developed any recurrence of NEC. More important, none developed feeding intolerance, a common occurrence after an episode of NEC.

Availability Dr Christensen and Dr Calhoun got approval from the Food and Drug Administration in the summer of 2003 to conduct more clinical trials on the solution, and they are now looking for a pharmaceutical partner to help fund the studies.

Sexual health

Search continues for **female Viagra**

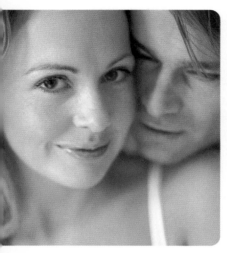

From the moment the male impotence drug sildenafil (Viagra) became available in 1998, scientists have been investigating whether it or a similar drug could also benefit women with sexual problems. Viagra's manufacturer, Pfizer, halted all trials of the drug for women in March 2004 because of disappointing results, but other companies are pursuing the quest. Among several products promising an answer to female sexual dysfunction is Viacrem, a cream applied directly to the clitoris, and Pleasure Plus, a herbal preparation. Testosterone implants and stick-on testosterone patches that need to be replaced twice a week have also been tested, but no satisfactory solution has yet been found.

The challenge of finding a drug to enhance women's libido is that women's sexual desire is governed by emotional as well as physical factors. In men, blood-flow to the penis is at the heart of the sexual response. But research has shown that for women, vaginal blood-flow may have little to do with feeling aroused. In women feelings of arousal and desire seem to be much more to do with the response of the brain than that of the sexual organs, leading some scientists to look into drugs that act on the brain as a treatment for female sexual problems. Promising results were obtained from a Scottish study involving ten women with reduced sexual desire who were treated with a drug called apomorphine. Apomorphine is active in the brain, where it mimics the effect of one of the brain's main chemical messengers, dopamine.

There is some scepticism, however, about the very existence of the condition called female sexual dysfunction. An article published in 2003 in the *British Medical Journal* suggests that drug manufacturers have defined the condition to create a new market for their products.

In the article, writer Ray Moynihan says, 'A cohort of researchers with close ties to drug companies are working with colleagues in the pharmaceutical industry to develop and define a new category of human illness at meetings heavily sponsored by companies racing to develop new drugs.'

Bacterial infections are more common than we think

If you have vaginal itching and odour, don't instantly assume that it's thrush. You could have a dose of bacterial vaginosis (BV), the most common cause of abnormal vaginal discharge among women in the UK. Left untreated, it may lead to health complications in pregnant women or women undergoing gynaecological surgery, including premature delivery, postnatal infections, endometriosis, infertility and increased vulnerability to HIV infection.

The condition has been considered by some to be a sexually transmitted disease, but a study published in the US journal *Obstetrics and Gynecology* found it to be prevalent in virgins as well as much more common overall than previous estimates suggested.

The study, which involved young women entering the armed forces, found that 27 per cent of the 2,000 women evaluated had BV. Among those who were sexually active, 28 per cent had the infection, as did 18 per cent of those who were virgins. The researchers also found lower rates of BV in women who were using hormonal contraception, such as birth control pills – which suggests that hormonal treatments may provide some protection against the infection.

BV is treated with antibiotics but often recurs. Symptoms include a change in the colour and consistency of vaginal fluid, itching and burning, and an unpleasant odour, but up to half of women have no symptoms.

Sexually transmitted diseases
Promising vaccine may wipe out herpes

Herpes is a sexually transmitted disease that never goes away. Once you have it, you will be vulnerable to painful flare-ups throughout your life. There is no cure for herpes, but a new vaccine that is undergoing clinical testing in the USA may eventually vanquish the virus for good by preventing new infections in uninfected women.

The problem 'Clearly, genital herpes is a huge problem,' says Dr Rhoda Sperling of the Mount Sinai School of Medicine in New York City, which is participating in the herpes vaccine trials. The National Institutes of Health estimates that genital herpes affects an estimated 67 million Americans, and, Dr Sperling notes, rates are rising.

Numbers are also high in other countries around the world. It is estimated that one in four people attending sexually transmitted disease clinics in the UK are suffering from herpes, and in various other European countries between 5 and 40 per cent of the population is infected. Another factor, says Dr Sperling, is that 'people express more worry and concern about herpes than any other sexually transmitted disease' – even more than HIV.

Herpes is caused by one of two forms of the herpes virus, HSV-1 and HSV-2, which cause either oral herpes – marked by sores and blisters on the lips, gums and in the mouth – or genital herpes – marked by painful sores in the genital area. HSV-1 typically causes oral herpes, but either form of the virus can cause either type of herpes.

The virus can be transmitted by means of sexual or other skin-to-skin contact and can spread even when the infected person shows no symptoms. It is particularly dangerous if a pregnant woman passes the virus to her infant, causing *herpes neonatorum*, an often fatal illness affecting the nervous system and internal organs. Herpes infection also increases the risk of HIV infection by providing easier entry for HIV through open sores. Only women who are not already infected with either type of herpes virus are eligible to participate in the current trial.

How the vaccine works Called Herpevac, the vaccine contains small amounts of the outer coatings of herpes viruses, together with other substances that are designed to boost the immune system. Once injected, the vaccine stimulates the immune system to create antibodies to the viruses. Therefore, if an immunized person ever encounters the real virus, the immune system is already primed to launch an all-out attack, staving off an infection.

The vaccine works differently in men and women, however. Previous studies of uninfected women and men who had infected partners concluded that, although Herpevac could prevent herpes in more than 70 per cent of women, the vaccine had no effect on men.

'It may be that herpes is a different disease in women than in men,' explains Dr Sperling. For instance, herpes in men may be largely a disease of the skin, while in women it may be predominantly a genital disease because women have more warm, damp areas in their genitals that make perfect viral breeding grounds.

The vaccine, if approved, would therefore be targeted at women. By vaccinating all uninfected women, researchers hope eventually to break the

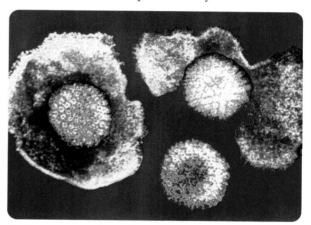

The three purple circles are herpes simplex viruses. A vaccine could provide protection for women who are not yet infected.

cycle of viral transmission and send HSV the way of the polio virus. The vaccine will be of no benefit to people who are already infected with herpes.

Availability The study, which will involve 7,550 women at 23 sites throughout the USA, is funded by the National Institute of Allergy and Infectious Diseases and the vaccine's manufacturer, Glaxo-SmithKline Biologicals. Results are expected in 2006 or 2007. It could be available in the UK from 2008.

RESPIRATORY
SYSTEM

Here's a good reason not to beg your doctor for antibiotics you don't need: they may contribute to **allergies and asthma**

That's the news according to recent research. There's also a new, simple blood test that will tell doctors immediately whether antibiotics are the right choice for symptoms that may or may not be caused by a bacterial infection.

You and the person sleeping next to you would love to put an end to your snoring – especially if it's a symptom of sleep apnoea, the rest-robbing breathing disorder. A simple orthodontic device could be the answer. Swedish research shows that it works as well for some people as more cumbersome breathing apparatuses.

There's also good news for people with cystic fibrosis. Researchers have confirmed that healthy genes can be safely sprayed into the lungs of people with the life-shortening disease. The new genes take over from the congenitally damaged ones, improving lung performance for about a month. The breakthrough is a major step towards the day when stem cell gene therapy will permanently restore healthy lung function.

Asthma and allergies
Three common nutrients
reduce asthma risk in children

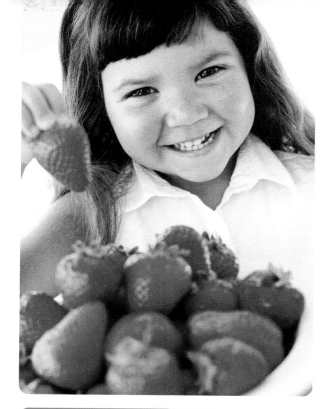

Are your children taking their vitamin C? Do they eat enough grains and fish? Do they eat orange and yellow vegetables? If not, they may be running an unnecessarily high risk of asthma, the most common serious chronic condition among youngsters under 18. Two new studies have shown a clear link between asthma risk and three nutrients: vitamin C, beta-carotene (the plant form of vitamin A, which gives carrots, squash and other vegetables their yellow or orange colour) and selenium (a trace mineral found in grains and fish). One of the studies found that children with low levels of vitamin C and beta-carotene in their bloodstreams were more likely to develop the airway disease. The other concluded that increased intake of vitamin C, beta-carotene and selenium reduce a child's risk of asthma.

Also, if anyone in your household smokes, you may want to be doubly sure that your children are getting plenty of vitamin C (in its recommendations for school meals, the Department of Health has suggested a daily intake of 30-35mg for children). The new studies show that children who are regularly exposed to secondhand tobacco smoke have as much as a 40 per cent lower asthma risk when they get enough vitamin C. The same is true for selenium and beta-carotene.

Why these nutrients might protect children from asthma is not clear, but all are antioxidants, which neutralize free radicals (unstable oxygen molecules that damage cells and contribute to disease).

The two studies, published in February 2004 in the *American Journal of Respiratory and Critical Care Medicine* and the *American Journal of Epidemiology,* follow several others in the UK and elsewhere in recent years which suggested that antioxidants help to combat asthma. One study even found improved lung function in children with asthma who were given antioxidant supplements, meaning that antioxidants may help to treat asthma

TOP trends

LAST GASP FOR CIGARETTES?

Smoking bans in public places are cropping up across the globe, from Norway to Australia and from Canada to the Netherlands. What's more, they are surprisingly popular. In Ireland, where a new policy outlaws smoking even in bar rooms, a survey found that two out of three Irish drinkers prefer smoke-free pubs. A similar ban in Scotland is imminent; and in July 2004 a report from Sir Liam Donaldson, Britain's Chief Medical Officer, showed that smoke-free public places would boost the hospitality business.

So is an outright ban on smoking – anywhere, any time – the next step? In the UK, it would be if the editors of *The Lancet* got their way. In an editorial published in December 2003, the prestigious British medical journal called for making possession of cigarettes a crime. Citing an estimated 1,000 yearly deaths from secondary smoking in the UK alone, the editors wrote, 'If tobacco were an illegal substance, possession of cigarettes would become a crime, and the number of smokers would drastically fall... We call on Tony Blair's government to ban tobacco.'

In an informal poll conducted by the online medical information service Medscape, 67 per cent of respondents (and 72 per cent of those who identified themselves as doctors) said that they would support criminalizing tobacco use in their own countries.

as well as prevent it. The researchers want to await the results of larger studies, now underway, on the asthma-antioxidant link before recommending that children take supplements of vitamin C, beta-carotene or selenium. One reason is that current studies don't indicate how much of each antioxidant is best for asthma prevention.

Meanwhile, experts agree that children should eat plenty of the fruits, vegetables and grains that provide antioxidants and are vital to healthy lungs. At a recent British Thoracic Society meeting, Professor John Britton from Nottingham City Hospital suggested that free fruit in schools would protect children from asthma and help to improve their general health.

TOP trends

ASTHMA LINK TO CLEANING PRODUCTS

Government estimates are that air pollution in the UK may cause between 12,000 and 24,000 people a year to die prematurely. As a result of poor air quality, more people suffer breathing problems and those with asthma are particularly vulnerable.

But while national and international strategies and targets are being devised to achieve a cleaner external environment, the air quality in your own home could be posing an asthma risk – especially if you're house proud. Research shows that the more enthusiastically you clean and decorate your home, the more you could be increasing the risk.

A variety of cleaning and DIY products, including polishes, paints, solvents and glues, contain chemical irritants called volatile organic compounds (VOCs). These are known to be triggers for many people with asthma. But a new Australian research study of 192 children aged from 6 months to 3 years, published in the journal *Thorax* in August 2004, shows that the chemicals might also cause asthma to develop in young children. The study findings identified the prime culprits as benzene, ethylbenzene and toluene. So be sure to read the product labels carefully and use low-VOC paints.

Dr Matthew Hallsworth, research manager of Asthma UK, welcomed the findings. 'Early infancy is a critical period in the development of a child's lungs and immune system,' he said, adding that although we already know that development of asthma depends on a complex interaction of genetic and environmental factors in early life, 'the study reminds us of the effect of indoor air quality on the lungs of young children, who can spend lots of time indoors'.

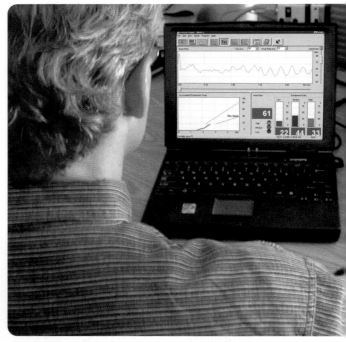

With a fingertip pulse sensor connected to his computer, a patient gets in touch with his breathing and heart rate to help him to control his asthma.

Asthma and allergies

Biofeedback is strong asthma medicine

Inhaled steroid drugs are an asthma patient's best bet for easier breathing and fewer serious attacks, yet 50 per cent of people who are prescribed these drugs for asthma don't use them as often as they should. They hate the routine, fear side effects or resent the cost.

If you are among them, take heart. An alternative to steroids may come from a surprising source: biofeedback training. Once seen as a 'fringe' therapy but now increasingly accepted, biofeedback may keep asthma symptoms under control so well that, for some, it can reduce the need for steroids.

In a recent US study, the largest yet conducted on biofeedback as an asthma treatment, 45 adult volunteers who practised the technique daily reported significant reductions in symptoms over the four-month study period. Doctors regularly examined the people who used biofeedback, as well as 48 asthma patients who didn't use it. Without knowing which patients fell into which category, the doctors consistently prescribed less steroid medication for those in the biofeedback group.

How it works Biofeedback uses machines – usually electronic monitoring devices – to give you information about physical changes in your body. The aim is to help you to achieve conscious control over factors of which you are not normally even aware, such as heart rate, muscle tension and electrical activity in the brain.

The biofeedback training given to the asthma patients in the study helped them to improve their heart rate variability (HRV), the periodic variations in the time between heartbeats. Such variations may not sound desirable but, in fact, high HRV is associated with good health. Asthma tends to lower HRV, and raising it seems to reduce asthma symptoms, although researchers are not sure why.

The type of biofeedback used in the study teaches people to breathe in a way that maximizes their HRV. Sensors, similar to the heart-rate monitors on exercise bikes, are connected to pulse points such as the chest or fingertips. A small read-out screen indicates HRV, usually in the form of a vertical bar that lengthens as HRV rises. By focusing on your breathing as you watch the screen, you eventually learn which subtle variations in breathing lengthen the bar. With enough training, you can carry that knowledge with you throughout the day, regularly breathing in a way that helps to control asthma.

Availability HRV biofeedback is thought to help with other conditions, such as stress and depression, but is not yet used in the UK to help treat asthma.

Home HRV biofeedback kits are available from internet sources. However, Paul Lehrer Ph.D., professor of psychiatry at Robert Wood Johnson Medical School in Piscataway, New Jersey, who published the biofeedback-for-asthma study in the August 2004 issue of the medical journal *Chest*, strongly suggests that beginners should seek professional assistance before practising biofeedback on their own.

Dr Lehrer also cautions against premature substitution of biofeedback for prescribed steroid medications. 'It looks as if biofeedback will be a good adjunct asthma therapy and may allow some people to go off steroids,' he says, 'but first we need larger studies that look at biofeedback's benefits for longer than four months.'

In 2004, Dr Lehrer applied to the US National Institutes of Health for funding for just such a study.

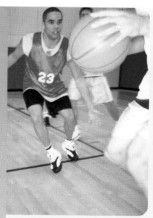

RESEARCH ROUND-UP

Basketball gets losing score

A recent US study shows that basketball is the deadliest sport for people with asthma.

Researchers at Drexel University, Philadelphia, investigated the sports-related asthma deaths over a seven-year period and found that more (21 per cent) occurred while playing basketball than any other sport. Almost all the victims had a known history of asthma, and most were under 20. Hardly any were using long-term control medications.

The study did not try to explain why basketball was associated with the most deaths, and the mechanics of exercise-induced asthma attacks are not yet fully understood. But when exercising you breathe faster, so there is less time for the nose to warm and add moisture to the air intake. It is thought that colder, drier air in the airways triggers asthma symptoms.

Should people with asthma sit on the sidelines and watch others score all the baskets? No, say the researchers in the February 2004 issue of the *Journal of Allergy and Clinical Immunology*. The benefits of regular exercise far outweigh the risks. After all, only 61 sports-related asthma deaths occurred in the USA from 1993 to 2000. Nevertheless, coaches, parents, doctors and athletes should be aware of the potential risks and be prepared to deal with emergencies.

Asthma UK also encourages people with asthma to indulge in exercise and sports, and can advise on how to reduce symptoms of exercise-induced asthma. Scuba diving, sky diving and parachuting can be risky for people with asthma, so consult your doctor first, and inform your instructor that you have asthma.

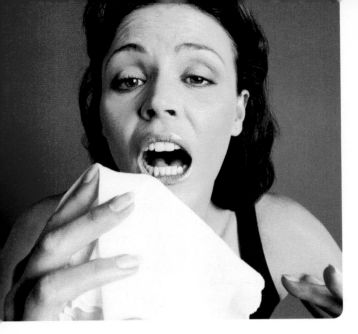

Asthma and allergies
Do **antibiotics** promote asthma and allergies?

The widespread use of antibiotics in the second half of the 20th century corresponded with soaring rates of asthma and allergies in the West that continue today. Coincidence? Dr Mairi Noverr and Dr Gary Huffnagle don't think so. The two Michigan University researchers released a report in April 2004 revealing strong evidence from a mouse study that antibiotic use promotes respiratory allergies.

These findings are consistent with earlier studies suggesting links between antibiotic treatment and childhood asthma. If they are borne out by further research on humans, doctors and patients will have at least three good incentives for restricting the use of antiobiotics, unless essential: to spare patients unnecessary side effects from the drugs, to slow the growth of drug-resistant strains of bacteria, and now, to avoid increased risk of asthma and allergies.

How it works Simultaneous increases in allergy cases and antibiotic use don't prove that one causes the other, but the Michigan team was able to establish a link between antibiotic use and allergies. When antibiotics kill harmful bacteria to clear up an infection, they also kill 'friendly' bacteria that live in the gut. Researchers think that the resulting imbalance in intestinal bacteria impairs the immune system's ability to distinguish harmless molecules in the body from true invaders. And that is what an allergic reaction is: a misguided immune system attack on benign visitors, such as mould spores.

The researchers administered antibiotics to a group of mice for five days and then exposed them to mould spores. The treated mice experienced much greater allergic immune responses to the spores than the untreated mice.

The message With these results, the study authors see additional incentive to use antibiotics responsibly. If they're needed, take them – but if they're not necessary, use an alternative treatment. When your course of antibiotics is complete, ask your doctor about 'probiotic' tablets that can help to restore proper bacterial balance in the intestines. You can also help to restore that balance by eating plenty of yoghurt, raw fruit and vegetables.

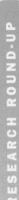

RESEARCH ROUND-UP

For many, aspirin and asthma don't mix

Up to now, about 5 to 10 per cent of adults with asthma were thought to be aspirin sensitive. For them, taking an aspirin for a headache may trigger an asthma attack that in extreme cases could be life-threatening. Now it turns out that the problem is worse than experts thought. After analysing data from 21 studies, British and Australian researchers have concluded that 21 per cent of adults with asthma are prone to aspirin-induced attacks. That's one in every five.

It's not only aspirin that carries a risk. The study results, published in February 2004 in the *British Medical Journal*, show that most adults with asthma who are sensitive to aspirin will also react to other over-the-counter pain relievers, including ibuprofen (Nurofen, Advil), naproxen (Naprosyn) and diclofenac (Voltarol). The findings, say the study authors, suggest that all adults with asthma should discuss the possibility of aspirin sensitivity with their doctor and, if necessary, decide on a pain-relief strategy that reduces the risk of reactions.

Eye drops for glaucoma and beta blockers are known to trigger asthma attacks in some people.

Asthma and allergies
A Chinese formula for solving peanut allergies

An ancient 11-herb Chinese formula for soothing stomach ailments may soon become the basis for a modern three-herb treatment for the growing problem of peanut allergies, which is thought to affect at least 1 in 200 people in the UK.

A research team at Mount Sinai School of Medicine in New York City became interested in the Chinese formula several years ago. An important breakthrough occurred in 2004, when the researchers announced that after they had eliminated two superfluous herbs from the formula, peanut-sensitive mice treated with the nine-herb combination had virtually no reaction when fed the offending peanuts.

The next step will be to whittle down the formula to the three most essential herbs. Such a streamlined formula has already shown early promise in protecting mice from peanut allergy reactions, but the researchers will not yet divulge which three herbs they are working with. Whichever they are, the pared-down version could pave the way for testing the herbs – or a new drug based on their properties – on humans who have peanut allergies.

Availability Four of the herbs from the original formula are well known in the West and are available at health food stores and Chinese markets. They are reishi mushrooms (called ling zhi), panax ginseng (ren shen), ginger root (gan jiang) and Chinese angelica (dang gui). The other herbs in the nine-herb formula are wu mei, chuan jiao, huang lian, huang bai and gui zhi. Of course, buying the herbs individually and blending them yourself is neither recommended nor likely to work. If you can't wait for the final version to be tested and approved, the original 11-herb formula is available through practitioners of Traditional Chinese Medicine. At present, however, it is still used only to treat stomach conditions.

Cystic fibrosis

Breathing in a long-awaited cure

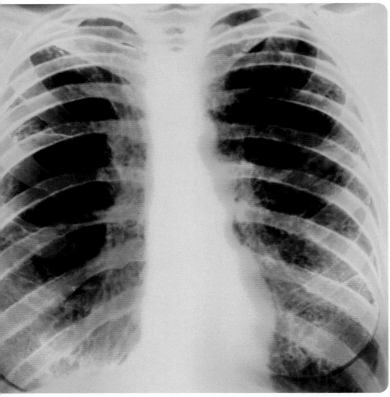

Repeated infection has thickened the air passages (orange, beside the spine) in this cystic fibrosis patient's lungs. A cure for the disease could be getting closer.

The most likely cure for cystic fibrosis – installing normal genes in a patient's lung cells to replace the defective genes that cause the life-shortening disease – is no longer a distant dream. In fact, such a cure may be only a year or two away, now that Stanford University researchers have successfully tested a treatment whereby cystic fibrosis patients can literally inhale healthy genes into their lungs.

Medical experts have long known that a flaw in a gene called CFTR (cystic fibrosis transmembrane-conductance regulator) is responsible for this condition – the UK's most common life-threatening genetically inherited disease, affecting some 7,500 babies, children and young adults. Previous attempts to deliver healthy CFTR genes by injection and other methods have had limited success, but the results of the latest test, involving 37 cystic fibrosis patients, represent a major step forward for two reasons. 'Inhalation is the only method that gets the genes to the lungs, where we want them,' says Dr Richard Moss, the lead study author. 'And there are far fewer side effects.'

The inhalation gene delivery method significantly improved lung function for about a month after each treatment. That is key, because lung damage from abnormal mucus production is what kills most cystic fibrosis patients, usually by the age of 30.

How it works In the Stanford study, published in the medical journal *Chest* in January 2004, the inhaled genes were carried into the lungs inside harmless viruses, known as AAV. Once there, the viruses inserted themselves into the cells lining the airways, giving the cells flawless copies of the CFTR gene.

It is thought that the 'good' genes then took over command of the lungs, sending out correct instructions for functions such as salt and water secretion and overriding the old instructions that caused mucus to become abnormally thick and sticky.

Availability A follow-up study of inhalant gene therapy involving 100 cystic fibrosis patients was under way in 2004, and results from a larger test (with 500 to 600 participants) could be available this year. If both confirm the treatment's safety and effectiveness, some cystic fibrosis patients may receive monthly gene therapy as soon as 2006.

Two hurdles will remain. The therapy has been tested only on patients aged 12 and older, so more research is needed before younger children can benefit. Also, since cell turnover in the lung tissue means that cells with the congenital bad gene reclaim control of lung function a month after each treatment, ongoing monthly treatments will be needed to improve and prolong patients' lives (This, however, is unlikely upset patients who are used to often daily therapy to remove secretions from the lungs.)

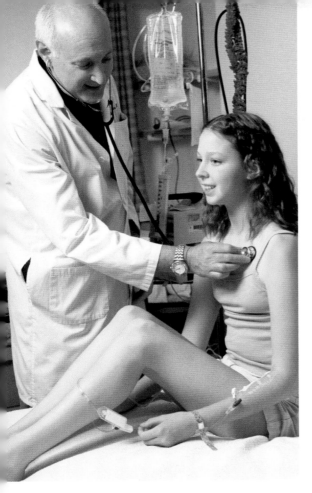

Researcher Dr Richard Moss examines a young cystic fibrosis patient. Inhaling healthy genes, he discovered, gives patients a month of improved lung function.

A true one-treatment cure for cystic fibrosis will come only when stem cells – the subject of so much debate – replace viruses as self-renewing gene delivery vehicles. Those special cells, widely thought to be the best hope for curing a host of diseases from Parkinson's to Alzheimer's, could multiply indefinitely in lung tissue once they are delivered, assuring a lifelong supply of healthy CFTR genes for the patient. Such a permanent cure is at least a decade away.

Meanwhile the UK Cystic Fibrosis Gene Therapy Consortium – possibly the largest focused group worldwide addressing the problem – is engaged in a five-year research programme into the use of gene therapy: the first clinical trials in the lungs are due to begin this year.

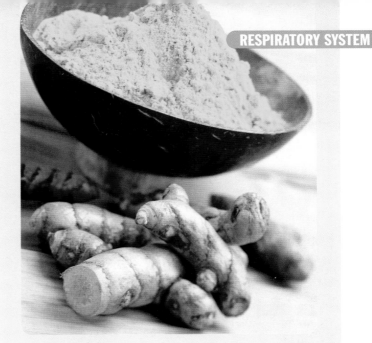

Is there a cure in curry?

Wouldn't it be nice if a treatment for cystic fibrosis were as close as the kitchen spice rack? That could be the case, say Yale University researchers, who fed curcumin, the main component in the common curry spice turmeric, to mice with cystic fibrosis.

According to the research team's report, published in the US journal *Science* in April 2004, curcumin helps a gene called CFTR to do its job correctly. In most cystic fibrosis patients, CFTR is rendered defective by the mutation responsible for the life-shortening genetic disorder. This causes the perpetual infection and inflammation that eventually lead to lung failure.

The mouse experiments were so successful that plans were under way in 2004 to begin testing curcumin in humans who have cystic fibrosis. The first phase will explore the safety of concentrated doses of the compound, and later studies will examine how well it works. The safety studies should be completed by the end of 2005.

A spokesman for the UK Cystic Fibrosis Gene Therapy Consortium welcomed the mouse study results as 'extremely promising', and said that many drugs being researched for cystic fibrosis do not produce such a dramatic correction.

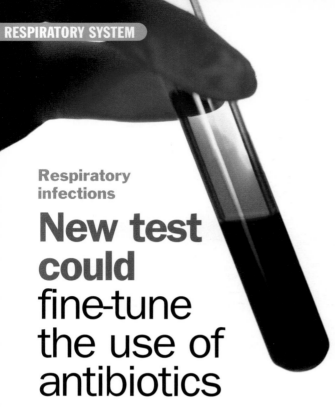

Respiratory infections

New test could fine-tune the use of antibiotics

You've been coughing for a week, your throat is sore and you're running a fever. Suspecting a respiratory tract infection, you visit your GP and are prescribed antibiotics. A week later, you're fine. Was it the antibiotics, or did your illness simply run its course?

The fact is that most respiratory tract infections are caused by viruses, and antibiotics – which work only on bacteria – are useless against them. Although some doctors are now beginning to adopt a more a delayed prescription strategy, (see Strategy to reduce antibiotic use, right), many GPs still err on the side of caution and prescribe antibiotics because they have no easy way of knowing whether they are dealing with a bacterial or a viral infection.

That may be changing. Swiss researchers announced in a February 2004 issue of the medical journal *The Lancet* that they have developed a safe and reliable blood test that reveals in less than an hour whether a respiratory infection is bacterial and therefore treatable with antibiotics. The test works so well that it could reduce the frequency of antibiotic treatments by 50 per cent worldwide.

Such a test would do much to undercut the growing problem of bacterial resistance to antibiotics. (The more antibiotics are prescribed, the greater the chance that bacteria resistant to those drugs will develop. Methicillin-resistant *staphylococcus aureus* (MRSA) is an oft-quoted

example.) It would also spare millions of people unnecessary antibiotic treatment and its potential side effects, such as diarrhoea and yeast infections.

In the study, researchers asked doctors to decide whether to prescribe antibiotics to 243 people who had symptoms of a lower respiratory tract infection. After the patients had the new blood test and the results were revealed to the doctors, the number of antibiotic prescriptions fell by half. Patients who were not given antibiotics because their infections were non-bacterial recovered just as well as those given antibiotics for their bacterial infections.

How it works The test measures blood levels of a protein called procalcitonin, which acts as a marker for bacterial infections. Levels are high in bacterial infections and lower when the cause is a virus.

Dr Beat Muller, a member of the Swiss research team, says that any medical professional who invests in the equipment needed to measure procalcitonin can use the test right away. And Roy Anderson, an expert on antibiotic resistance at Imperial College, London, hailed the new test as 'very promising'. But more research is needed to determine whether it is safe to withold antibiotics from high-risk patients,

Strategy to reduce antibiotic use

Prescribing antibiotics for viral illnesses is a common but ineffective practice. Overuse of antibiotics leads to the development of resistant bacteria strains, making the drugs less effective against the germs they are designed to fight.

Evidence shows that antibiotics continue to be used to treat upper respiratory tract infections. despite Cochrane reviews indicating minimal or no benefit from antibiotics for sore throat, acute bronchitis, the common cold and otitis media. This is a major issue for some doctors, who advocate a strategy of delayed prescriptions – written with a proviso that they not be used immediately and only if symptoms do not improve. Research shows this reduces antibiotic use – and it has the added advantage of avoiding side effects, reducing the drugs bill, educating patients and involving them in decision making.

A recent postal survey of 605 patients in general practice in Grampian, north-east Scotland, showed that under half (45 percent) were concerned about antibiotic resistance.

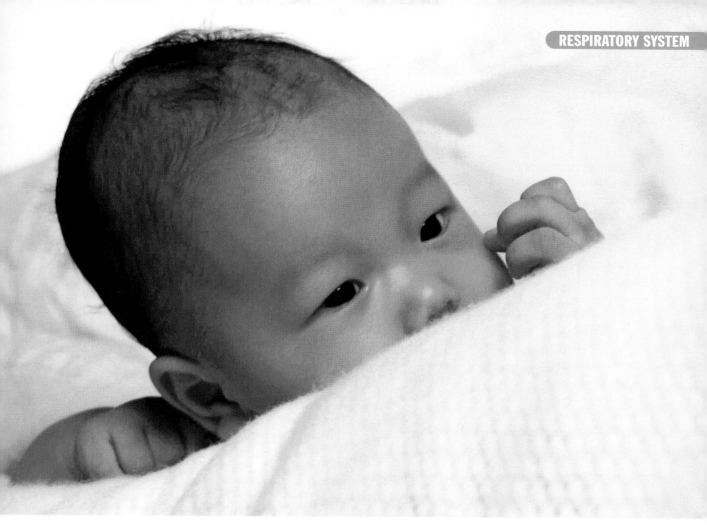

Respiratory infections

Bronchitis?
Pneumonia?
Think zinc

If your young child comes down with a lower respiratory tract infection such as bronchitis, you may want to ask your GP about zinc supplements. While zinc, critical to a healthy immune system, had already been shown to help the body resist such infections, two recent US studies found that the trace mineral also helps children under the age of 2 to recover faster from them.

One study, led by an Indian researcher and published in the March 2004 issue of the *American Journal of Clinical Nutrition*, found that boys between 2 and 24 months old who were given 10mg of zinc daily in a syrup recovered from their illness 2.6 times faster than those who did not receive zinc. (For unknown reasons, the zinc did not speed recovery for girls.)

Another study, conducted in Bangladesh and published in a May 2004 issue of the British medical journal *The Lancet*, found that treatment with 20mg of zinc a day in addition to the usual antibiotics helped boys and girls under 2 years old to recover faster from the most serious lower respiratory tract infection, pneumonia.

The doses administered in the studies were far higher than those found in over-the-counter zinc lozenges taken to help ward off colds. In fact, 10mg a day is more than double what is normally considered the safe upper limit for zinc in children under two, so this is definitely not a home treatment. If you are interested in zinc as a possible therapy for your child, you should talk to your doctor.

Spray away sleep problems

A simple nasal spray may be the solution to the serious sleep problems of millions of adults worldwide. Sleep apnoea – short, frequent breathing interruptions during sleep – often requires the use of mechanical devices to assist breathing, or even surgery to clear airway blockage. Now, Irish researchers have found that for certain people, spraying a steroid called fluticasone into the nose twice a day can cut down on apnoea episodes.

The medication is already frequently prescribed for rhinitis, an inflammation of the mucous membranes in the nasal passages that causes a stuffy, itchy or runny nose. About 26 per cent of people who suffer from sleep apnoea also have rhinitis. The new study confirms that fluticasone's anti-inflammatory, nose-clearing action seems to help those people to sleep better.

Researchers at St Vincent's University Hospital, Dublin, treated 13 such patients twice a day for a month with a nasal spray containing fluticasone. According to results published in the January 2004 issue of the medical journal *Thorax*, the frequency of sleep interruptions (apnoeas) decreased by 40 per cent in those patients compared with a group of 10 apnoea-and-rhinitis patients who received no fluticasone. Those given the medication also reported less nasal congestion and more daytime alertness.

Sleep apnoea

A 'splint' for snore-free sleep

What's worse: night after night of poor sleep, or having to don a cumbersome face mask before bed and spend the night hooked up to a breathing machine? That's the choice for many people with sleep apnoea, a disorder that causes frequent breathing interruptions during the night. But there is a third option, which new research from Sweden confirms can improve sleep without much fuss or discomfort.

How it works The device, which resembles a gum shield, is called a mandibular advancement splint because it holds the lower jaw (mandible) in a forward position, which opens the airway from the nose on down the throat. That is critical, since both snoring and sleep apnoea are a result of tissues partially obstructing the flow of air from the mouth and nose to the lungs. While snoring may bother your sleeping partner more than it does you, sleep apnoea can trouble your sleep so severely that you are unable to perform well during the day.

The standard treatment for people with severe apnoea is nasal CPAP (continuous positive airway pressure): at night you wear a tightly fitting face mask connected to a machine that pumps in air at a steady pressure to keep the airway open. However, many people are unwilling or unable to tolerate that set-up, says Marie Marklund, D.D.S., Ph.D., of Umea University in Sweden. So she and her research team tested an alternative – the mandibular

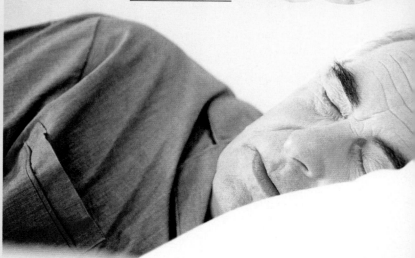

Wear this device and you could banish sleep apnoea.

advancement splint – on 619 volunteers who snored and had sleep apnoea. The device is smaller and easier to use than the CPAP machine and has the added advantages that once fitted , it can't be seen when the lips are closed, and you can speak, drink water and give a goodnight kiss with it in place.

Air interrupted

In a person with sleep apnoea, tongue and throat tissues relax, blocking the airway.

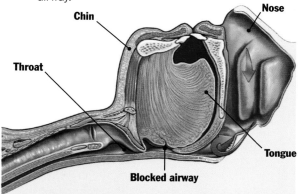

More important, the device improved sleep for a significant number of the study volunteers who used it throughout the one-year test period. According to the study results, women are most likely to get relief from the device because a more forward jaw position opens their airways more effectively than men's airways, but the men in the study whose apnoea occurred when they slept face-up also benefited significantly.

Not everyone liked the device, though, and nearly a quarter of the study volunteers stopped using it before the end of the test period. Some cited its orthodontic appearance, and others objected to side effects that included excessive salivation and discomfort associated with having the set of their jaws determined by a foreign object. But Dr Marklund maintains that, 'Once you get used to it, you'll improve your well-being, at night and during the day.'

Availability Mandibular advancement splints are widely available; many are offered on the Internet. Don't buy one on your own, though, warns Dr Marklund. The doctor who is treating your apnoea or snoring first needs to determine whether you are likely to benefit from it, and then the device should be prescribed and fitted to your mouth.

INBrief

▶ Antibacterial cleaners let many illnesses thrive

If you wash your hands with antibacterial soap, you're just as likely to come down with a variety of common illnesses as people who use regular cleaning agents.

That's the conclusion of researchers who provided either regular soap and cleaners or antibacterial versions to 238 New York City households, then tracked their rates of illness for nearly a year. Both groups reported similar rates of coughing, runny noses, sore throats and conjunctivitis.

Why was there no difference? These common symptoms are typically caused by viruses, which are not affected by antibacterial cleaners.

▶ Bug zappers reduce illness

Blasting germs with ultraviolet light deep in the ventilation ducts of office buildings may lead to a healthier workforce, according to new Canadian research.

Researchers equipped the ventilation systems in three Montreal office buildings with germ-killing UV lights. The lights shone on air-conditioning coils and drip pans – hotbeds of mould and bacterial growth.

The lights were turned on for 4 weeks then off for 12 weeks over 48 weeks. On questionnaires, nearly 800 workers reported if they had symptoms such as congestion, headache, fatigue and difficulty breathing. When the UV lights were on, workers reported 20 per cent fewer symptoms that started after they arrived at work. In addition, microbe concentrations in the ventilation systems fell by 99 per cent.

In tests at the Health Protection Agency, Porton Down, a UV air filtration unit made by Energy Technique proved 99.8 per cent effective in killing MRSA, the hospital superbug, and other germs. The company hopes to sell to the NHS, and a couple of units are on trial at a Basingstoke hospital.

SKIN
HAIR AND NAILS

Can you change the skin you're in?
Maybe not, but new drugs and
discoveries can **improve it**

If it's acne prone, there's a new laser treatment to keep outbreaks at bay. If itchy, inflamed skin caused by atopic eczema is your problem, a nonprescription vitamin B_{12} cream could help. For the face-reddening condition rosacea, a new soothing gel could soon be available. And there's a revolutionary new 'living bandage' that can actually help burn victims grow new skin, speeding healing and possibly reducing scarring.

When it comes to the hair on your head – or an unfortunate lack thereof – stay tuned for stem cell transplants in the scalp that grow brand-new hair-producing follicles.

Finally, two cosmetics companies have agreed to remove from their nail polish a substance that some consumer advocates believe could be dangerous to your health. The ingredient is still found in some other companies' nail polish.

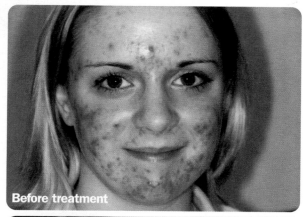

Before treatment

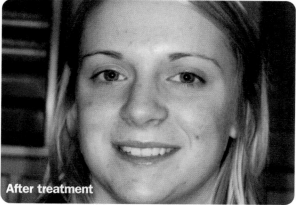

After treatment

Acne

NLite laser goes into NHS hospitals

A new UK laser treatment for acne, whose success was reported in *The Lancet* in October 2003, is gaining increasing acceptance in British dermatology. A dozen NHS hospitals are now using the NLite technology, at locations including Bradford and Leeds in Yorkshire and Hammersmith in London. The treatment is also available privately at clinics in the UK and abroad.

Designed and produced in Llanelli, South Wales, NLite is a low fluence laser therapy. It was originally conceived as a treatment for wrinkles and acne scarring but it has also been found to be dramatically effective at reducing active outbreaks of acne. The research published in *The Lancet* in October 2003 described how more than 87 per cent of the patients studied at London's Hammersmith

Hospital saw a marked improvement after a single treatment, with a 50 per cent reduction in spots on average per treatment. Courses of three treatments are typical and side effects are reportedly minimal.

According to the manufacturers, Euphotonics Ltd: 'NLite treatments can be used for all skin types and takes typically 20 minutes for a full face. Patients can expect to see noticeable results within three to four weeks.' Consultant dermatologist Dr Tony Chu who led the Hammersmith research says: 'This is the first major advance in acne treatment in 30 years.'

How it works Acne occurs when the sebaceous glands in the skin overproduce an oily substance called sebum and skin pores become blocked. In this oxygen-free environment, bacteria multiply and the skin quickly becomes inflamed causing unsightly spots. The condition is closely associated with hormonal changes, which is why it often first appears in puberty when the body begins to produce large amounts of sex hormones. The NLite treatment triggers naturally occurring porphyrin to release oxygen which attacks the bacteria, and prompts a localised immune response to heal the skin naturally. The laser technology uses a unique frequency and pulse length to achieve the desired results. NLite has also been shown to treat thread veins and rosacea without bruising.

TOP trends

DO-IT-YOURSELF DERMABRASION KITS – HERE'S THE RUB

In search of younger-looking skin, many women have been visiting dermatologists or plastic surgeons for microdermabrasion, the skin-renewing technique that uses a device not unlike a fine sandblaster to smooth out skin. Now the treatment is increasingly available at beauty salons and even as 'DIY kits' over the internet. Dermabrasion promises to soften wrinkles, reverse sun damage, fade acne scars and lighten age spots. But be warned, in untrained hands the results can be far from beautifying. A recent US survey revealed that patient complications were primarily associated with 'non-physician operators' (such as cosmetic technicians and beauty salon employees), performing the procedure outside their scope of practice. So before you order a DIY kit, think about the possible consequences of a slip up. It may be more expensive, but ultimately best to find a fully qualified practitioner. After all, your face is your fortune.

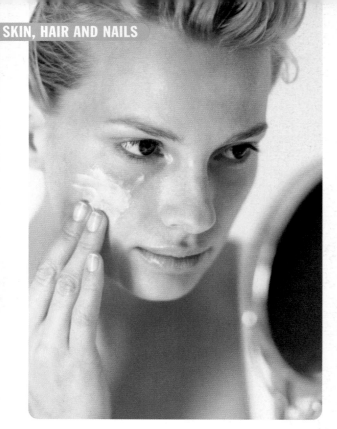

Dermatitis
Vitamin cream heals common skin rash

Atopic eczema is a distressing and incurable skin condition that causes itching and inflammation. The cause is unknown, but a combination of inherited, environmental and immunity-related factors seems to be at work. Topical steroids and oral cortisone are two of the most common treatments, but both of them carry a risk of side effects, particularly when used over a long period. Another, safer answer may be vitamin B_{12} cream.

How it works Compared with normal skin, the skin of people with atopic eczema contains elevated levels of a chemical called nitric oxide. When rubbed into the skin, vitamin B_{12} prevents further build-up of the chemical, according to Dr Markus Stücker, a dermatologist at Ruhr-University Bochum in Germany and lead author of the study. Previous research has shown that other substances that inhibit nitric oxide can reduce the itching and swelling of atopic eczema. Vitamin B_{12} is also thought to prevent immune system cells from releasing cytokines, chemicals that are associated with inflammation.

Researchers in past studies have tried giving vitamin B_{12} by mouth for the skin condition psoriasis, with no success (the vitamin leaves the body too quickly in the urine to yield any benefit). However, vitamin B_{12} is known to be absorbed through the skin, notes Dr Stücker, and since it's water soluble – which means it doesn't build up in the body's tissues – it is generally regarded as safe.

In the new study, researchers found that the B_{12} cream relieved symptoms much better than a placebo (dummy) cream and had no serious side effects. One small drawback was the natural red colour of the vitamin, which isn't a problem if the cream is rubbed into the skin thoroughly. The study results were published in the May 2004 issue of the *British Journal of Dermatology*.

Availability Vitamin B_{12} is available without a prescription, and government approval of its use is not necessary in Europe. Vitamin B_{12} cream is not yet widely available. It is probably best to seek advice from your GP or dermatologist if you are interested in trying out this treatment.

TOP trends

NO MORE TOXIC TIPS AND TOES

Two major cosmetics companies have agreed to phase out the use of a common – and, according to some consumer advocates, potentially dangerous – nail polish ingredient. Chemicals called phthalates are regularly used in the manufacturing industry to make plastics more flexible. One type of phthalate, DBP, an ingredient that prevents nail polish from chipping, has been linked to birth defects in the male offspring of female laboratory mice exposed to high levels of the chemical.

The cosmetics industry as a whole insists that the chemicals used in their products pose no danger to people, despite the fact that the European Union voted to ban phthalates as of September 2004. In view of this, some companies have decided to discontinue use of DBP as a precautionary measure including Procter & Gamble, makers of Max Factor and Cover Girl, and Estée Lauder.

Hair loss
Stem cells used to grow new hair

Stem cells, those 'master' cells that can become just about any other type of cell, have been found in the hair follicles of mice and may hold the key to effective treatments for baldness. When scientists removed these cells, grew them in the laboratory, and transplanted them back in the mice, the mice grew hair where none had been before the treatment.

The discovery of the stem cells in mouse hair follicles provides researchers with important clues that should help them to identify and manipulate similar cells in human hair, perhaps leading to a cure for baldness.

'Very simplistically, one could envision a process in humans whereby we isolate stem cells from the scalp [grow them in the laboratory], and transplant them back to areas that need hair,' says Dr George Cotsarelis, a researcher from the University of Pennsylvania Medical School in Philadelphia, who took part in the study. The implanted stem cells would develop into new, functioning hair follicles, which could produce new hair.

The researchers also hope that their stem cell discovery will teach them more about the skin ageing process in general. They suspect that increasing the amount of stem cells in the skin would have visible rejuvenating effects. 'In ageing, we believe that there is a decrease in the number of stem cells in the skin,' says Dr Cotsarelis, 'so if we know more about stem cells, we will be able to modify their number and behaviour.'

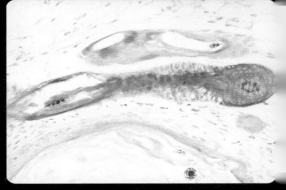

In blue, a new hair follicle grows from donor stem cells that were isolated from the skin of a mouse.

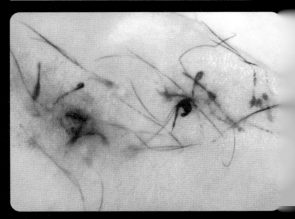

Thanks to the new hair follicles, this mouse is growing hair where it had none before.

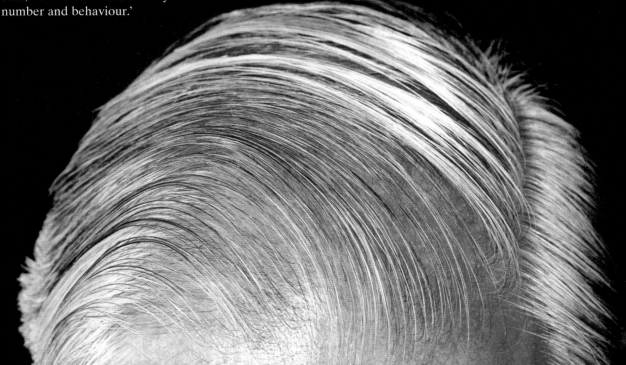

Rosacea
New drug wins face-off in rosacea study

There's a new topical drug for treating rosacea, and a recent study showed it does a better job of alleviating the face-reddening condition than an older medication called metronidazole (MetroGel).

Rosacea generally strikes people after the age of 30, beginning as flushing redness on the face that repeatedly flares up, then goes away. The condition can progress to cause longer episodes of flushing and noticeable blood vessels in the skin. Rosacea can also cause itching and burning on the face as well as raised bumps that are solid or contain pus. It's sometimes called acne rosacea, and its symptoms may be confused with those of plain old acne.

The new gel, azelaic acid (Finacea), was approved in the USA for rosacea in 2003. Research published in the *Archives of Dermatology* found that it did a better job of reducing the number of lesions on study volunteers' faces than metronidazole. It also reduced more patients' facial redness, and researchers and patients gave it better overall ratings for improving the condition. Azelaic acid cream is available in the UK as Skinoren, although it is currently only licensed for use in treating acne. In the light of this new research this could soon change.

How it works Azelaic acid may relieve rosacea by reducing skin inflammation, the authors suggest. Metronidazole is a germ-killing medication. Why it would help to treat rosacea is unknown, but other antibiotic preparations have also been used to alleviate the condition. According to the maker of MetroGel, it may also have an anti-inflammatory effect.

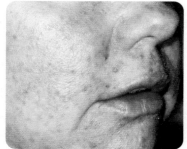
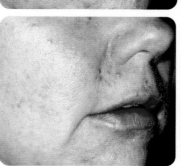

A 54-year-old woman with mild to moderate rosacea before treatment (top) and after eight weeks on Finacea.

Wounds
Biological bandages speed burn healing

More than 14,000 people are hospitalized with serious burn injuries every year in the UK, which can lead to scarring and disfigurement. Now a special high-tech bandage, developed by researchers at Sheffield University, is able to promote speedier, more complete healing. The 'living' bandages deliver new skin cells right to the site of the injury.

In a process that takes about one week, a small skin sample is removed from the patient (usually from the thigh or buttock) and treated in the laboratory so it develops into a supply of new skin cells. The fledgling cells are secured onto a specially prepared, disc-shaped bandage, which is then placed on the wound. The cells move from the bandage to the injury, where they begin prompting new layers of skin to grow. They also encourage undamaged skin cells at the edges of the burn to migrate to the injured site and

IN*Brief*

▶ Smokers left out in the cold
We know smoking is bad for your lungs, heart, skin and most other organs in the body. Now, a study of Finnish men has shown that smoking puts your fingers and toes at risk, too. Research published in the March 2004 issue of the *International Journal of Circumpolar Health*, involving 5,839 men (aged 17–30), showed that those who smoked were much more susceptible to frostbite. The result is related to the way that smoking impairs the circulatory system.

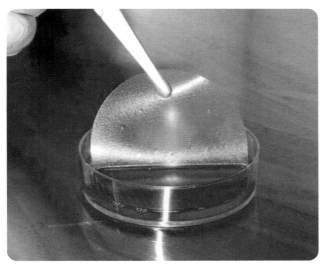

A Myskin bandage is lifted out of the petri dish where new skin cells were grown. The bandage promotes faster healing of wounds and appears to leave less scarring than traditional treatments.

begin to grow. Burn patients are often too badly hurt for their bodies to jump-start this kind of healing on their own. Standard treatments for serious burns, including skin grafts, take longer and are much more complicated to administer. Grafting also carries the risk of rejection in some cases.

The bandage, called Myskin, is also useful for difficult-to-heal, longstanding wounds, such as stubborn foot ulcers caused by diabetes that can lead to toe and foot amputations. Myskin also apparently leaves behind much less scarring than traditional treatments, researchers say, although additional testing is required to confirm that.

Availability Myskin, manufactured by CellTran, was launched at the British Burns Association meeting in April 2004 and is available to doctors and patients throughout the UK.

▶ A dab of pain relief

Dread the stab of a needle? A new device developed at the Massachusetts Institute of Technology could make that pain a thing of the past. Called SonoPrep, it uses ultrasound to open tiny, temporary channels in the skin to allow an anaesthetic cream to pass through. Together, the device and cream numb skin in just five minutes, compared with an hour for the cream alone. SonoPrep was approved for use in the USA in August 2004, and in time may become standard equipment in doctors' offices and hospitals in the UK, too.

Psoriasis

Skin that heals from within

In February 2004 the University of Glasgow announced the creation of a new biotechnology company, Grannus Biosciences, that hopes to revolutionize treatment for psoriasis and other inflammatory-related diseases. Until now, people with psoriasis, a common skin disease characterized by thickened patches of inflamed red skin, had little choice but to be treated with steroids, which can cause some unwelcome side effects such as osteoporosis and diabetes. The new approach, developed by Grannus, is based on a substance that is produced naturally by the body.

Thymosin beta 4 sulphoxide – or TB4 for short – is a potent anti-inflammatory substance that acts to prevent the immune system from racing out of control. Thymosin beta 4 is present in most cells of the body but when it is released in a modified form, it signals to the body that the processes used to destroy bacteria have started to damage host tissues and so must be switched off.

Professor Iain McInnes, one of the founders of Grannus, says 'The treatments that Grannus is developing will revolutionize inflammation therapy, providing sufferers with effective alternatives.' If successful the drug will have applications in a whole host of inflammatory diseases.

URINARY
TRACT

Doctors are using microwaves to zap enlarged prostates and offer older men **new relief**

If you're taking medication for this condition – which affects one in three men over 50 – talk to your doctor. New research shows that taking two different drugs together works better than taking one, both in relieving symptoms and preventing disease progression. And a small preliminary study in the USA has found that Botox, the wrinkle cure, may also help (although you may not like the injection).

For women who are distressed to find that they 'leak' a bit every time they laugh or cough, help is at hand. A new drug available in the UK holds significant promise for treating stress urinary incontinence and improving quality of life.

Lastly, a new study should put the final nail in the coffin of the pervasive 'calcium causes kidney stones' myth. The study confirms a wealth of earlier evidence that consuming calcium actually reduces the risk of developing kidney stones – so drink your milk!

Kidney stones

Drink your milk to prevent kidney stones

For decades, researchers and doctors believed that too much calcium was to blame for kidney stones, the often painful mineral deposits that form in the kidney from substances concentrated in the urine. Now, though, a new study published in the journal *Archives of Internal Medicine* has found that the more calcium women get from their diets, the lower their risk of developing kidney stones. The study builds on other, similar research in older men and postmenopausal women.

Many studies since the 1970s have shown that dietary calcium prevents kidney stones, yet a number of women who developed stones during the new study were still being told by their doctors to reduce their calcium intake, says the study's lead author, nephrologist

Dr Gary C. Curhan, associate professor of medicine at Brigham and Women's Hospital in Boston. 'Many ideas take a long time to change,' he says. He hopes this study will finally put the record straight.

Calcium/kidney stone theory wrong The idea that calcium contributed to kidney stones made sense in a simple way, says Dr Curhan, because most kidney stones are partly composed of a salt called calcium oxalate. For years, doctors thought that reducing calcium intake would reduce production of this salt, but the scientific picture is more complex. People on low-calcium diets actually have *higher* oxalate levels because calcium binds with oxalate in the intestine, preventing it from being absorbed by the body. So the more calcium you eat, the less oxalate you absorb from food. The less oxalate you absorb, the less likely you are to develop kidney stones.

Also, notes Dr Curhan, 'There may be some unidentified factor in calcium products that reduces the likelihood of stones forming.'

Dietary guidelines The study, which evaluated the dietary habits of 96,000 women aged 27 to 44, also found that eating whole grains and vegetables reduced the risk of kidney stones. Dr Curhan thinks that is due to naturally occurring phytate in these foods. Additionally, the more fluids –

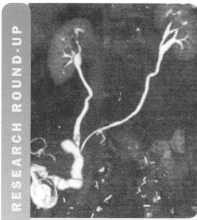

Better than an X-ray: the MDCTU scan is a special type of CT scan that reveals kidney stones and other urinary tract problems.

RESEARCH ROUND-UP

Detecting kidney stones and bladder cancer

Between bladder and kidney cancer, kidney stones and other urinary tract problems, it can sometimes seem as if that part of your body is a minefield of health problems. But detecting the mines may be easier now that researchers at the University of Michigan Health System in Ann Arbor have developed a simple, 15-minute CT (computed tomography) scan that they say can find tiny cancers, stones and other urinary tract problems.

The researchers used a special CT technique called multi-detector CT urography, or MDCTU, to find problems in the tiny tubes of the body's urine collection system as well as to detect bladder cancer, bladder stones, kidney stones, kidney cysts and kidney cancer. The technique, which creates three-dimensional urograms and provides an overview of the whole genito-urinary tract, was tested with more than 1,000 patients and proved much more accurate than the typical X-ray conducted on patients who are at high risk of such problems. Already available at certain hospitals in the USA, the MDCTU scan is still under investigation and not yet in use in the UK.

of any type – that the women drank, the lower their risk of developing stones. By contrast, the study found that sugar increased the women's risk. This may be because the more sugar in your diet, the more calcium you excrete in your urine, which could increase the amount of oxalate you absorb.

Dietary advice based on recent UK research is to maintain normal calcium intake, drink plenty of fluids (cranberry juice is good), and to cut down on animal protein, salt, soya-based foods and oxalate-rich foods (spinach, rhubarb, chocolate and nuts).

Lose the weight, lose the stones

As if increased risks for cancer, heart disease and diabetes weren't enough, now comes further research showing that being overweight also increases your risk of developing uric acid kidney stones. Results of a study published in April 2004 confirm earlier findings that the more you weigh, the more likely you are to develop this type of kidney stones, found in about 5 per cent of people with kidney stones and in about 30 per cent of people with diabetes who have kidney stones.

One reason, the researchers speculate, is that overweight people tend to have more acidic urine – which is not diet related. Instead, says lead researcher Dr Khashayar Sakhaee, professor of internal medicine at the University of Texas Southwestern Medical Center in Dallas, it is probably related to insulin resistance, a condition common in overweight people in which cells become resistant to insulin, leading to high blood sugar. 'When you have this defect, the kidneys can't produce and excrete sufficient amounts of a buffer chemical to neutralize the acid,' he says. The cure? Lose weight and exercise more to reduce insulin resistance.

Prostate enlargement
Zapping prostates with microwaves

For men who get up several times in the night to urinate and feel they're never quite able to empty their bladders, there's a new (if somewhat scary-sounding) treatment to solve the problem. In February 2004, the US Food and Drug Administration (FDA) approved Prolieve, a microwave-based procedure to treat enlarged prostate, or benign prostatic hyperplasia (BPH).

The procedure adds to the current treatment options, which all have drawbacks as well as benefits. Medications leave four out of six men dissatisfied with the results because they don't always work and can have side effects, such as hot flushes, dizziness and impotence. Surgical

The Prolieve thermodilation system

In this procedure, approved in the USA, microwaves destroy excess prostate tissue that blocks urine flow.

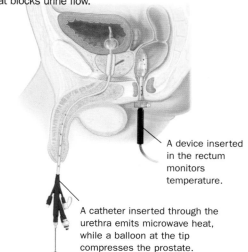

A device inserted in the rectum monitors temperature.

A catheter inserted through the urethra emits microwave heat, while a balloon at the tip compresses the prostate.

The bulb-shaped tip of the temperature monitor (top) rests near the prostate. The catheter inserted through the urethra (bottom) delivers microwave heat and protective warm water.

removal of part of the prostate may leave men incontinent, impotent or subject to retrograde ejaculation, in which semen flows back into the bladder during ejaculation.

Using microwaves to shrink enlarged prostates is not new, notes Dr Jonathan Henderson, a urologist in Shreveport, Louisiana, but older microwave treatments are very painful, requiring high levels of anaesthesia. Also, patients need to have urinary catheters in place for a few weeks after the procedure and it can take up to six weeks before the patients feel any relief. By contrast, men who undergo Prolieve rarely need catheters and usually feel significant relief from symptoms within a week or two.

How it works The Prolieve procedure combines microwaves that destroy excess prostate tissue with a balloon device that circulates warm water through the urethra to prevent any damage to its lining. The warm water and balloon are keys to the treatment's success, says Dr Henderson, and differentiate Prolieve from other microwave techniques, some of which use cool water to protect the urethra.

Cool water, says Dr Henderson, can decrease the effectiveness of the microwave-induced heat. In addition, he notes, the balloon keeps the urethra open while it's warm, then stays inflated during the 'cooldown' period of the procedure, so it stays open. 'It's like heating up plastic, bending it, and then, when it cools down, it maintains its new shape,' he explains. This often removes the need for a postoperative catheter; in one study, only 16 per cent of the men required catheters after the procedure, most of them for no more than three days. Prolieve also prevents permanent damage to the urethra, which may occur with other microwave devices.

Clinical trials on Prolieve found that 75 per cent of men who had the treatment experienced fewer BPH-related symptoms two weeks afterwards than those who took finasteride (Proscar), the drug commonly prescribed for BPH. Side effects included soreness and some blood in the urine, both of which disappeared within a few days. The treatment takes about 45 minutes and requires no anaesthesia. Patients stay awake and can inform the doctor if they feel any pain or heat.

Availability Now that the FDA has approved Prolieve, its manufacturer, Celsion, is training urologists across the country in its use. As yet the procedure is available only in the USA. In the UK, various microwave treatments for enlarged prostates are available, but not widely used. A new radio wave therapy called Transurethral Needle Ablation (TUNA) is being evaluated at multiple centres across Europe.

RESEARCH ROUND-UP

Two drugs are better than one

A five-year US study of more than 3,000 men found that taking two drugs commonly used to treat benign prostatic hyperplasia (BPH) relieves symptoms more effectively than taking either drug individually, and greatly reduces the risk that the condition will worsen and need surgery.

The drugs, which are used individually in the UK, are doxazosin (Cardura) and finasteride (Propecia). Cardura relaxes the muscle cells in the prostate that tend to choke off urine flow and is usually the first drug given for BPH, while Proscar shrinks the prostate by 15–20 per cent within 6–18 months. Taken individually, the drugs reduce the risk that symptoms will worsen by one-third; but taken together, they cut it by two-thirds. The combined drugs also caused fewer side effects, such as impotence and dizziness.

Professor Roger Kirby of the British Association of Urological Surgeons welcomed the study's finding as 'something to be taken on board by doctors in the UK'. But as two pills cost more than one, there are cost implications for the NHS.

Prostate enlargement

Older men may have a use for Botox

Along with migraine headaches, facial wrinkles, urinary incontinence and cerebral palsy, benign prostatic hyperplasia (BPH), or enlarged prostate, is now on the list of health conditions that can be treated with botulinum toxin A, more commonly known as Botox.

Dr Michael Chancellor, professor of urology and gynaecology at the University of Pittsburg's school of medicine, had spent years researching the use of Botox to treat incontinence. Since Botox works on smooth muscles, and the prostate gland contains smooth muscle cells, he thought it was time to try Botox to treat BHP, the condition that is so common in older men.

A 10-minute procedure Dr Chancellor, along with colleagues in Pittsburgh and at Chang Gung Memorial Hospital in Taiwan, tried the paralysing poison on 11 men aged between 50 and 82. The men, all of whom had BPH symptoms that did not improve with medication, each received a single injection directly into the prostate via a needle inserted through the rectum. The procedure took about 10 minutes.

The men's symptoms improved within a few days, says Dr Chancellor. The

Enlarged prostate

Enlargement of the prostate gland is common in men over 50. If symptoms are bothersome, it is usually treated with drugs or surgery.

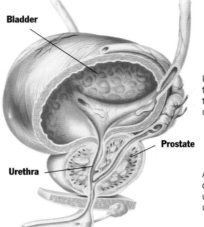

Bladder

Urine travels from the bladder down through the urethra.

Prostate

Urethra

A swollen prostate constricts the urethra, inhibiting urine flow.

participants found it easier to urinate, had improved urinary flow, and got up less often during the night to urinate. At the same time, they had none of the side effects that sometimes occur with medication or surgery, such as impotence, urinary incontinence and retrograde ejaculation (in which semen leaks into the bladder). Dr Chancellor presented the results of his study at the annual meeting of the American Urological Association in April 2004.

'We have good treatments available with pills and surgery, but if the pills don't work, many men don't want to have the surgery because it's irreversible,' says Dr Chancellor. 'Botox provides an option. It seems just as effective as surgery.' He said the results should last for at least six months.

Availability The use of Botox in this way is currently confined to the USA where, technically, any doctor could begin using Botox for BPH as an 'off-label' use (a use other than the one for which it was originally intended and approved). However, it is doubtful that insurance companies would reimburse for the treatment, which costs up to $1,000 for the medicine alone.

Dr Chancellor hopes that the drug's manufacturer will eventually begin larger clinical trials on its use as a treatment for BPH.

Botox can relax muscle cells in the prostate, making urination easier.

Drug stops embarrassing 'leaks'

Think how annoying and humiliating it would be if every time you sneezed, coughed, jumped up and down, or laughed hard, you also wet your pants. Yet that is a fact of life for an estimated one in five women who suffer from stress urinary incontinence.

Current treatments for the condition include pelvic exercises called Kegels, which strengthen the muscles that hold in urine; biofeedback; and medications that calm an overactive bladder. Now a new drug that may provide significant relief has undergone trials in 10 studies across five continents.

How it works The drug, called duloxetine, takes advantage of a relatively new understanding about the role of serotonin in the urinary tract. Yes, serotonin – the chemical that plays such a large role in depression and the workings of antidepressant drugs called selective serotonin reuptake inhibitors (SSRIs), such as fluoxetine (Prozac).

Serotonin and another chemical, norepinephrine, released by nerves, signal muscles in the bladder

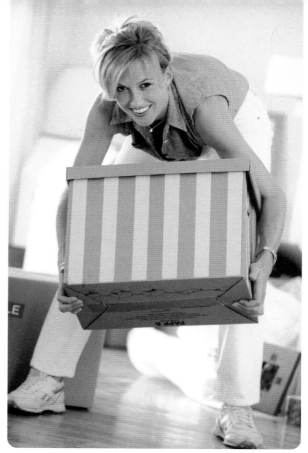

Hold it! If daily physical stresses bring on bladder leaks, the new drug duloxetine may help to solve the problem.

FUTURE BREAKTHROUGHS

A pacemaker for incontinence

Imagine being able to control your bladder with the push of a button. Crazy? Not necessarily. Australian researchers are working on a device called a urinary pacemaker which would let you do just that. An implanted electrical stimulator, operated by remote control, would activate a ring of muscle created from a patient's own body and transplanted to the bladder. On command, the stimulator would send a signal telling the muscles to relax, thus allowing the release of urine when the person is ready. The research team from the University of Melbourne is currently raising money to begin clinical trials in 2005.

area to contract, helping to control the urge to urinate, explains Dr Roger Dmochowski, professor of urology at Vanderbilt University in Nashville. Duloxetine prevents the spinal cord from reabsorbing these chemicals from the bladder neck, allowing them to continue their job of stimulating the sphincter (valve) muscles to contract. This is similar to the way SSRIs work in the brain.

In a major study on duloxetine, the researchers found that in half of the women taking the drug, their condition was 50 to 100 per cent improved, compared with one-third of women taking placebos (dummy pills). Those who took the drug were also able to go longer before needing to urinate. In the world of stress incontinence, notes Dr Dmochowski, these are significant improvements, and the women confirmed this in patient surveys that assessed the treatment's effect on their quality of life.

Availability In August 2004 the drug duloxetine hydrochloride (Yentreve), made by Eli Lilly, was granted approval for treatment of stress urinary incontinence throughout the European Union. It became available in the UK a month later.

RESOURCE DIRECTORY

For a wealth of information on a particular ailment or other medical topic, turn to the organizations listed here. Call, write, or log on to their web sites to find out what type of news, information, and services they provide. Many offer advice, newsletters and publications, details of events and also support groups.

GENERAL RESOURCES

British Dental Health Foundation
Smile House
2 East Union Street
Rugby
Warwickshire CV22 6AJ
0870 7704000
www.dentalhealth.org.uk

Carers UK
20-25 Glasshouse Yard
London EC1A 4JT
020 7490 8818
www.carersuk.org

Department of Health
Richmond House
79 Whitehall
London SW1A 2NL
020 7210 4850
www.dh.gov.uk

Disabled Living Foundation
380-384 Harrow Road
London W9 2HU
0845 1309177 or
020 7432 8009
www.dlf.org.uk

General Chiropractic Council
44 Wicklow Street
London WC1X 9HL
020 7713 5155
www.gcc-uk.org

Health Protection Agency
Floor 11
The Adelphi Building
John Adam Street
The Strand
London WC2N 6HT
020 7339 1300
www.hpa.org.uk

Medicines and Healthcare products Regulatory Agency
Market Towers
1 Nine Elms Lane
London SW8 5NQ
020 7084 2000
www.mhra.gov.uk

National Blood Service
0845 7711711
www.blood.co.uk

NHS Direct
0845 4647
www.nhsdirect.nhs.uk

Royal Society for the Prevention of Accidents
RoSPA
Edgbaston Park
353 Bristol Road
Edgbaston
Birmingham B5 7ST
0121 248 2000
www.rospa.co.uk

World Health Organization
Avenue Appia 20
1211 Geneva 27
Switzerland
011-41-22-791-2111
www.who.int

AGEING

Age Concern
Astral House
1268 London Road
London SW16 4ER
0800 009966
www.ageconcern.org.uk

Alzheimer's Society
Gordon House
10 Greencoat Place
London SW1P 1PH
020 7306 0606
www.alzheimers.org.uk

Help the Aged
207-221 Pentonville Road
London N1 9UZ
020 7278 1114
www.helptheaged.org.uk

National Osteoporosis Society
Camerton
Bath BA2 0PJ
01761 471771 or
0845 4500230
www.nos.org.uk

BRAIN AND NERVOUS SYSTEM

British Psychological Society
St Andrews House
48 Princess Road East
Leicester LE1 7DR
0116 254 9568
www.bps.org.uk

Epilepsy Action
New Anstey House
Gate Way Drive
Yeadon
Leeds LS19 7XY
0113 210 8800 or
0808 8005050
www.epilepsy.org.uk

Headway – The brain injury association
4 King Edward Court
King Edward Street
Nottingham NG1 1EW
0115 924 0800
www.headway.org.uk

MENCAP – Understanding learning disability
123 Golden Lane
London EC1Y 0RT
020 7454 0454
www.mencap.org.uk

Meningitis Trust
Fern House
Bath Road
Stroud
Gloucestershire GL5 3TJ
01453 768000
www.meningitis-trust.org

Migraine Action Association
Unit 6
Oakley Hay Lodge Business Park
Great Folds Road
Great Oakley
Northants NN18 9AS
01536 461333
www.migraine.org.uk

Motor Neurone Disease Association
PO Box 246
Northampton NN1 2PR
01604 250505
www.mndassociation.org

Multiple Sclerosis Resource Centre
7 Peartree Business Centre
Peartree Road
Stanway
Colchester
Essex CO3 5JN
01206 505444
www.msrc.co.uk

Multiple Sclerosis Society
MS National Centre
372 Edgware Road
London NW2 6ND
020 8438 0700
www.mssociety.org.uk

Muscular Dystrophy Campaign
7-11 Prescott Place
London SW4 6BS
020 7720 8055
www.muscular-dystrophy.org

National Autistic Society
393 City Road
London EC1V 1NG
020 7833 2299
www.nas.org.uk

Pain Concern
PO Box 13256
Haddington EH41 4YD
01620 822572
www.painconcern.org.uk

Parkinson's Disease Society (PDS)
215 Vauxhall Bridge Road
London SW1V 1EJ
020 7931 8080 or
0808 8000303
www.parkinsons.org.uk

Scope (Cerebral Palsy)
6 Market Road
London N7 9PW
0808 8003333 or
020 7619 7100
www.scope.org.uk

Stroke Association
240 City Road
London EC1V 2PR
020 7566 0300 or
0845 3033100
www.stroke.org.uk

CANCER

Breast Cancer Care
Kiln House
210 New Kings Road
London SW6 4NZ
020 7384 2984
www.breastcancercare.org.uk

CancerBACUP
3 Bath Place
Rivington Street
London EC2A 3JR
0808 8001234
www.cancerbacup.org.uk

Cancer Research UK
PO Box 123
Lincoln's Inn Fields
London WC2A 3PX
020 7009 8820
www.cancerresearchuk.org

Leukaemia Research Fund
43 Great Ormond Street
London WC1N 3JJ
020 7405 0101
www.lrf.org.uk

Macmillan Cancer Relief
Macmillan Cancerline
89 Albert Embankment
London SE1 7UQ
0808 8082020
www.macmillan.org.uk

CHILDREN'S HEALTH

Hyperactive Children's Support Group
Dept W
71 Whyke Lane
Chichester
West Sussex PO19 7PD
01243 551313
www.hacsg.org.uk

National Deaf Children's Society
15 Dufferin Street
London EC1Y 8UR
020 7490 8656 or
0808 8008880
www.ndcs.org.uk

DIGESTION AND METABOLISM

British Liver Trust
Portman House
44 High Street
Ringwood BH24 1AG
01425 463080
www.britishlivertrust.org.uk

Coeliac UK
PO Box 220
High Wycombe
Buckinghamshire HP11 2HY
01494 437 278
www.coeliac.co.uk

Diabetes UK
10 Parkway
London NW1 7AA
020 7424 1000
www.diabetes.org.uk

Digestive Disorders Foundation
PO Box 251
Edgware
Middlesex HA8 6HG
020 7486 0341
www.digestivedisorders.org.uk

IBS Network (Irritable Bowel Syndrome)
Northern General Hospital
Sheffield S5 7AU
0114 261 1531
www.ibsnetwork.org.uk

NACC (National Association for Colitis and Crohn's Disease)
4 Beaumont House
Sutton Road
St Albans
Hertfordshire AL1 5HH
0845 1302233
www.nacc.org.uk

EYES AND EARS

British Deaf Association
1–3 Worship Street
London EC2A 2AB
020 7588 3520
Text phone: 020 7588 3529
www.bda.org.uk

Eyecare Trust
PO Box 131
Market Rasen
Lincolnshire LN8 5TS
0845 1295001
www.eyecare-trust.org.uk

International Glaucoma Association
108C Warner Road
London SE5 9HQ
020 7737 3265
www.glaucoma-association.com

National Federation of Families with Visually Impaired Children (LOOK)
Look National Office
c/o Queen Alexandra College
49 Court Oak Road
Harborne
Birmingham B17 9TG
0121 428 5038
www.look-uk.org

Royal National Institute for Deaf People (RNID)
19-23 Featherstone Street
London EC1Y 8SL
020 7296 8000
www.rnid.org.uk

Royal National Institute of the Blind (RNIB)
105 Judd Street
London WC1H 9NE
020 7388 1266
www.rnib.org.uk

HEART AND CIRCULATORY SYSTEM

Arterial Disease Clinic (North)
32 Bolton Road, Atherton
Manchester M46 9JY
01942 886644
www.chelationuk.com
(South)
3rd Floor
57a Wimpole Street
London W1M 7DF
020 7486 1095
www.chelationuk.com

Blood Pressure Association
60 Cranmer Terrace
London SW17 0QS
020 8772 4994
www.bpassoc.org.uk

British Heart Foundation
14 Fitzhardinge Street
London W1H 6DH
020 7935 0185
www.bhf.org.uk

British Vascular Foundation
Fides House
10 Chertsey Road
Woking
Surrey GU21 5AB
01483 726522
www.bvf.org.uk

Cardiomyopathy Association
40 The Metro Centre
Tolpits Lane
Watford WD18 9SB
01923 249 977
www.cardiomyopathy.org

Raynaud's & Scleroderma Association
112 Crewe Road
Alsager
Cheshire ST7 2JA
01270 872776
www.raynauds.org.uk

MUSCLES, BONES AND JOINTS

Arthritis Care
18 Stephenson Way
London NW1 2HD
020 7380 6500
www.arthritiscare.org.uk

Brittle Bone Society
30 Guthrie Street
Dundee DD1 5BS
01382 204446
www.brittlebone.org

General Osteopathic Council
176 Tower Bridge Road
London SE1 3LU
020 7357 6655
www.osteopathy.org.uk

Lupus UK
St James House
Eastern Road
Romford
Essex RM1 3NH
01708 731251
www.lupusuk.com

ME Association
4 Top Angel
Buckingham Industrial Park
Buckingham
Buckinghamshire
MK18 1TH
0870 4448233
www.meassociation.org.uk

National Ankylosing Spondylitis Society
PO Box 179
Mayfield
East Sussex TN20 6ZL
01435 873527
www.nass.co.uk

National Association for the Relief of Paget's Disease
323 Manchester Road
Walkden
Worsley
Manchester M28 3HH
0161 799 4646
www.paget.org.uk

REPRODUCTION AND SEXUAL HEALTH

Family Planning Association
2–12 Pentonville Road
London N1 9FP
020 7837 5432 or
0845 3101334
www.fpa.org.uk

Infertility Network UK
Charter House
43 St Leonards Road
Bexhill on Sea
East Sussex TN40 1JA
08701 188088
www.infertilitynetworkuk.com

Marie Stopes International
153–157 Cleveland Street
London W1T 6QW
020 7574 7400
www.mariestopes.org.uk

Maternity Alliance Educational and Research Trust
Third Floor West
26 Northburgh Street
London EC1V 0AY
020 7490 7638
www.maternityalliance.org.uk

National Aids Trust
New City Cloisters
196 Old Street
London EC1V 9FR
020 7814 6767
www.nats.org.uk

National Childbirth Trust
Alexandra House
Oldham Terrace
Acton
London W3 6NH
0870 7703236
www.nctpregnancyandbabycare.com

RESPIRATORY SYSTEM

Action on Smoking and Health (ASH)
102 Clifton Street
London EC2A 4HW
020 7739 5902
www.ash.org.uk

Allergy UK
No 3 White Oak Square
London Road
Swanley
Kent BR8 7AG
01322 619898
www.allergyfoundation.com

Asthma UK
Providence House
Providence Place
London N1 0NT
020 7226 2260
www.asthma.org.uk

British Lung Foundation
73-75 Goswell Road
London EC1V 7ER
020 7688 5555
www.lunguk.org

British Thoracic Society
17 Doughty Street
London WC1N 2PL
020 7831 8778
www.brit-thoracic.org.uk

Cystic Fibrosis Trust
11 London Road
Bromley
Kent BR1 1BY
020 8464 7211
www.cftrust.org.uk

NHS Smoking Helpline
0800 1690169
www.givingupsmoking.co.uk

Quit – Helping Smokers to Quit
Ground Floor
211 Old Street
London EC1V 9NR
020 7251 1551 or
0800 002200
www.quit.org.uk

243

SKIN, HAIR AND NAILS

Acne Support Group
PO Box 9
Newquay
Cornwall TR9 6WG
0870 8702263
www.m2w3.com/acne/home.html

British Association of Dermatologists
4 Fitzroy Square
London W1T 5HQ
020 7383 0266
www.bad.org.uk

British Association of Plastic Surgeons
The Royal College of Surgeons
35-43 Lincoln's Inn Fields
London WC2A 3PE
020 7831 5161
www.baps.co.uk

Institute of Trichologists
24 Langroyd Road
London SW17 7PL
08706 070602
www.trichologists.org.uk

Psoriasis Association
Milton House
7 Milton Street
Northampton NN2 7JG
0845 6760076
www.psoriasis-association.org.uk

URINARY TRACT

British Kidney Patient Association
Bordon
Hampshire GU35 9JZ
01420 472021/2
www.britishkidney-pa.co.uk

Cystitis and Overactive Bladder Foundation
76 High Street
Stony Stratford
Buckinghamshire MK11 1AH
01908 569169
www.interstitialcystitis.co.uk

National Kidney Research Fund
Kings Chambers
Priestgate
Peterborough PE1 1FG
0845 0770 7601
www.nkrf.org.uk

UK National Kidney Federation
6 Stanley Street
Worksop S81 7HX
01909 487795 or 0845 6010209
www.kidney.org.uk

WELLNESS

Alcoholics Anonymous
PO Box 1
Stonebox House
York YO1 7NJ
01904 644026
www.alcoholics-anonymous.org.uk

BackCare
16 Elmtree Road
Teddington
Middlesex TW11 8ST
020 8977 5474 or 0870 9500275
www.backcare.org.uk

British Acupuncture Council
63 Jeddo Road
London W12 9HQ
020 8735 0400
www.acupuncture.org.uk

First Steps to Freedom (Phobias)
1 Taylor Close
Kenilworth
Warwickshire CV8 2LW
01926 864476 or 0845 1202916
www.first-steps.org

Institute for Complementary Medicine
PO Box 194
London SE16 7QZ
020 7237 5165
www.i-c-m.org.uk

Keep Fit Assocation
Astra House
Suite 1.05
Arklow Road
London SE14 6EB
020 8692 9566
www.keepfit.org.uk

National Institute of Medical Herbalists
Elm House
54 Mary Arches Street
Exeter EX4 3BA
01392 426022
www.nimh.org.uk

Society of Chiropodists and Podiatrists
1 Fellmonger's Path
Tower Bridge Road
London SE1 3LY
020 7234 8620
www.feetforlife.org

Vaccine Information Service (VAN UK)
PO Box 6261
Derby DE1 9QN
0870 4440894
www.vaccine-info.com

Weightwatchers
Millenium House
Ludlow House
Ludlow Road
Maidenhead
Berkshire SL6 2SL
0845 3451500
www.weightwatchers.co.uk

INDEX

CREDITS

Photo Research by Jeanne Leslie